THE BLOOMSBURY ENCYCLOPEDIA OF AROMATHERAPY

THE BLOOMSBURY ENCYCLOPEDIA OF

AROMATHERAPY

Chrissie Wildwood

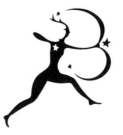

BLOOMSBURY

First published in 1996 by
Bloomsbury Publishing Plc
2 Soho Square
London W1V 6HB

A copy of the CIP entry for this book is available from the British Library.

ISBN 0 7475 2085 2

10 9 8 7 6 5 4 3 2

Designed by Amanda Hawkes
Typeset by Hewer Text Composition Services, Edinburgh

Printed in Italy by Graphicom Srl

NOTICE

The author and publisher cannot be held responsible for misadventure resulting from the misuse of essential oils, or any other therapeutic method mentioned in this book. Where there is doubt about how to use essential oils, or if there is concern regarding the suitability of home-treatment for a particular ailment, do seek the advice of a professional aromatherapist. Should symptoms persist despite sensible use of essential oils, it is important to seek medical advice and to mention that aromatherapy has been used.

ACKNOWLEDGEMENTS

I would like to thank everyone who contributed in some way towards the birth of this book, especially Howard Crabbe (horticulturalist) for researching the aromatic profiles section and advising on suitable plants for the aromatherapeutic garden. I am also grateful to Tim Couzens for his recipes and advice; Nick Webley of Kittywake Oils, for his enfleurage drawing; Shirley Whitton for allowing me to make use of her article entitled *Wild about the Rose*; Amanda Wilde and Dr Peter Wilde for further information on the Phytonics process and for correcting the relevant part of the manuscript; Harold Gaier, naturopath and researcher for *What Doctors Don't Tell You*, for pointing me in the right direction regarding phytohormones; Séza Eccles for recommending some very helpful people; Dr Thelma Moss of Anglia Foods and Mrs Colquhoun of the Hyperactive Children's Support Group for some interesting facts on evening primrose oil; Andrew Jedwell of Meridian Foods for explaining the process of vegetable oil extraction; Thrity Engineer for the fascinating information on bio-feedback imaging; Francezca Watson for permission to make use of *A Safety Guide on the Use of Essential Oils*; Evelyn Matthew (nursing lecturer) for kindly reading the menopause section and for supporting this project despite disagreeing with my views on HRT! A big thank you to Dr Viviane Lunny for ploughing through the manuscript and for writing the foreword; to my editors Rowena Gaunt and Isabelle Auden for supporting me when the going got tough; Amanda Hill, Andrew Syer and Polly Napper for seeing the book through the production process. Thanks also to Isabelle Auden, Kate Bouverie, Tom Drake-Leigh, Alison Emmett, Mike Jones and Muriel Rooney, for their contributions to the massage section, and to Paul Lawrence for his hard work and photographic skill. And finally, I would like to thank Martin Watt of the Medical Aromatherapy Training Services for responding so speedily and so generously to my requests for further information about essential oils, and for allowing me to glean from *Plant Aromatics: Effects on the Skin of Aromatic Extracts* and especially for letting me make use of certain unpublished material.

CONTENTS

CONTENTS

CONTENTS

CONTENTS

PART 6
HOME AND GARDEN

PART 5
AESTHETIC AROMATHERAPY

PART 7
AROMATIC PROFILES

FOREWORD

The Bloomsbury Encyclopedia of Aromatherapy takes the reader on a voyage of discovery into the various applications of aromatherapy. Divided into seven almost self-contained parts, this comprehensive reference book gives the reader a complete overview of the many fascinating uses of aromatherapy, both for self-help and the home.

Part 1 is essential reading for those who are less familiar with the use of essential oils, explaining the main terms and principles. Exploring the history of this healing art, it reveals that, contrary to popular opinion, aromatherapy is not a new age therapy, but in fact a practice which has its roots in ancient traditions.

Part 2 is concerned with the main systems of the body and conditions which affect them, as seen from the point of view of the aromatherapist. Aimed at giving general information (but not intended to replace a visit to a qualified medical practitioner) it gives practical advice about the home treatment of many common ailments.

The various healing philosophies and theories which can play an important role in aromatherapeutic treatments and aromatherapy in general, are discussed in Part 3. It is a very enlightening section for the discerning seekers of natural remedies.

The role of aromatherapy and the techniques used in massage are covered in Part 4. This section invites the reader to explore the world of touch therapies and illustrates their positive benefits.

Part 5 gives some very interesting insights into the world of beauty and perfumery. It also inspires the reader to create their own fragrances using essential oils.

Part 6 is packed with suggestions and ideas for various ways in which to use aromatics around the home and garden.

In the final section, the aromatic profiles of the most commonly available essential oils are listed with some safety precautions related to their uses.

Chrissie Wildwood's background as a holistic aromatherapy practitioner, as well as her widespread writing experience, has enabled her to present a clear and informative overview of the varied and complex facets of aromatherapy. She gives the reader a flavour of what can be achieved by this healing art. The Bloomsbury Encyclopedia of Aromatherapy will most certainly fulfil the expectations of any reader who has a thirst for information about this remarkable art.

Dr Vivian Lunny
MD, DIPL SCB - ESIPF, MIFA REG., MIACT CERT. ED., DMS.

INTRODUCTION

Aromatherapy is a multifaceted healing art which uses the essential oils of aromatic plants and trees to promote health of body and serenity of mind. Although the roots of this beautiful therapy are ancient, this book sets out to prove that the basic principles on which aromatherapy is based are no less valid today. It is also a practical guide to the many uses of plant essences – from the symptomatic treatment of everyday ailments through to the holistic approach to healing body, mind and soul. There are also a few intriguing diversions; an introduction to the art of natural perfumery, the making of cosmetic lotions and potions, and an exploration of sensual aromatherapy – for those wishing to enhance their love life through the alchemy of fragrance and the magic of touch.

With the current plethora of books on aromatherapy, what makes this one different? It is the first to explore the many aspects of aromatherapy in a single, highly illustrated volume. Gentle massage, however, is the mainstay of the art (at least in Britain and in countries to which it has spread since) and therefore the focus of this book. Included is a full-body massage routine accompanied by illustrated step-by-step instructions, with advice on massaging pregnant women, babies, children and elderly people. There is also a helpful section on dealing with sports injuries.

Although aimed at lay people wishing to employ aromatic plant essences for pleasure and to promote health and vitality in themselves and their families, *The Bloomsbury Encyclopedia of Aromatherapy*, is an invaluable guide for the aromatherapy student and a useful addition to the qualified aromatherapist's library. Moreover, it should serve as a comprehensive reference for other health care specialists, and beauty therapists, wishing to know more about aromatherapy – perhaps with a view to incorporating at least one aspect of this versatile therapy as an adjunct to their work.

Although aromatherapy has been around for a long time, only within the last few years has it achieved popular awareness. What makes it so special? Apart from the undeniable therapeutic properties of plant essences (the subject of ongoing medical research), aromatherapy appeals to our sense of the aesthetic. And, with the current upsurge of interest in anything that could be remotely categorised as 'stress-reducing', 'natural', or 'holistic', aromatherapy certainly resonates in harmony with the mood of the times.

Nevertheless, while most people are familiar with the word 'aromatherapy', not everyone is aware of the true nature of the art. For some, aromatherapy is associated with a luxurious beauty treatment. Then there are those who believe that it is simply a relaxing massage with aromatic oils. To those drawn to the esoteric, aromatherapy is a sojourn into the realms of the deep psyche – triggered by the soul-caressing properties of nature's ethereal essences. Other more down-to-earth people regard aromatherapy as a pleasant way to maintain health and vitality.

Aromatherapy is indeed all of these things, and much more besides.

WHAT ARE ESSENTIAL OILS?

Essential oils, or 'essences' as they are also called, are highly concentrated substances extracted from various parts of aromatic plants and trees. They are usually captured by steam distillation, a process whose origins can be traced back to ancient Mesopotamia. Unlike ordinary vegetable oils, such as corn and olive, plant essences are highly volatile and will evaporate if left in the open air.

The chemistry of essential oils is complex. Most consist of hundreds of components, such as terpenes, alcohols, aldehydes, and esters. For this reason a single oil can help a wide variety of disorders. Lavender, for instance, is endowed with antiseptic, anti-bacterial, antibiotic, anti-depresssant, analgesic, decongestant and sedative properties. Moreover, due to their tiny molecular structure, essential oils applied to the skin can be absorbed into the bloodstream. They also reach the blood as a result of the aromatic molecules being inhaled. In the lungs, they pass through the tiny air sacs to the surrounding blood capillaries by the process of diffusion. Once in the bloodstream the aromatic molecules interact with the body's chemistry.

A PLEASURABLE THERAPY

Quite apart from their medicinal properties, just smelling an essential oil can uplift the spirits and make us feel better. This is because the sense of smell is an interrelated aspect of the limbic system – an area of the brain which is primarily concerned with emotion and memory. And herein lies the mysterious potency of the art. Indeed, this influence of aroma on the psyche has led some aromatherapists to practise what is now called 'psycho-aromatherapy', whereby oils are used solely as mood-enhancing substances.

Aromatherapy is one of the few healing arts which could be described as creative, for much of the skill of an aromatherapist lies in their ability to create wonderful aromatic blends. Unlike more clinical therapies, such as homoeopathy and acupuncture, the efficacy of aromatherapy stems from its power to stir the imagination and to engender an immediate sense of joy or tranquillity.

There is nothing new about the sensuous approach to healing body and mind. It was adopted by the ancient Greek physician Asclepiades who advocated the use of massage, aromatic baths, music and perfume to soothe away the stresses and strains of life – even wine had a place in his Elysian regime!

Similarly, aromatherapy gives pleasure by nurturing the sense of smell and touch. Add gentle music and a pleasing decor, and we also heighten our senses of hearing and sight. Apply with tender loving care, and we are nurtured physically, emotionally and spiritually.

Just in case you are beginning to think that all this sounds too good to be true, the concept of the healing power of pleasure is grounded in the new science of psychoneuroimmunology. It has been confirmed that pleasing experiences such as falling in love, listening to music, receiving nurturing massage, and inhaling pleasant fragrances actually strengthen the body's immune defences. Unhappiness, on the other hand, lowers our resistance to all manner of physical ills – be it colds, flu, shingles or something much more serious. We also know that people can truly die of a broken heart, such is the power of emotion.

THE HOLISTIC APPROACH

Holistic healing is concerned with looking to the causes and the prevention of illness rather than solely quelling symptoms. It is also about taking responsibility for our own health. So for lasting benefits, aromatherapy should complement a healthy diet and lifestyle. Aromatherapy is also a marvellous adjunct to most other forms of treatment – psychotherapy, nutritional counselling, medical herbalism, or even orthodox medicine. For aromatherapy reigns supreme as a means to buffering the adverse effects of 'stress' – the bane of modern living.

Emotional disharmony in its many guises can eventually manifest as physical illness. The joy of aromatherapy massage, however, can help redress the balance. By enabling a person to relax deeply, to let go of all their cares – even for just a while – it is potentially powerful enough to activate the body's own innate self-healing ability. An amazing achievement!

A GENTLE HEALING ART

One approach to aromatherapy is as a hands-on therapy. It combines the physical and emotional effects of gentle massage with the medicinal and psychotherapeutic properties of plant essences. Not only does aromatherapy alleviate stress and improve mood, it is a successful treatment for all manner of minor disorders for which doctors cannot always find a gentle solution. That is to say, a solution free of the potentially harmful effects of drugs.

Massage with essential oils is especially helpful for women's problems, including pre-menstrual syndrome (PMS) and menopausal distress. It can also soothe away moderate anxiety and depression, sleeping problems, emotionally induced sexual difficulties, digestive disorders, headaches and muscular aches and pains. Many essential oils are also superb skin care agents. They help to balance sebum (the skin's natural oil secretion), and to tone the complexion by supporting capillary function, Similarly, plant essences can be used in hair and scalp formulas to improve the circulation of the scalp, prevent dandruff and promote healthy hair growth. Applied without massage, essential oils can heal skin problems such as athlete's foot, cold sores, ringworm and scabies. Used in steam inhalations, they can alleviate cold and flu symptoms. They are also efficacious for problems such as coughs, tonsillitis, sore throats, sinusitis and acute bronchitis.

Aromatherapy is beneficial in more serious conditions, but an aromatherapist (or the home user of essential oils) should always seek the co-operation of a doctor before treating people with long-term health problems. Many doctors are now sympathetic to complementary therapies. This approach to aromatherapy is popular in Britain and many other parts of the world, including Italy, Spain, Norway, Denmark, the USA, Canada, Australia, New Zealand, South Africa, and even Saudi Arabia, Japan and Singapore.

AROMATHERAPY AROUND THE WORLD

In France (and in many other European countries), essential oil massage is employed by beauty therapists – rarely by those involved with the curative effects of essential oils. In many European countries it is against the law to practise any form of therapy (i.e. that which aims to cure) without a medical qualification. As a result, most European aromatherapists are also doctors. Since few aromatherapy doctors hold certificates in massage therapy, the majority employ essential oils in the treatment of infectious illness, and oral dosage is the principle method of administration. In this instance, it could be argued that the word 'aromatherapy' is something of a misnomer, since the oils are chosen for their pharmacological action rather than the subtle effect of the aroma upon the emotions.

Due to the work of the aromatherapy pioneers, a number of medical schools in France now include the study of essential oils as part of their curriculum. Moreover, a branch of herbal medicine, which includes the use of essential oils, is also widely practised in France. Nevertheless, there is one drawback; even when essential oils are prescribed by a doctor (most pharmacies stock a wide range of essences), patients cannot reclaim the cost of the oils through health insurance. In Germany and Switzerland, however, health insurance does cover the cost of complementary treatment, but only if carried out by a medically qualified practitioner.

TAKING IT FURTHER

Having read so far, you may be interested in finding out about training in aromatherapy and massage. Listed in the Useful Addresses section (see page 00) are a number of schools and colleges offering some excellent courses. All include the study of anatomy and physiology as part of their curriculum – an essential requirement for all therapists. Although the majority of accredited aromatherapy courses are primarily aimed at those intending to gain professional qualifications, most schools also conduct short introductory workshops for those wishing to learn how essential oils can be used safely at home. Aromatherapy is sometimes included as an 'extra' on beauty culture courses, but beauty therapists often decide to follow separate aromatherapy classes.

If you are already qualified in massage therapy, or perhaps in some other healing art, and wish to employ essential oils as an adjunct to your work, an aromatology course may satisfy your needs. Aromatology is the study of essential oils without massage. At the time of writing, very few schools offer such courses. However, with the growing demand for more detailed theoretical courses on essential oil pharmacology, especially within the nursing and medical professions, it seems likely that many more training establishments will be offering this route

Chrissie Wildwood

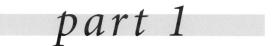

part 1

BASIC
PRINCIPLES

> *What is understood by essence,*
> *in the pure sense as used by the*
> *mediaeval alchemists,*
> *for example, is the actual*
> *energy, the 'soul' of the plant.*
>
> MARGUERITE MAURY

A BRIEF HISTORY OF AROMATICS

EARLIEST DAYS AND THE ANCIENT EGYPTIANS

The aromatic oils known to ancient civilizations were very different from the vast array of highly refined essences captured by modern methods of distillation. Be that as it may, the ancient Egyptians are generally regarded as the true founders of aromatherapy, even though, according to many archaeologists, they had no knowledge of distillation. Most of their healing oils and unguents were prepared by placing aromatic plant material in a vegetable oil or animal-fat base and leaving the mixture to infuse in the sun for several weeks.

It seems strange that a technologically advanced civilization like the ancient Egyptians – builders of the pyramids, practised astronomers, mathematicians and master embalmers – adopted such basic methods for capturing the essences of aromatic plants. And indeed, according to the ancient Greek historian Dioscorides, the Egyptians did eventually acquire the knowledge of distillation – albeit a relatively primitive version compared to that of later civilizations. Water was poured into large clay pots over the plant material (cedarwood resin, for example) and the pot openings were covered in woollen fibres. The pots were heated and the essential oil rose in the steam which saturated the wool. This was later squeezed to obtain the essence. Oil of cedarwood was highly prized because it was used in embalment, medicine and perfumery. It was one of the most expensive and sought after aromatics in the whole of the ancient world.

Another Egyptian method for extracting aromatic oils from exotic flowers, such as lilies, was by squeezing. A bas-relief, now in the Louvre in Paris, depicts women gathering blooms into a large cloth bag, while two men hold sticks attached to the sides of the bag. These sticks would be twisted round until the bag was tightly pressed and the essential oil oozed out of the petals.

Moving even further back through the mists of time we might imagine our very early ancestors gathered around a ritual fire breathing in the holy smoke of woods and resins. Certain aromas were credited with the power to drive out demons which would sometimes possess the minds and bodies of unfortunate people. Aromatics were also burned on the sacred altar to appease the wrath of the gods and to facilitate the channelling of divine knowledge. Echoes of such practice can still be heard, for the word 'perfume' is derived from the Latin *per fumen*, meaning 'through the smoke'.

In the light of scientific research, the ancient idea that incense and perfume elevates the human spirit to other dimensions of awareness is not as primitive or as superstitious as it once may have seemed. The phenomena associated with altered states of consciousness, such as out of body sensations, feelings of euphoria, religious or sexual ecstasy – experiences known to those practising advanced methods of tantric yoga and meditation, or as a result of taking certain hallucinogenic drugs – arise from the limbic system. The limbic system is the area of the brain which is closely connected with the sense of smell. Interestingly, scientists in Germany have recently discovered that frankincense resin, one of the most ancient of incense materials, contains trahydrocannabinole, a psychoactive substance which is released when the resin is burned as incense.

On the physical level, we also know that the aromas of natural aromatics such as pine, cedarwood, myrrh and cinnamon have the power to retard putrefaction and decay. Indeed, the survival of the Egyptian mummies bears witness not just to the embalmers' skills, but to the extraordinary preservative powers of plant essences. When Tut'ankhamun's tomb was opened in 1922, archaeologists discovered a pot of ointment which was still redolent with the fragrance of frankincense. More recently, when forensic scientists unwrapped a 3,000-year-old mummy, the aromas of myrrh and cedarwood wafted from the inner bandages.

Moreover, the odorous matter found on the Egyptian mummies may still be potent. In mediaeval times, for example, apothecaries employed a macabre drug called 'elixir of mommie', prepared from the sticky aromatic exudate which resulted from embalment. It was said to be efficacious for all manner of infectious illness due to its antiputrid and energising virtues.

Embalment was just one of many uses of aromatics employed by the ancient Egyptians. Aromatics were also burned as fumigants and as mood-altering incense, blended into luxurious and heady perfumes, incorporated into skin care preparations, compounded into medicinal brews, made into healing unguents and aromatic massage oils. The formulae for many medicinal and psycho-active concoctions were carved into the stone walls of the temple 'laboratories' (chambers where the priest-healers created their fragrant prescriptions), thus allowing us partial access to some of the most potent of aromatic blends. Unfortunately, the botanical origin of some of the listed aromatics is unknown, for their local names cannot be deciphered. Until pollen samples and other residues of the mystery aromatics are found and analysed by modern techniques, the compounds cannot be replicated.

We do know that one concoction, Kyphi, was a luxurious and heady brew consisting of at least 16 ingredients, including calamus (which contains a narcotic and hallucinogenic substance called asarone), saffron, cassia, spikenard, cinnamon and juniper, bound together with honey, raisins and wine. Dioscorides called it a perfume welcome to the gods. As well as being burned as a soporific incense, it was taken as medicine, or applied externally as a treatment for wounds and skin disorders.

Then there was Theriaque, said to banish anxiety. It was also a sovereign remedy against every kind of poison or pestilence; including the bites of wild animals, and even the plague. It comprised between 57 and 96 ingredients (temple recipes vary), which included myrrh, cinnamon, sweet flag, juniper and cassia and, less aesthetically, serpent skin, crocodile dung and spittle! The ancient Greek physicians, who gleaned much of their knowledge of the healing power of aromatics from the Egyptians, were especially enamoured of Theriaque. In fact, it was considered a panacea right up until the early-nineteenth century, or until the emergence of mainstream Western medicine.

THE GREEKS AND ROMANS

The Greeks, more than any other peoples, had a penchant for decorating their heads with fragrant flowers – a form of psycho-aromatherapy. Indeed, the physician Marestheus wrote a treatise on the making of chaplets and garlands, mentioning those that tended to lower the spirits, causing depression and fatigue, and those which exerted an uplifting or exhilarating effect. The rose, the

hyacinth with its balsamic fragrance, and most fruity or spicy scents were shown to invigorate a tired mind; whereas the lily and narcissus were deemed oppressive, causing feelings of lassitude if inhaled too frequently.

Hippocrates extolled the virtues of a daily aromatic bath and scented massage to prolong life. So effective were his recommended treatments that Plato is said to have reproached Herodicus (one of Hippocrates' teachers) for protracting the miserable existence of the aged!

The perfumes and healing balms so popular with the Greeks soon became fashionable in Rome. Pliny describes the costly unguent called susinum, which originated in Athens. He tells us it was composed of extracts of white lilies, roses, saffron and myrrh. As well as its cosmetic value, susinum was employed as a diuretic and to soothe vaginal inflammations.

The Romans were the world's greatest bathers, not only appreciating cleanliness, but also the health-giving properties of naturally warm spa waters. They were also fond of aromatherapy massage. Wealthy families would while away their days at the baths being massaged with aromatic oils by unfortunate eunuch slaves whose sole function in life was to knead and pummel their masters.

EASTERN CIVILIZATIONS

In ancient China, herbal medicine was used in conjunction with acupuncture and massage to treat a myriad of ailments. The Chinese were also involved with the quest for immortality through the practice of alchemy. The alchemist would burn incense and douse himself in specially prepared perfumes before carrying out his experiments. He believed that the perfume or quintessence of plants held magical forces and plant spirits whose power would help him concoct the elixir of life. The alchemical task was also about spiritual transformation and the perfecting of the soul.

The Persian physician Avicenna is credited with having perfected the art of distillation in the eleventh century AD. So advanced was his method that the apparatus for distillation has barely altered in 900 years. He also advocated massage, traction (for broken limbs) and a detoxifying all-fruit diet as part of his healing regime. As for perfume, the essential oil of red roses (attar of rose) and the less costly rosewater became an all-consuming passion with the Persians. Legend has it that some of the caliphs had fountains of rosewater dancing in their palaces.

Following the recommendations of Hippocrates, the Arab physicians harnessed the power of aromatic oils and floral waters to purify the air and to protect themselves from disease. Although they had no knowledge of microbial germs, they were well aware of the prophylactic capabilities of perfume. They disinfected their bodies and clothes with aromatics such as sandalwood, camphor and rosewater. The psychotherapeutic effects were also recognised. Avicenna believed that plant essences fortified body and spirit. He also promoted the idea that pleasing aromas combated baser passions like fear and sorrow, which lowered vitality and contributed to the development of disease.

EARLY EUROPE

The legendary 'perfumes of Arabia' were brought back to Europe by the crusading knights, along with the knowledge of distillation. Some of the wealthy households installed their own still for capturing essential oils which were used as medicine as well as perfumes. People smothered their unwashed bodies and clothes with perfume and carried little bouquets of aromatic herbs (tussie mussies) to prevent catching infectious illness and to mask the stench of filthy city streets.

It was also the custom in mediaeval Europe to strew sweet-smelling plants, such as lavender, thyme and chamomile, on the floor, which gave off pervasive scents when crushed underfoot. Since most aromatic plants have insecticidal and bactericidal properties, they must have played a significant role in helping to counter the spread of infectious illness. Their scents also deterred lice and fleas.

But could aromatics combat the greatest scourge of all – the bubonic plague?

AROMATHERAPY VERSUS THE PLAGUE

The discovery of the bubonic plague bacillus and the role of fleas and rats in propagating the disease was not made until the latter part of the nineteenth century. Prior to this, a variety of causes were suggested: bad smells, deadly breezes from hell – God's punishment for the sins of mankind. The pestilence was believed to enter the body through the pores of the skin or by breathing in its fetid odour.

Yet Chinese medicine had long recognised a correlation between rats and human plague. And in 50 BC, the Greek physician Lucretius almost hit the nail on the head when he attributed the origin of infections in general to 'atoms' of disease sometimes present in the atmosphere, in the air we breathe. In the second century AD, Galen postulated that there had to be a combination of two imbalances in order for the plague to strike: contaminated air 'excessively different from the norm', comple-

mented by a body weakened by such things as overindulgence in erotic pleasures, gluttony, indolence, overwork and emotional upset. Centuries later, the English physician Thomas Sydenham attributed the plague that decimated the population of London in 1655–6 to a 'miasma' or a 'virus' from some infected site: from the emanations of rotting bodies in cemeteries sited too close to inhabited areas.

Throughout the history of the world, aromatic wood fires, along with the copious use of incense and perfume, were employed to halt the spread of infectious disease. Since pleasant aromas were associated with all that was good, it made sense to counter the evil stench of the plague with sweet-smelling vapours (one of the earliest symptoms of bubonic plague was fetid breath reminiscent of rotting flesh).

It is said that when the plague struck, perfumers, who were pervaded with essential oils, remained immune. This discovery led to the development of the famous 'Four Thieves' Vinegar', a potion so called because a quartet of robbers in Marseilles during the Great Plague in 1722 would rub themselves all over with it before plundering the bodies of stricken victims. The ingredients of this remarkable prophylactic compound included a concentration of garlic along with extractions of rosemary, camphor, lavender, nutmeg, sage and cinnamon, suspended in vinegar.

The seventeenth-century French plague doctor protected himself by covering his body from head to toe in an ensemble of garments made out of Moroccan leather – including a grotesque beaked mask. The bird-like beak through which he breathed was permeated with the scents of ambergris (a substance excreted by the sperm whale), cloves, cinnamon and other spices. To enable him to keep a safe distance from stricken victims, he also carried a wand which he placed on the wrists of his patients in order to feel the vibration of their pulses.

From the Middle Ages onwards, bathing (at least with hot water) was generally regarded as dangerous. In fact, the fear of bathing led in the sixteenth century to the closing of public baths in many parts of Europe. Since the plague was believed to enter the body through the pores of the skin as well as through inhalation, the 'no bathing' decree was grounded by a certain logic. Hot water opened the pores of the skin; it was thought that this allowed pestilential air to enter the body more easily. Physicians of the day recommended washing only the hands and face with aromatic lotions. The plague doctors themselves sponged their whole bodies with tepid aromatic vinegar twice daily.

Although pleasant odours were reasonably effective as prophylactics against the bubonic plague, they were apparently powerless in effecting a cure. In a desperate bid to rout the enemy once and for all, the French physician Henri de la Cointe in 1634 decided to go against the grain of contemporary medical practice. He proposed to fight stench with stench. The smell of goat urine was perhaps the least objectionable of Henri de la Cointe's foul weapons; decaying bodies, the worst. In fact, modern research has revealed that the odour of goat has the power to repel the lice and fleas which spread bubonic plague. Surprisingly, the same is true of the odours of certain vegetable oils, namely olive, walnut and peanut.

Not surprisingly, many of Henri de la Cointe's contemporaries rejected the 'hawkish' medicine of foul odours, preferring the 'dovish' medicine of pleasant aromas. The majority eventually chose to compromise. A system was developed in which violent odours like sulphur and antimony were combined with pleasant aromas such as cinnamon, cloves and ambergris, and used to fumigate houses, clothing and persons. But they did not always get it right. Tragically, many healthy people died of asphyxia as a result of overzealous fumigation with caustic substances.

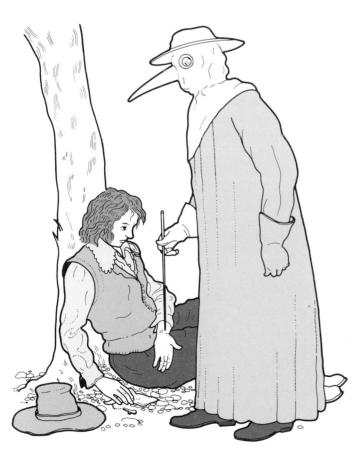

The seventeenth century French plague doctor

THE EMERGENCE OF CHEMICAL DRUGS

By the late seventeenth century the emergence of synthetic and chemical drugs began to sideline the use of herbs and essential oils in medicine. Mercury, for example, proved especially popular for the treatment of syphilis. The horrific side-effects of this treatment included copious salivation (several pints of it a day), tooth loss, disintegration of the jaw, tremors and occasionally even total paralysis. Although in some cases the disease was eradicated, the treatment certainly killed great numbers of patients. In retrospect, dying of the disease itself would seem infinitely preferable to the agonies of death from mercury poisoning. Incidentally, the French aromatherapy doctor Jean Valnet cites essential oil of lemon as having the power to quell syphilis. If only they had known this in the seventeenth century!

It was during the nineteenth century, however, that a pattern was established that continues today; chemists were intent on sifting out the so-called impurities of plants in order to isolate their 'active principles'. But those components which are regarded as impurities are often a necessary part of the whole. According to herbalists, the numerous trace elements work in harmony with the active principle, thus reducing the possibility of side-effects. Nevertheless, it is important to point out that not all substances in nature are benign. Take laurel leaves, from which cyanide is derived, and the foxglove, which contains the heart tranquilliser digitalis – both plants in quantity can be lethal.

THE TWENTIETH-CENTURY PIONEERS

THE FRENCH

The word 'aromatherapy' was first used in 1937 by the French cosmetic scientist Rene-Maurice Gattefossé, whose research revealed that the volatile extracts distilled from certain aromatic plants had a profound effect on the skin. His interest in the healing potential of essential oils was aroused by the work of DríChaberies, another Frenchman who in 1838 had written a treatise on the therapeutic properties of aromatic plants. Gattefosse®'s own research was confined to the cosmetic uses of essential oils, but he soon realised that many had powerful antiseptic and painkilling properties as well. The most remarkable instance of this was demonstrated to

Gattefossé after his hand was severely burned in a laboratory explosion. He treated the wound with neat lavender essence, which immediately eased the pain. The wound healed remarkably well, with no sign of infection, or even a scar to remind him of the accident.

Gattefossé also discovered that essential oils applied to the skin could be absorbed into the bloodstream where they interact with the body's chemistry.

A great deal of interest in aromatherapy was kindled in France as a result of Gattefossé's work. Not only were the oils found to heal skin, but also to strengthen the body's immune defences. The ex-army surgeon DríJean Valnet is credited with having contributed most to the medical assessment and acceptance of aromatherapy. Inspired by Gattefossé, he used essential oils to treat battle wounds of soldiers during the Second World War. Later, he described how he successfully treated several long-term psychiatric patients with essential oils. These people also had physical symptoms caused by the side-effects of drugs they had been given to control their depression and hallucinations. They were gradually weaned off the drugs and treated with essential oils both externally, with aromatic baths and liniment rubs, and internally, by mouth or interdermal injections, (through the upper layers of skin rather than into a vein). The treatment was reinforced with herbal remedies and a strict dietary regime. Both physical and mental symptoms were relieved, sometimes within days of discontinuing the drugs.

PSYCHOTHERAPEUTIC AROMATHERAPY

In the 1920s two Italian doctors, Gatti and Cajola, demonstrated the psychotherapeutic effects of smelling essential oils. They concluded: 'The sense of smell has, by reflex action, an enormous influence on the function of the central nervous system'. Still on the psycho-aromatherapy track, professor Paolo Rovesti of Milan University in the early 1970s employed the essences produced from locally grown fruits such as bergamot, orange and lemon as psychotherapeutic agents. He passed bits of cotton wool soaked in essential oils under the noses of his patients. The aromas, he said, helped to evoke and release suppressed memories and emotions that had detrimental effects on the psyche of these people. Other anxiety-relieving essences listed by Rovesti include: marjoram, cypress, rose and lavender.

AROMATHERAPY MASSAGE

In the 1950s, the Austrian-born cosmetologist Marguerite Maury introduced the idea of combining essential oils with massage. She was not happy with administering essential oils by mouth but preferred to dilute them in vegetable oil and to massage them into the skin. Inspired by the methods used in traditional Tibetan medicine, she developed a special massage technique of applying the oils along the nerve centres of the spine. She also devised the 'individual prescription' – essences were chosen according to the physical and emotional needs of the recipient. As the mental and physical pattern altered, so too the aromatic prescription.

Her clients, mainly wealthy women seeking rejuvenation, reported dramatic improvement in their skin condition as a result of her treatments. To their delight, there were also some interesting side-effects; many experienced relief from rheumatic pain, heightened sexual pleasure, deeper sleep, and a generally improved mental state.

Marguerite Maury opened an aromatherapy clinic in London in the early 1960s. Although her treatments were geared to beauty therapy she knew that aromatherapy went much deeper. Indeed, she had discovered an important key to the art of true healing. Marguerite Maury was totally dedicated to her work and, in 1962 and 1967, was rewarded with two international prizes for her research. Soon after, at the age of 73, she died of a stroke, thought to be due to overwork. Her achievements are best described by her husband and colleague, the French homoeopathic physician Dr E.A. Maury, who says: 'She continues to show the way for those who have been willing to recognise her and will long do so for those who seek a new way of achieving moral and physical well-being.'

However, it could be argued that it was the British aromatherapist, author and researcher Robert Tisserand, who really put aromatherapy on the agenda. He is the author of *The Art of Aromatherapy*, one of the first books in English on the subject, which was published in 1977. Although inspired by Marguerite Maury, it would be fair to say that this book above any other has sparked the greatest interest, worldwide, in the therapeutic properties of essential oils and aromatherapy in general. Tisserand has also helped to found two aromatherapy associations and is the editor of the *International Journal of Aromatherapy*.

2
THE ESSENCE OF AROMATHERAPY

The majority of essential oils produced are used as food flavouring agents and perfume materials. They are also of some interest to the pharmaceutical industry, but usually in order for chemists to isolate their 'active principles'. However, some continue to be employed in their natural state by practitioners of aromatherapy and herbal medicine. In this chapter we shall take a closer look at plant essences, including their chemistry, therapeutic properties and the various methods of extraction.

THE NATURE OF PLANT ESSENCES

Essential oils, also known as 'essences' or 'volatile oils', are the highly odoriferous liquid components of aromatic plants, trees and grasses. The word 'essential' is derived from *quintessence*, which the Oxford English Dictionary defines as 'An extract of a substance containing its principle in its most concentrated form'. In ancient philosophical or alchemical terms, quintessence was related to *ether* or the fifth element and was thought to be the spiritual aspect of matter. It is also interesting to mention that essential oils are sometimes called 'ethereal oils', a Germanic term which aptly describes their otherworldly nature; for if left in the open air they disappear without a trace, evaporating into the ether like a mist.

WHERE ARE THEY FOUND?

Essential oils may be found in different parts of the plant: in the petals (rose), leaves (eucalyptus), roots of grass (vetiver), bark (cinnamon), heartwood (sandalwood), citrus rind (lemon), seeds (caraway), rhizomes (valerian), bulbs (garlic), the aerial or top parts of the plant (marjoram) or resin (frankincense), and sometimes in more than one part of the plant. Lavender, for instance, yields oil from both the flowers and the leaves, while the orange tree produces three different smelling essences with vary-

ing medicinal properties; the heady bitter-sweet neroli (flowers), the similar though less refined scent of petitgrain (leaves) and the cheery orange (rind of the fruit).

Although sometimes denigrated as 'waste products' of plant metabolism, studies have shown that plants utilise essential oils for such purposes as attracting pollinating insects, repelling predators and protecting themselves from disease – quite a significant survival mechanism. Yet essential oils are not vital to the life of plants as a whole, as the word 'essential' may suggest. Indeed, while it is true that most plants have an odour to a sensitive nose, not all plants produce volatile oils.

Essential oils accumulate in specialised plant tissues, harbouring oil glands. The more oil glands present in the plant, the cheaper the oil, and vice versa. For instance, 100 kilos of lavender yields almost 3 litres of essential oil, whereas 100 kilos of rose petals can yield only a half a litre. Essential oils are highly concentrated substances and therefore rarely used neat, though certain essences, such as lavender and tea tree, are sometimes used undiluted as an antiseptic. For aromatherapy massage, however, they are diluted in a 'carrier' oil such as sweet almond or olive (see Chapter 4). As well as being soluble in ordinary vegetable oil, essential oils will dissolve in alcohol, egg yolk and waxes (melted beeswax or jojoba for example). However, they are only partially soluble in water – and a little more soluble in vinegar.

COLOUR AND CONSISTENCY

Even though they are technically classified as oils, plant essences are quite different from 'fixed' or fatty oils such as sunflower seed, corn or sweet almond. They are highly volatile, which means they evaporate when left in the open air, and they do not leave a permanent mark on paper. While many essences are virtually colourless (peppermint), yellowish (lavender), greenish (bergamot), amber (patchouli) or dark brown (vetiver), a few are endowed with an idiosyncratic hue. Tagetes, for example, is dark orange or yellow, whereas German chamomile is a splendid inky-blue. Many essences have the consistency of water or alcohol – lavender, peppermint and rosemary, for example. Others, such as myrrh and vetiver, are viscous, or thick and sticky, whereas rose otto is semisolid at room temperature, but becomes liquid with the slightest warmth.

ENVIRONMENT

The quantity and quality of essential oil produced by a plant is determined by many interrelated factors. As well as climate and altitude, the type of soil and its fertility is significant: German chamomile, for instance, produces a higher yield of oil when grown on soils rich in calcium. There are also special vintage plants whose essential oil quality supercedes that produced in different locations only a few kilometres apart, where soil and climatic conditions are apparently identical. Moreover, the time of year and day has a major influence on the quality and abundance of essential oil, which moves around the plant according to both a daily and a seasonal cycle – individual plant species having their own characteristic rhythm.

While the concentration of essential oil in flowering plants is generally highest at midday during warm dry weather, there are a few exceptions. The oil of jasmine, for instance, is most concentrated in the petals at night, which means the flowers must be picked before dawn. The oil of the damask rose, on the other hand, is most concentrated in the petals after the morning dew and before the greatest heat of the day.

And, just like wine, the quality and 'bouquet' of an essential oil will vary from year to year. To the commercial perfumer, who demands a standardised product, such variability is regarded as a distinct disadvantage. But to the aromatherapist and natural perfumer, it simply adds to the charm of using aromatics from the earth rather than from the laboratory. The fragrances of organic essences are very different from the highly synthetic scents to which many of us have become accustomed. Newcomers to aromatherapy may need to acquire a 'nose' for natural aromatic oils. Similarly, it takes time for a junk-food-laden digestive system to adapt to a wholefood diet. But once weaned on to natural essences, synthetic fragrances may even be perceived as a nostril-stinging assault!

THE PROPERTIES OF ESSENTIAL OILS

While each essential oil has its own unique properties, many also share some common therapeutic actions. All plant essences are antiseptic to a greater or lesser degree; good examples being eucalyptus, tea tree and thyme. Some oils are endowed with antiviral properties as well; garlic and tea tree being two of the most powerful. For obvious reasons, garlic essence is not usually employed in aromatherapy massage (though it has been known!) but instead, is taken as a medicine in the form of garlic capsules. Many essences, notably rosemary and juniper, are also antirheumatic. When rubbed into the skin, they stimulate blood and lymphatic circulation and increase oxygen to the painful areas, which in turn aids the elimination of tissue wastes (uric and lactic acids, for example) which contribute to the pain of arthritic and rheumatic complaints.

MEDICINAL AROMATHERAPY

Another interesting property of many essential oils (and also herbal remedies) is their adaptogenic or 'normalising' ability. Researchers in eastern Europe have found that garlic has the ability to raise abnormally low blood pressure, and to lower blood pressure that is too high. Essential oil of hyssop is cited as having the same action. Studies have shown that it causes blood pressure to go up, then down, then back to normal, as if testing out the required pressure! A phenomenon which is totally alien to a synthetic or chemical drug.

Valnet and other doctors in the field of medical aromatherapy have also discovered that blends of certain essences are not only more powerful than when used singly, but that the mysterious factor of synergy is at work – the effect of the whole becoming greater than the sum of its equal parts. This is particularly noticeable with the anti-bacterial action of essential oils. A blend of clove, thyme, lavender and peppermint, for example, is far more powerful than the chemist might expect of the blend, taking into account the combined chemical constituents of the oils. Curiously, mixing more than five essences is counter-productive. The anti-bacterial action is weakened. But even as loners, certain plant essences are remarkable aggressors against microbial germs. According to Valnet, essential oil of lemon neutralises typhoid, diphtheria and pneumonia bacteria in less than three hours.

To ascertain the most efficacious oils for a particular person, French aromatherapy doctors usually employ the *aromatogram*. This involves taking a swab from an infected area of the patient, culturing it in the laboratory and then testing as many as fifteen different essences to find out which blend of oils would be the most effective for that particular person's infection. The most potent oils are then encapsulated and administered orally. It may come as a surprise to learn that a different patient suffering from the same named bacterial invasion will need a different blend of oils in order to combat the infection. From this we may conclude that even our germs carry the essence of our individuality!

A great many essential oils also have a cicatrising effect: they stimulate the growth of healthy skin cells. One of the most remarkable is calendula essence (pot marigold). Unfortunately, the distilled essence is not generally available because the plant produces too little volatile oil to make distillation commercially viable. However, aromatherapists tend to use the infused oil, made by macerating the flower heads in vegetable oil, thus capturing a dilution of the essential oil (see page 38). As testimony to the skin-healing properties of calendula, herbalists warn that the oil causes skin to 'knit' back so rapidly that it can actually seal dirt into the body. It is very important therefore to clean wounds thoroughly before applying calendula in any shape or form – whether it be an ointment, tincture or oil. Another renowned cicatrisant oil is lavender, a marvellous healing agent for scar-tissue, burns, wounds and ulcers.

AROMATHERAPY FOR HORMONAL IMBALANCES

A major area of influence is the effect of essential oils upon the female reproductive system. Essences such as chamomile, cypress, sage and rose are cited as especially helpful in regulating the menstrual cycle. In my own experience, frankincense is perhaps the most efficacious essential oil for irregular or heavy periods, yet it is rarely acknowledged as significant in this respect.

Just how hormone-balancing essences work their special magic is open to conjecture. Even though sage (the herb and the essence) is known to contain hormone-like substances called phyto-oestrogens, there is no scientific evidence to suggest that all hormone-balancing essences contain such substances. However, studies have shown that frankincense and myrrh contain resin alcohols which have a similar chemical structure to human steroids – the male and female hormones. Whether resin alcohols exert a hormonal influence on humans has not been proven, but anecdotal evidence amongst aromatherapists suggests the affirmative. Of course, much more research into this area is needed before we dare jump to any firm conclusions.

Interestingly, plants such as rhubarb, hops, soya beans, fennel, gingseng and red clover have been found to contain phyto-oestrogens. Hops and fennel also produce an essential oil which might possibly contain the same substances. There is evidence that plant oestrogens extracted from rhubarb and hops (available in tablet form and marketed as Phytoesterol) can be used successfully to treat menopausal symptoms and also to minimise oestro-gen withdrawal symptoms for women who have had problems on Hormone Replacement Therapy.

But rather than being a form of HRT from the plant kingdom, it is thought that most other hormone-balancing essences (and herbal medicines) have a precursory influence; that is to say, they enhance the body's ability to balance its own hormone secretions.

AROMATHERAPY FOR BREASTFEEDING

A hormonal influence is also recognised in those aromatics which for centuries have been used to promote the flow of mothers' milk – fennel and caraway, for example. If, for some reason, the milk supply needs to be stopped, others such as sage and peppermint will have the opposite effect and will help to diminish the supply. But there are differing opinions regarding the oils' mode of action: herbalists sometimes argue that galactagogues (substances which promote lactation) do not work unless taken internally, in the form of an infusion from the plant. Similarly, Valnet advocates oral doses of fennel essence for promoting the flow of milk in nursing mothers, and sage essence to dry up the supply.

When essential oils are applied externally, it is difficult to ascertain whether it is the oil or the massage itself which influences lactation. For even without essential oils, breast massage can stimulate the flow. As for diminishing the supply, in India jasmine flowers are traditionally applied as a poultice to the breasts to suppress excess lactation after childbirth (the petals contain the essential oil). British aromatherapy midwives successfully employ peppermint compresses for the same purpose. In fact, external applications of essential oils are employed by aromatherapists for all manner of conditions, not just for stimulating or suppressing lactation. Because aromatherapy is so popular, many thousands of people can testify to the efficacy of the treatment.

AROMATHERAPY FOR THE CENTRAL NERVOUS SYSTEM

Aromatherapists believe that enough essential oil is absorbed through the skin and into the systemic circulation to exert a pharmacological action. However, inhalation of the aromatic molecules (which is virtually impossible to avoid, whatever the application) is another significant pathway. In regard to balancing sex hormones, inhalation may, in fact, turn out to be the most important route of all – because of the influence of plant pheromones on the libido (see Chapter 27). Furthermore, it has been found that essential oils reach the bloodstream more speedily via inhalation than by oral administration.

There is no doubt whatsoever that the aromas of essential oils (and also synthetic fragrances) act on the central nervous system, and this can be measured by EEG (electroencephalograph) scanning equipment. If perceived as pleasant, essences such as chamomile, neroli and clary sage produce alpha, theta and delta brainwave patterns. This translates into feelings of relaxation and inner ease. Other essences such as black pepper, rosemary and coriander produce beta brainwaves, indicating a state of alertness and well-being. Then there are those oils which have been credited with exerting a balancing effect – they gently stimulate people who feel lethargic, and lower anxiety levels in those who feel tense and nervy – bergamot and lavender are especially helpful. If an aroma is disliked, however, its effect on the central nervous system is effectively blocked.

An essence may also have the ability to exert seemingly paradoxical actions. A person suffering from exhaustion as a result of hyper-anxiety, for example, can be both calmed and stimulated by sniffing peppermint. This may be easier to understand if we consider a common response to the oil. Its piercing aroma gives an initial charge (rather like the shock of cold water) which clears the head and awakens the senses. This feeling gradually gives way to an expansive sensation which may also be perceived as a sense of quietude. If this seems unlikely, sniff it and see!

MODES OF ABSORPTION

When essential oils are applied externally (the recommended method for lay people and medically unqualified aromatherapists), there are two main routes by which they may reach the bloodstream: by skin absorption and by diffusion across the tiny air sacs in the lungs.

SKIN ABSORPTION

The skin is a two-way system, capable of both absorption and excretion. When we eat spicy or garlicky foods, the odour will be noticeable on our breath; the odoriferous molecules will also be secreted through the pores of the skin with the sweat. While it is true that water cannot be absorbed into the bloodstream through the skin, the upper layers of skin will temporarily hold a little water. This is particularly noticeable after a long soak in the bath; the pads of your fingertips and toes will take on a wrinkled appearance. The skin can, however, convey certain substances to the systemic circulation, provided that their molecular structure is small enough. Essential oils are good examples of such substances.

It is thought that the tiny molecules of essential oils pass through the hair follicles, which contain sebum, an oily liquid with which essential oils have an affinity. From here the oils diffuse into the bloodstream or are taken up by the lymph and interstitial fluid (a liquid surrounding all body cells) to other parts of the body. If the skin is healthy, the aromatic molecules will be easily absorbed into the bloodstream, though different essences are absorbed at varying rates. The fastest travellers include eucalyptus and thyme, which reach the systemic circulation within half an hour of application; the slowest include coriander and peppermint, which can take up to two hours to reach the bloodstream. A classic test of the skin's ability to absorb substances is to rub a clove of garlic into the soles of the feet; the odour will be detected on the breath an hour or two later.

If the skin is congested, or if there is much subcutaneous fat, absorption of plant essences is greatly hindered. Even so, people with congested skin often benefit from aromatic baths because warmth and moisture facilitate penetration of the aromatic molecules. The skin also becomes more receptive to essential oils when warmed and frictioned by the action of massage. Moreover, when we take an aromatic bath or receive a full-body massage, essential oils will come into contact with sensitive areas such as the abdomen, inner thighs and upper arms: the skin in these places is softer and therefore more permeable.

Even though essential oils are sometimes given orally, they can often be even more effective when applied to the skin. This can also be seen with other substances such as evening primrose oil; though not an essential oil, it appears to work better when applied externally for the treatment of hyperactivity in babies and children. Oral doses are not always successful because absorption from the gut is often impaired in these children. In fact, the skin of the very young child is especially permeable, which is why I no longer advocate skin applications of essential oils for babies and young children (see Chapter 18).

Critics would argue that external applications of evening primrose oil, and indeed any other fixed oil, cannot be absorbed through the skin because the oil's molecules are too large. It would seem that this argument is born of a misunderstanding, for it is not the molecules of the vegetable oil itself which slip through the skin, rather it is the oil's *nutrients*. Substances like vitamin E and essential fatty acids (found in unrefined vegetable oils) have a tiny molecular structure which can indeed diffuse into the bloodstream, just like an essential oil.

Similarly, empirical evidence would suggest that the skin can also absorb the medicinal properties of aromatic decoctions (water-based medicines) by osmosis or diffusion. Herbal baths and compresses can, it seems, be used to treat all manner of internal ailments, although experts argue about whether such treatment is truly effective. As with vegetable oil, it is not the carrier itself (i.e. the water or the vegetable oil) which is absorbed, but the medicinal substances suspended in the carrier – their passage through the skin being facilitated by warmth and moisture.

Despite advances in administering drugs by inunction (applying to the skin), many physicians underestimate the ability of the skin to convey nutrients to the bloodstream. It is often forgotten that vitamins (suspended in an oily base) were applied to the inner thighs of malnourished ex-prisoners who were too ill to take them by mouth after the Second World War. Even more remarkable, it was not only the fat-soluble nutrients which were found to enter the bloodstream by this method, but also the water-soluble molecules, vitamin C and B-complex vitamins. It is my own belief that in serious conditions, especially in life-or-death situations such as the example given, the skin becomes super-efficient at absorbing substances: becoming a kind of emergency 'digestive system'. Therefore, it would seem that 'feeding' by inunction would also benefit sufferers of anorexia nervosa, for impaired absorption from the gut is a well-known complication of this distressing illness.

There is nothing new about administering drugs by inunction. Indeed, it is well known that the 'witches' of antiquity anointed their bodies with hallucinogenic 'flying ointments' impregnated with extracts of hemlock, deadly nightshade and the poisonous toadstool known as fly agaric. Since these plants are without an essential oil, their active principles being crystalline alkaloids, this must surely counter the notion that it is only the oil-soluble, highly volatile essential oil of a plant which is capable of travelling across the skin. The use of the nicotine patch (nicotine is an alkaloid) to help smokers kick the habit is a more modern example of the effect.

Administering drugs by inunction has been made safer recently with the introduction of a measured dose. For example, oestrogen and trinitrin can be administered through a patch applied to the skin. The advantage of transdermal applications over oral dosage is that much smaller quantities of the drug may be administered because none is lost in the digestive processes, nor broken down by the liver. This method also avoids irritation of the gastrointestinal tract (a common side-effect of many drugs). Likewise, smaller doses of essential oils applied externally may be just as efficacious as larger quantities of the same essences taken by mouth.

ABSORPTION VIA THE LUNGS

When inhaled, the aromatic molecules of essential oils reach the lungs from where they diffuse across tiny air sacs (alveoli) into the surrounding blood capillaries and eventually find their way into the systemic circulation from where they exert their therapeutic effect.

A Japanese experiment carried out in 1963 concluded that the effect of peppermint oil on the digestive system was stronger if inhaled than when the same oil was taken by mouth. Interestingly, aromatherapists often comment upon the appetite-stimulating 'side-effect' of working with essential oils in general. To the weight conscious, this could be regarded as something of an occupational hazard. But to the epicurean, the aromas of essential oils sharpen the senses, and thus enhance all of life's pleasures, not just the enjoyment of food.

It is also interesting to note that a common side-effect reported by female hop pickers is menstrual change as a result of inhaling the aroma of hops. Some women experienced heavier menstrual flow; others whose menstrual cycles were jerky discovered the efficacy of hops in regulating the cycle. Although a certain amount of oestrogen-like substances found in hops may be absorbed through the skin of the hands, it seems much more likely that inhalation is the most important route. Indeed, herbalists generally agree that it is the volatile aromatic element (the essential oil) of hops that appears to be the most active.

HOW CAN SO LITTLE DO SO MUCH?

Whether absorbed through the skin or inhaled, once in the bloodstream and body fluids, the essences may have a pharmacological effect – even though the amount absorbed is very small indeed. According to Gattefossé®, essential oils diluted to a degree at which they no longer have any effect on living cultures in the laboratory still have a clear, rapid and beneficial action on the body. This indicates that essential oils are immuno-stimulants or bio-catalysts. Having triggered their healing effect, the aromatic molecules are rapidly excreted from the body – via the skin, sweat, urine, faeces, or, in the case of certain essences, such as eucalyptus and garlic, mainly through exhalation – and yet the aromatic molecules remain almost unchanged in themselves. Therefore, if used correctly as described in this book, there is little danger of toxicity. The efficacy of the treatment is also due to the fact that aromatherapy treatments are given once or twice weekly over a period of not less than one month, thus repeatedly stimulating the body's self-healing processes.

Of course, there is also the psychotherapeutic aspect of aromatherapy which, so far, we have only touched upon. As this is a subject worthy of much more space than can be afforded here, a whole section is devoted to the mysteries of smell and the psycho-spiritual aspect of healing (see Part Three). Here we shall continue our exploration by taking a closer look at the chemistry of essential oils.

ESSENTIAL OIL CHEMISTRY

The known chemical constituents of plants are of two kinds: products of primary metabolism and products of secondary metabolism. The first are chiefly carbohydrates, amino acids and fixed oils, produced by light-absorbing (photosynthetic) processes. The latter group of chemicals arise from the primary metabolites. They include glycosides, terpenoids, alkaloids and essential oils.

The chemistry of essential oils is elaborate. An individual oil may have hundreds of ingredients, the principle components being a group of complex substances known as terpenes and their compounds or derivatives. This explains why a single essence has a wide range of therapeutic actions.

HERBAL MEDICINE AND PHARMACEUTICAL DRUGS

Medicinal plants prepared as herbal remedies, or distilled to extract their essential oils, contain certain 'active principles'. It is these substances which the chemist is intent on isolating, purifying and even synthesising from simpler substances in the preparation of powerful pharmaceutical drugs. Some of the most familiar isolates are morphine, a pain-killing alkaloid from the opium poppy, atropine, a narcotic derived from the deadly nightshade, and the heart tranquilliser digitalis, extracted from the foxglove.

No one would argue that such drugs represented a major advance in the early part of the nineteenth century when they were first isolated. Indeed, they continue to save lives and ease pain. Nevertheless, there are those who would think that we have moved too far down the synthetic drug road. As well as the enormous cost of pharmaceutical drugs, the side-effects of many of these preparations can sometimes be severe. Indeed, drug-induced illness known as *atrogenic* disease, may be far more widespread than is generally realised.

A chemical drug may contain a single, therefore unbalanced and very powerful, active principle. As a result, it acts in the manner of the proverbial sledge-hammer to crack a nut. An essential oil or herbal remedy, on the other hand, contains numerous trace chemicals which the chemist may regard as pharmacologically inactive. To the natural healer, however, it is these very substances which serve to increase the efficacy of the active principle. At the same time, they act to buffer the harmful side-effects of the same chemical when used as an isolate or produced synthetically. This action is known as synergism. An example of the potential risks of isolating the active principle can be seen with lemongrass essence.

When its major chemical constituent citral is isolated and applied to the skin, there is a high chance that it will cause an allergic reaction. The whole oil is much less likely to cause such a reaction, even though citral is present at levels of around 80 per cent.

The main difference between conventional drug treatment and natural medicine is that conventional treatment aims to suppress symptoms as quickly as possible. Side-effects are regarded as the inevitable price we must pay for an instant cure, no matter how temporary. Natural healing requires more time and effort on the part of the recipient, for it aims to stimulate gently the body's immune defences, thus creating the right conditions for lasting health. From an ecological perspective, the overuse of antibiotics (especially over the last thirty years) has created highly resistant strains of bacteria, so that problems become even more unyielding to treatment. Yet, by cultivating a stronger immune system through a balanced lifestyle and diet (see Chapter 16), we become more responsive to the relatively gentle healing actions of herbs and essential oils, which means antibiotics can often be avoided.

Moreover, we need to adopt a balanced viewpoint and accept that the use of drugs cannot be totally ruled out; everything has its place in the holistic scheme of things. If, for example, a person fails to respond to natural treatment and is in a great deal of discomfort, or in a life-or-death situation (road accident, congenital organ dysfunction, and so on) drug intervention may be vital.

BUT ARE ESSENTIAL OILS WHOLE?

Although essential oils have been credited with possessing almost all of the plant's therapeutic properties in a concentrated form, the word 'almost' needs some clarification. Essential oils lack the water-soluble constituents such as tannins, bitter compounds, sugars, mucilages and pectins, all of which play an important role in the medicinal action of the plant. With the exception of cold expressed citrus essences, the heat of distillation (and other warm extraction methods) causes changes in the natural chemical composition of the essential oil, resulting in substances not found in the plant. Having taken these things into account, some herbalists believe that the term 'natural' is something of a misnomer when applied to an essential oil.

While it is true that the essential oil lacks certain chemical compounds found in the raw plant material, it is still a highly complex substance, so complex that it cannot be replicated in the laboratory. Even though high-tech processes such as gas-liquid chromatography (GLC) can separate out the main components of essential oils by looking at the chemical 'fingerprint' produced, it is impossible to isolate the numerous trace elements – including a number of unidentified compounds – which make up the whole. For this reason, synthetic or 'nature identical' aromatic oils are never quite the same as organic essences. Even the most skilfully composed 'nature identical' will smell a little different. This is because the characteristic fragrance of an essential oil is often found in the minute traces of odoriferous chemicals, not in the major components. The fragrance of rose essence, for instance, is so complex that in order for the synthetic counterpart to be convincing, it has to contain a tiny amount of the real thing. In the same way, jasmine cannot be successfully synthesised, at least not to the highly discerning nose.

Moreover, it is impossible to create a 100 per cent pure chemical. Every chemist knows that any synthetic chemical will carry with it a small percentage of undesirable substances which are not found in the essential oil. For this reason, synthetic aromatic oils are much more likely to provoke allergic reactions.

It should also be pointed out that most herbal medicines are 'incomplete' in the sense that they are extracted from various parts of a plant – not the 'whole' plant – each part having a different chemical composition. Sometimes the difference is so great that while one part of the plant may be safe to use, another may be highly poisonous. A good example of this can be seen with the opium poppy. While the seeds are nutritious, all other parts of the plant are extremely poisonous. Similarly, while the rhizomes of rhubarb can be used as a remedy for diarrhoea, the leaves contain a high level of oxalic acid which is potentially lethal.

As soon as plant material is collected, its chemical composition begins to alter, eventually leading to a loss of potency. But in the case of some plants, chemical change is desirable. Chamomile oil, for example, contains the valuable anti-inflammatory agent *chamazulene* which occurs as a direct result of distillation. The laxative result of the herbal medicine cascara (*Rhamnus purshiana*) is the result of chemical changes brought about during the drying process. Heat, of course, brings about further chemical changes; but fibrous material such as barks and roots need to be simmered in water for some time in order to extract the medicinal compounds and make them readily available for absorption. If carried out with care, the remedy remains effective.

THE MAIN CHEMICAL COMPONENTS OF ESSENTIAL OILS

While it is interesting to take a closer look at the individual components of essential oils, it is important not to lose sight of the whole. Assigning actions to an essential oil based on its chemical composition can be misleading. As we have seen, the therapeutic properties of the whole oil is the result of synergism: an interaction of all its chemical constituents working harmoniously together so that the whole becomes more potent than the sum of its individual parts. Bearing this in mind, here is a brief survey of the main chemical compounds found in essential oils.

Terpenes
This is a vast group of chemicals with widely varying properties, so it is impossible to generalise about their therapeutic actions. However, common terpenes include limonene (an antiviral agent found in 90 per cent of citrus oils), and pinene (an antiseptic found in high concentrations in pine and turpentine oils). Others, such as chamazulene and farnesol (found in chamomile essence), possess remarkable anti-inflammatory and bactericidal properties.

Esters
The most widespread group found in plant essences, which includes linalyl acetate (found in clary sage and lavender), and geranyl acetate (found in sweet marjoram). Esters are fungicidal and sedative, usually with a fruity odour.

Aldehydes
These substances are found notably in lemon-scented essences, such as lemongrass and citronella. Aldehydes generally have a sedative, though uplifting, quality.

Ketones
Certain ketones are known to be toxic, so this chemical group is regarded with a degree of caution. However, it is misleading to generalise about the toxicity of individual chemical components without knowing the exact ratio of the substance in relation to other chemicals in the whole oil. Certain essences, however, do contain appreciable quantities of toxic ketones, so should be avoided by lay people. Mugwort, tansy, wormwood and common sage contain the potentially risky thujone, while pennyroyal contains pulegone. Non-toxic ketones include jasmone, found in jasmine, and fenchone in sweet fennel. Ketones ease congestion and aid the flow of mucus, which is why plants and essences containing relatively large quantities

of these substances are usually helpful for upper respiratory complaints.

Alcohols

Some of the most common alcohols include linalol (found in abundance in lavender), citronellol (rose, lemon, eucalyptus and geranium) and geraniol (geranium and palmarosa). These substances tend to have good antiseptic and antiviral properties and an uplifting quality.

Phenols

These are bactericidal with a strong, stimulating effect on the central nervous system. Essential oils containing relatively large quantities of certain phenols are potentially irritant to skin and mucous membranes. Common caustic phenols include eugenol (found in clove essence), thymol (thyme) and carvacrol (oregano). However, anethole (from fennel) and estragole (tarragon) are not at all caustic.

Oxides

These are found in a wide range of essences, especially those of a camphoraceous nature, such as rosemary, eucalyptus, tea tree and cajuput. Oxides tend to have an expectorant effect; for example, eucalyptol (eucalyptus).

CHEMOTYPE OILS

At one time it was thought that there was no difference between the concentration of active principles in individual plant species. However, recent research has revealed the existence of 'chemical races'. Certain specimens can have the same external appearance and yet have chemical compositions which differ considerably. Evidently, these differences are inherited and are not solely due to differences in environment. This has enabled certain strains to be selected which are high yielding in desirable chemical constituents. These are bred and cultivated for medicinal purposes. The essential oils obtained from such plants are known as chemotypes.

Take tea tree oil, for example; the botanical name appearing on the bottle of essential oil will be *Melaleuca alternifolia*. However, there are a number of sub-varieties of this strain having wildly differing chemical compositions. For this reason, the Australian government's standard for tea tree oil does not just specify *M. alternifolia*, but adds 'Oil of Melaleuca, Terpinene-4-ol Type'. In fact the botanical names given to essential oils are not always the name of the plants from which the oil was obtained. The botanical name is often just a trade term.

The situation is a little more straightforward with thyme essence. Even though few essential oil companies specify the exact chemotype (as illustrated by the tea tree

example) we can safely assume that those oils labelled 'Red Thyme' are high in caustic phenols and are therefore more likely to irritate sensitive skin. Thymes containing a higher ratio of alcohols are labelled 'Sweet Thyme' and these are much safer to use (refer to the Aromatic Profiles, Chapter 31).

FRACTIONATED OR FOLDED OILS

These are oils which have had a part of their chemical composition removed. There are three categories: those which have been re-distilled at low pressure in order to remove all their terpenes; those which have had varying amounts of terpenes removed (known as singlefold, twofold – up to fivefold, depending on the percentage of terpenes removed); and those which have been fractionated to remove certain 'undesirable' substances. A good example of a fractionated oil commonly used in aromatherapy is bergamot FCF, which has had the non-volatile, photo-toxic substance bergaptene removed. With the exception of bergamot essence (and perhaps one or two others) fractionated or folded oils are not generally used in aromatherapy, but are mainly employed by the perfume and flavours industries.

The danger with removing the terpenes from essential oils is that the whole chemistry is radically altered (terpenes form the major part of many plant essences) and the natural synergy is lost. De-terpenated thyme oil, for example, becomes very much more hazardous than the natural oil because it contains a higher concentration of thymol and carvacrol. The terpenes act to quench (at least to a degree) the caustic effects of these two phenols.

ADULTERATION OF ESSENTIAL OILS

Unfortunately, adulteration of essential oils is common. They may be tampered with at source or somewhere else along the line before reaching the retail outlets. Essences may be diluted with an alcohol, for example, or perhaps blended with a less expensive oil that has a similar-smelling aroma. Or they may be extended with an isolate obtained from other essential oils, or perhaps with the colourless and odourless synthetic chemical DPG (dipropylene glycol).

It is essential to buy your oils from reputable suppliers, preferably those companies whose oils carry a recognised certificate of purity (see page 26).

GAS-LIQUID CHROMATOGRAPHY

It is possible to assess the purity of individual essences using high-tech methods such as gas-liquid chromatography (GLC). But the *precise* chemical nature of essential oils is still largely unknown. Moreover, different batches of the same type of essential oil, for example *Lavandula augustifolia*, will show variations in chemical composition. With GLC analysis there is a good chance that any adulteration of the oil can be discovered, for the oil's fingerprint (which allows for a wide range of variation in the natural chemical composition) will show chemical imbalances which cannot possibly occur in the natural essential oil.

Despite complicated high-tech methods of assessing the purity of individual essences, the final decision regarding its quality is made by organoleptic analysis. This is the technical term describing the work of the 'nose' – a person with a highly trained sense of smell employed by the perfume and flavours industries.

3
CAPTURING ESSENTIAL OILS

Strictly speaking, the term 'essential oil' describes an aromatic oil captured by distillation and composed entirely of volatile molecules. Nevertheless, the term is often stretched to include aromatic extractions of every conceivable origin, including those captured by volatile solvents, liquid carbon dioxide and the recent phytol method. As well as volatile elements, the oils obtained by processes other than distillation also contain larger molecules of non-volatile matter (waxes, for example). Let us take a closer look at the various extraction methods and the resulting aromatic oils.

DISTILLATION

Although the roots of this method can be traced back to the Mesopotamians nearly 5,000 years ago, distillation as we know it today was initially developed by the Arabian mediaeval alchemists and perfected in Grasse, the home of the perfume industry in the south of France. Generally, soft plant material such as leaves and flowers may be placed in the vessel of a still without prior treatment; fibrous material such as wood, bark, seeds and roots must be cut up, crushed or grated to help release the

volatile oil. Certain plants, such as melissa (lemon balm) and rose, need to be distilled immediately after harvesting because enzymes present in the plant cells will start to break down the essential oil. Other essential oil-yielding plants are not so fragile; chamomile flowers, for instance, need to be dried prior to distillation; and patchouli undergoes a drying and fermentation process before it is ready to give up its precious liquid.

Once in the still, the plant material is subjected to concentrated steam, which releases the aromatic molecules from the plant cells. The aromatic vapour passes along a series of glass tubes surrounded by cold water which act as a condenser. The released essence is then separated from the water by siphoning it off through a narrow-necked container known as a Florentine.

Some distillers employ *direct* distillation which is similar to the former method, except that plant material comes into direct contact with the water. However, 'burning' of the distillate is much more likely to occur with this process, something which must be avoided if the oil is to retain its potency and characteristic aroma.

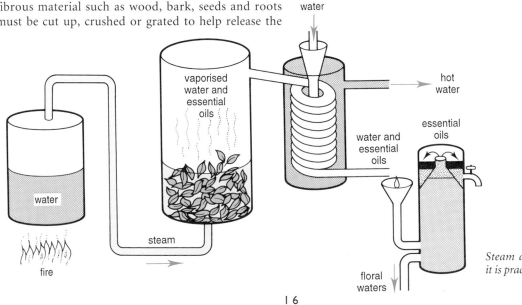

cold water

hot water

vaporised water and essential oils

essential oils

water and essential oils

water

steam

fire

floral waters

Steam distillation as it is practised now

Essential oils, for instance cajeput, have to be re-distilled or rectified in order to remove impurities such as plant dust or resinous matter. Certain essences such as ylang ylang are fractionated to capture several grades. The first distillate is called ylang ylang extra, with the distillation process continuing until three successive lower-grade distillates are also isolated. Another example of a fractionated oil is bergamot FCF, which has been rectified to remove its furocoumarin content. Furocoumarins are responsible for the photo-toxic side-effect of bergamot.

Unfortunately, the heat and water employed in distillation is to some degree harmful to the fragile constituents of the essential oil, as reflected in the aroma which is never identical to that contained in the plant cells. This is especially noticeable with the essential oils of black pepper and ginger. The more pungent notes which emanate from the freshly grated spice cannot survive the heat of distillation.

HOME DISTILLATION OF ESSENTIAL OILS

Although many old herbals (and a few aromatherapy books) extol the virtues of distilling essential oils at home, I am far from convinced that this would be a practicable option. For a start, to obtain a 'kitchen table' still would be an amazing accomplishment in itself since they are so hard to come by. Modestly sized distillation apparatus can be bought from laboratory equipment suppliers *only* if you have a special commercial licence.

For the determined kitchen alchemist, it is possible to rig up your own equipment for producing usable floral waters such as lavender water or rosewater which can be employed as skin tonics – or even as a base for home-made eau de cologne (see page 229). But home-distillation is extremely time consuming with little return for one's efforts.

EXPRESSION

The oils of citrus fruits such as bergamot, lemon and lime are much easier to obtain. Indeed, the essence (the zest of the fruit) is found in such profusion that it sprays the surrounding air when the fruit is peeled. If the zest comes into contact with a candle flame or lighted match, the oil droplets will ignite into a cascade of tiny sparks, albeit for a fraction of a second.

The highest quality citrus essences are captured by a simple process known as expression. Although this was once carried out by hand (by squeezing the rind and collecting the oil in sponge), machines using centrifugal force are now used instead. Since no heat is employed in this process, the aroma and chemical structure of expressed oils is almost identical to that contained within the skin of the fruit. Unlike distilled oils, expressed essences also contain non-volatile substances such as waxes. The drawback with expressed oils is their relatively short shelf-life. Even though producers usually add tiny amounts of a preservative at source, the oils will still deteriorate within six to nine months, whereas most distilled essences will keep for upwards of two years (see Caring For Your Oils page 26).

In the USA, the production of citrus essences is a profitable side-line of the fruit juice industry. There are many low-grade citrus oils with an inferior aroma obtained by steam distillation of the citrus skins after the best oil has been expressed. Unscrupulous suppliers may extend an expressed oil by 'bulking' it with such a product (see Adulteration of Oils page 14).

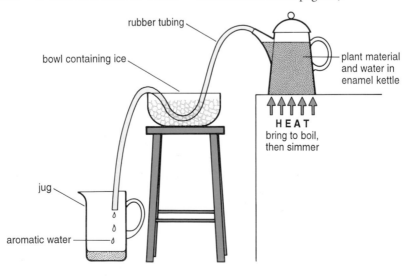

rubber tubing

bowl containing ice

plant material and water in enamel kettle

HEAT bring to boil, then simmer

jug

aromatic water

Home distillation

ENFLEURAGE

The enfleurage method of extraction was once widely used in the perfume industry to capture the fragrances of flowers such as jasmine, orange blossom and tuberose, whose exquisite fragrances would be spoiled by the intense heat of distillation. Except for the tiny amount of enfleurage oils produced for tourists visiting the distilleries in Grasse, this method of extraction is no longer commercially viable.

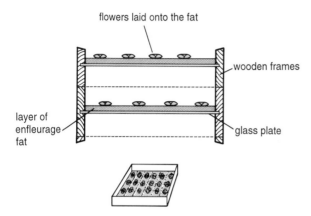

flowers laid onto the fat

wooden frames

layer of enfleurage fat

glass plate

Each "chassis" is a rectangular wooden box of 24"× 18" × 3". Set into each box is a plate of glass. Purified lard is spread onto each sheet and raked into parallel ridges like a ploughed field. The flowers are carefully laid onto the fat, then the chassis are stacked up on top of each other so that the flowers are enclosed by the chassis above.

The enfleurage method of extraction

VOLATILE SOLVENT EXTRACTION

The high cost of the labour-intensive and time-consuming enfleurage method has led to the wide use of volatile solvents such as petroleum ether, hexane and benzene as a means for capturing the essences of certain plants and resins – yet the enfleurage process gives a higher yield. Solvent extraction is employed a great deal in the perfume industry because it produces superb fragrances which are closer to the aromas contained within the plant. Nevertheless, these oils may not be suitable for aromatherapy as they often contain solvent residues and other non-volatile substances which can cause skin reactions in sensitive individuals when the oil is applied directly to the skin. They are also extremely vulnerable to adulteration.

Having been subjected to the volatile solvent (usually hexane) the aromatic plant material produces a waxy substance known as a *concrete*. Although concretes are used in the perfume and fragrance industries, as they still contain appreciable amounts of non-volatile substances and residues of solvent, they are more likely to provoke allergic reactions in those with sensitive skin. To obtain the aromatic liquid the concrete undergoes repeated treatment with alcohol which is finally recovered by evaporation under a gentle vacuum. The resulting viscous oil is known as an *absolute*.

With the exception of benzoin, the essential oils found in resins, such as frankincense, myrrh and galbanum, can be obtained by steam distillation of the dried resinous exudations. These are to be preferred for aromatherapy. The solvent extracted versions commonly employed by the perfume industry are known as *resinoids*. Unfortunately, benzene (a potentially carcinogenic volatile solvent) is, on occasions, used in the extraction of benzoin and other resins.

LIQUID CARBON DIOXIDE EXTRACTION

This process was hailed as nothing less than revolutionary when it was introduced at the beginning of the 1980s. Although a potentially excellent method of extraction, producing oils whose aromas are closer to those of the living plant, the apparatus required for this operation is not only massive, but also extremely costly. It will also take years for the equipment to pay for itself; until such time, the cost of carbon dioxide extracted oils will remain very high.

Although the method is much more complicated than described here, suffice it to say that carbon dioxide gas at exceedingly high pressure (pressures which are only found three miles under the sea) is employed to dissolve the aromatic oils from the plant material. When the pressure is allowed to fall (to one hundred times atmospheric pressure) the oils form a mist and can be collected. The resultant oils are free of the potentially harmful residues associated with solvent extraction, but there are those who would argue that carbon dioxide is an acidic gas and therefore detrimental to the chemical structure of essential oils.

Generally, carbon dioxide extracted oils have fewer terpenes, a higher proportion of esters and contain other substances whose molecules are too large to come through the distillation process. Since a great many terpenes are formed as a result of distillation, the lower terpene content of carbon dioxide oils (and the related difference in ratio of other constituents) means their chemistry is a little closer to nature. Surprisingly, this is not always beneficial. Take ginger, for example; the carbon dioxide extract has a superior aroma to that of the distilled oil, but it is also more likely to irritate sensitive skin. A major drawback with carbon dioxide extracts in general, apart from their high price, is that very few suppliers stock these oils.

HYDRODIFFUSION OR PERCOLATION

Although introduced more recently than carbon dioxide extraction, hydrodiffusion is similar to steam distillation, except that the steam is produced above the plant material and percolates down through it. The advantage of hydrodiffusion over distillation is that the process is quicker, especially for fibrous material such as woods and barks whose cells do not give up their oils easily. The resultant oils are reported to have a superior aroma and a richer colour than those obtained by ordinary distillation. At the time of writing, oils captured by the hydrodiffusion process are not widely available.

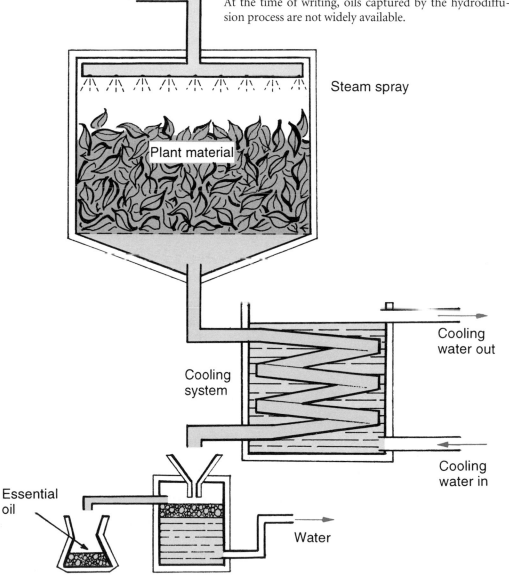

The process of hydrodiffusion

THE PHYTONIC PROCESS

The Phytonic Process was recently developed by British microbiologist Dr Peter Wilde in collaboration with the multinational chemical company, ICI. Proponents of phytonics technology believe that it heralds the biggest breakthrough in aromatic oil extraction since the discovery of distillation.

The process has been developed around a family of new solvents collectively known as phytosols, whose unique character ensures that the aromatic oils of plants can be captured at (or below) room temperature. This means that the exceptionally fragile, heat-sensitive components of an aromatic oil are not lost, or radically altered, in the extraction process.

Oils extracted using the Phytonic Process cannot, strictly speaking, be called essential oils, but neither can they accurately be called absolutes. Indeed, chemical analysis reveals phytonic – extracted oils to be somewhat different from other aromatic oils. English rose phytol oil, for instance, contains over 290 separate, identifiable components (including the water soluble phenylethyl alcohol), whereas the best available rose absolutes contain only 210 components.

MASQUERADE

A few oils are not quite what they seem. For example it is extremely difficult to obtain the true essence of melissa oil (distilled from lemon balm) because so little is produced. When it is available, the oil is costly, for the plant yields such a tiny amount of oil. Most of the so-called melissa oils on the market are actually blends of infinitely cheaper essences such as lemongrass, lemon and citronella. Only when you have smelled true melissa essence and compared it to the falsified versions will you be better able to tell the difference. Honest suppliers will highlight the difference, perhaps by labelling the blended version 'Melissa Type' and the genuine oil, 'Melissa True'. A word of warning: unfortunately, there are also a number of 'Melissa Type' blends on the market which are partly or wholly compounded using aroma chemicals.

If you come across an oil labelled 'Amber', be suspicious. It is certain to be a synthetic compound or a blend of clary sage and benzoin (a resinoid with a vanilla-like aroma). As far as I am aware, true amber oil, from the fossilised resin, is unobtainable. Ambergris (a substance excreted by the sperm whale and sometimes found floating on the sea) is also known as 'amber', an extremely costly fragrance material used in high-class perfumes. Ambergris is not generally available to the public. However, there is a genuine essential oil of ambrette seed, sometimes labelled 'ambre' (note the spelling). Ambrette essence is a popular, though very expensive, perfume material which is also occasionally used in aromatherapy.

ORGANICALLY PRODUCED OILS

Not all essential oils are produced by organic methods, that is to say, extracted from plants grown without the use of chemical fertilizers and poisonous sprays. Oils labelled 'organic' are often of the herb variety, such as lavender, rosemary, marjoram and chamomile, though some oils are distilled from wild plants, extracted from disease resistant trees such as frankincense and cypress, or produced in countries where chemical sprays and fertilizers are not in general use. Organic growers meeting the required standards are awarded certificates by bodies such as the Soil Association in Britain, Biofanc in France and Demeter in Germany.

Organisations such as EOTA (the Essential Oil Trade Association UK) are taking steps to establish reliable sources of pure, unadulterated essential oils for therapy. It is hoped that aromatherapy will benefit from this in two ways: that the purity of an oil can be guaranteed and that there will be a greater choice of organic oils more widely available. Essential oil suppliers have also established a form of certification known as AROMARK Grade for essential oils which can be guaranteed natural (usually tested by gas-liquid chromatography). In India, the government has given the term AGMARK (Agricultural Guarantee Mark) to some of their oils, mainly sandalwood and lemongrass. Although not necessarily organically produced, any oil carrying the AROMARK or AGMARK signature is guaranteed to be a pure unadulterated plant essence.

The problem is that not all essential oil suppliers are honest. Some will charge an inflated price for an 'organic' oil – ylang ylang is a good example, where most, if not all, of the ylang ylang oil on the market is organic in the sense outlined above. (However, ylang ylang is especially vulnerable to adulteration.) Or you may be hoodwinked into paying extra for an 'organic' jasmine or rose absolute, when no such oil exists. True, all essential oils are organic in the sense that they are obtained from living plants rather than produced in the laboratory, but the word 'organic' is open to abuse. It is extremely difficult to obtain totally uncontaminated medicinal and food plants, even when they are gathered from the wild.

A WORD ABOUT TREE OILS

Many people are deeply concerned about the capturing of essences from trees, especially if the tree has to be felled in order to do so, for example, rosewood (also known as bois de rose) and sandalwood. At present the principle supplies of rosewood essence come from trees torn down from the rapidly diminishing rainforests of Brazil. The production of essential oil (obtained by steam distillation of the wood chippings) is actually a side-line of the lumber industry, with most of the wood going to US furniture makers. Even though a re-planting programme has been attempted, the new trees are unable to grow healthily in the impoverished soil whose nutrients have been leached by exposure to the elements. So for sound ecological reasons it is advisable to avoid this oil – including supplies of rosewood from other areas of South America and also Africa.

The situation regarding Mysore sandalwood oil is apparently much healthier. The Indian government controls almost all the total output of sandalwood in the world. It has ordered that for every tree felled, two more must be planted in its place – and this is actually happening. However, the repeated demands of the perfume industry, combined with clandestine cutting, have caused the destruction of many trees, with disturbing results in some parts of India. For these reasons it might be advisable to use other oils with similar therapeutic properties, such as frankincense and galbanum. But the aromas of these two oils are totally different from that of sandalwood whose soft fragrance is unique.

There are those who feel that the essential oils distilled from resins and gums, such as frankincense and myrrh, are unsuitable for healing purposes because they are 'pathological' in origin. That is to say, the tree must be wounded (usually an incision is made in the trunk) before it will produce a milky exudation, which eventually hardens to seal the fissure. It is the hardened exudations which are collected for distillation. Having just outlined the alarming de-forestation situation, it is surely a case of misplaced sentiment to believe that the collection of gums and resins may be 'cruel' to the tree. In fact, trees are never felled in order to collect their exudations; and so long as they are not over 'milked' (highly unlikely as this would be uneconomical) they are not destroyed by the process.

4
ESSENTIAL OIL SAFETY

> *Essential oils are marvellous healing substances, but they are also highly concentrated and potentially hazardous if misused. So before you begin to experiment with essential oils, do please read the safety guidelines given here.*

SIMPLE SKIN TEST

When using an essential oil for the first time, it is advisable to carry out a skin test, especially if you have sensitive skin. Mix one drop of the test essence in a teaspoonful of almond oil. Rub a little of the mixture behind the ears, the crook of the arm or on the inside of the wrist (supersensitive spots). Leave uncovered and unwashed for 24 hours. If there is no redness or itching, the oil is safe for you to use. In fact, you can test up to six oils at the same time using this method. But you will need to keep a record of the oils used and where they were applied. For example, ginger behind the right ear, ylang ylang in the crook of the left arm, and so on.

A WORD ABOUT ALLERGIES

If you suffer from hay fever, food allergies, allergic rhinitis, eczema, asthma, wool or animal intolerance (or have a family history of any of these complaints), you are much more likely to develop contact dermatitis (redness or itching as mentioned above) as a result of using certain aromatic oils. This means the skin will react sometimes within seconds, certainly within 24 hours, of contact with the offending substance.

People in this group are also more likely to develop a *sensitivity* to a particular essence, or to a specific chemical component present in a number of oils. The last problem is known as *cross sensitivity* in which there may be no adverse reaction on first contact with the allergen, for it takes at least five to seven days for sensitivity to develop.

However, continual exposure to the same essence for prolonged periods may provoke sensitivity in anyone, even in those who have 'normal' tolerance levels to plant essences. Those most at risk are aromatherapists themselves. Indeed, I have met several practitioners over the last few years who have developed dermatitis of the hands as a result of using lavender essence almost every day for upwards of three years.

Once sensitised the body will *always* react to *any amount* of that substance, no matter how tiny the quantity. Symptoms can vary from an itchy rash (as in contact dermatitis) through to more widespread symptoms such as streaming and stinging eyes, swollen tissues and wheezing (see Patch Test for Allergy Sufferers).

However, it is vital to get the allergy scare into perspective. In reality, a full-blown allergic reaction to essential oils is rare. Moreover, the majority of tests for sensitivity have been conducted by the perfume and fragrance industries. This means that much of the available safety data reflects the testing of synthetic aroma chemicals, isolated chemical components of essential oils, or modified essential oils – not the *whole* oil as used in aromatherapy. With a few exceptions, unmodified oils are generally much safer to use due to their natural synergy.

Another point, it is possible to be allergic to almost anything, even to water or the seemingly innocuous sweet almond oil. If you fall into this high risk category, it would be wise to avoid all essential oils and to try another therapy instead, perhaps homoeopathy or acupuncture. Aromatherapy can, however, be of enormous benefit in less extreme cases.

Listed in the panel are the essential oils which are *more likely* to trigger allergic reactions in susceptible individuals. In fact, you may find that only a few of these potentially problematic oils are incompatible with your own body. Everyone is different. Although the list may appear to be alarmingly long, in fact less than half the oils listed are used by the average aromatherapist. Nevertheless, a few of the potentially harmful oils, such as aniseed and bay, are sometimes available from retail outlets.

OILS TO BE AVOIDED
IF YOU SUFFER FROM ALLERGIES OR HAVE
HIGHLY SENSITIVE SKIN

IMPORTANT *The following oils may have to be avoided if you are prone to allergies or have highly sensitive skin. Even if you have 'normal' skin, it is advisable to use these oils in the lowest recommended dilutions (at least until you are sure the essence suits your skin) e.g. one drop to every two teaspoonfuls of vegetable oil for massage, and no more than one or two drops in the bath.*

All absolutes, resinoids and balsams, for example Benzoin Resinoid, Rose Absolute, Jasmine Absolute, Peru Balsam*, Tolu Balsam*, and all of the following essences:

Allspice (Pimento)	Cinnamon (bark and	Juniper	Peppermint
Aniseed	leaf)*	Lemon	Pine
Basil	Citronella	Lemongrass	Sage
Bay	Clary Sage	Lime	Spearmint
Black Pepper	Clove (bud, stem and	Litsea Cubeba	Tagetes
Cedarwood	leaf)*	Lovage	Tea Tree
Celery Seed	Costus Root	Melissa***	Thyme
Chamomile (Roman and	Fennel	Nutmeg	Ylang Ylang
German)**	Ginger	Orange	
	Hops	Parsley	

* In my opinion these oils should never be applied to the skin or used in steam inhalations as they can be extremely irritant to skin and mucous membranes. Use in low dilution as room scents only.

** Although the chamomiles are actually recommended for allergies, they are highly odoriferous and may provoke skin rashes unless used in very low dilution.

*** There are two types of melissa: genuine melissa oil (a costly essence distilled from lemon balm) and a 'melissa type' oil (an inexpensive blend of lemon-smelling essences such as lemongrass and citronella). Both versions may cause skin irritation, especially if used in high concentration.

UNUSUAL ESSENTIAL OILS

Aromatherapy authors sometimes promote unusual oils, many of which are beginning to appear on essential oil suppliers' lists. Unfortunately, the majority have not been extensively tested for possible adverse reactions on human skin. Therefore, no adequate safety data has been published. Although I am unaware of any evidence to suggest that people have been harmed by these newcomers, it would seem appropriate to include a cautionary note just in case. According to recent research the following essences should be regarded as suspect for the time being: chamomile moroc, ravensara, inula (also known as elecampane), true melissa, spikenard (also known as 'nard'), valerian, yarrow, amyris (also known as West Indian sandalwood) and elderflower absolute.

PATCH TEST FOR ALLERGY SUFFERERS

Unlike the simple skin test described earlier, the patch test requires a great deal of patience. Nevertheless, it is a highly reliable test for allergy sufferers. You may discover that you can benefit from a number of essential oils, though three essences would suffice e.g. lavender, chamomile Roman, eucalyptus. However, it is important to avoid prolonged use of the same essence because you may develop a sensitivity to the oil even though a patch test has assured you of its safety. It is also important to ascertain that you are not allergic to the chosen base oil, for example almond or olive. So unless you know that the oil is safe for you to use, skin test it (the simple test should suffice) before mixing with your chosen essential oil.

Test only one essence at a time. Mix one drop of the test essence into one teaspoonful of base oil. Rub a little of the oil into the upper chest or forearm. Apply a piece of gauze followed by a waterproof dressing. Leave in place for 24–48 hours, then remove and examine the area for any redness or itching. If there is no reaction, apply a little more oil and replace the patch. Repeat the test daily for seven days. Following a period of 10–14 days' rest, challenge the skin once more with the same base oil and essence, covering with another waterproof patch. At this stage of the test, any sensitivity will become apparent within 24 hours. If so, the oil should be avoided at all costs.

SUBTLE TESTING OF OILS

There are two other methods for determining which oils are safe and beneficial for different people – muscle testing and pendulum dowsing. In the right hands, these subtle methods of diagnosis can be remarkably accurate – and certainly much speedier than the skin tests given above. However, their mode of action cannot be explained in scientific terms. They rely entirely on the user's ability to access their intuitive powers. But it can take a very long time to perfect such skills. For this reason, the novice is advised never to use subtle methods of diagnosis on atopic (allergy-prone) people, pregnant women, babies and children. But if you would like to learn the basics, instructions are given in Chapter 20.

PHOTOSENSITISING OILS

Certain aromatic oils can cause skin pigmentation when applied shortly before exposure to sunlight or other types of ultraviolet light, such as a sunbed. The most powerful oil in this respect is bergamot. In fact, I have discovered that bergamot can cause skin reactions without the presence of sunlight; for example, when applied immediately before working in a hot and steamy kitchen. For this reason, I no longer advocate the use of bergamot oil on the skin. However, it is possible to obtain a furocoumarin free oil called bergamot FCF (furocoumarins are responsible for the oil's photosensitising effect). Although shunned by some aromatherapists (on the grounds that it is not a whole oil), bergamot FCF is non-photosensitising.

The following essential oils are also photosensitising: angelica root, grapefruit, lemon, lime, mandarin, orange and tagetes.

PREGNANCY

Due to their tiny molecular structure, plant essences (and some synthetic perfume chemicals) can slip through the skin and find their way into the bloodstream and other body fluids. Normally, this is an important aspect of the treatment. However, the skin becomes more permeable during pregnancy and also more sensitive, and a number of essential oils (especially citrus essences) are able to cross the placental barrier. It should be pointed out that there is no evidence to suggest that unborn babies have been harmed as a result of their mothers using *therapeutic* applications of essential oils, indeed according to the aromatherapy associations, it is the citrus essences which are among the safest to use during pregnancy.

Nevertheless, a number of oils stimulate menstruation and are therefore potentially hazardous, especially during the first three months of pregnancy when miscarriage is more of a threat than the following months. Other oils potentially hazardous to pregnant women are those containing stimulating substances which have a strong effect on the nervous system, or those which have a stimulating effect on the liver or kidneys.

In reality, however, a woman would need to apply (or take by mouth) a very high concentration of the potentially risky essential oils to cause miscarriage or toxicity (as the few reported cases in the USA of attempted abortion by ingestion of essential oils would verify). However, it is always best to err on the side of caution. Before using any essential oil, do please check that it is safe to do so. Refer to the aromatic profiles (see Chapter 31). Where appropriate, a CAUTION note is included at the end of a specific profile.

For the record, my own approach is to avoid the use of essential oils on the skin during pregnancy (because of increased sensitivity) and to use mood-enhancing room scents instead. However, gentle massage with plain extra virgin olive oil is beneficial to both mother and baby (see page 37). The oil is also a wonderful preventative of stretch marks. Favourite essential oils can be vaporised into the room during the massage and at other times according to need, though much lower dilutions are usually preferred. During pregnancy, many women experience a heightened sense of smell and taste, especially in the first trimester. No doubt, this is a natural safety mechanism to deter the mother from ingesting (or inhaling) potentially toxic substances which may harm the unborn baby.

A great many of the potentially hazardous oils are not commonly used in aromatherapy. So rather than offer a long list of oils which should be avoided during pregnancy it would seem more helpful at this stage to offer an at-a-glance list of the beneficial essences.

RECOMMENDED ESSENTIAL OILS DURING PREGNANCY

Although I do not advocate the use of essential oils on the skin during pregnancy, other aromatherapists recommend the following essences in half the recommended dilution *but only after the first trimester.* However, it may still be advisable to carry out a skin test beforehand.

Geranium	Mandarin
Neroli	Grapefruit
Ylang Ylang	Bergamot
Petitgrain	Lemon
Frankincense	Coriander
Sandalwood	Black Pepper
Patchouli	Ginger
Chamomile (German	Pine
and Roman)	Cypress
Rose Otto	Peppermint
Lavender	Orange

NURSING MOTHERS

It is advisable to avoid the use of perfume-strength blends directly on the skin while breastfeeding. As mentioned in the notes on pregnancy, plant essences rubbed into the skin can find their way into the bloodstream and other body fluids (including breast milk). Moreover, the aromas of some essential oils (geranium for instance) can be stimulating to young babies and may interfere with natural sleep patterns. Remember to wash off all traces of essential oil before feeding the baby. (For more detailed advice on aromatherapy for nursing mothers, see pages 131–5.)

BABIES AND YOUNG CHILDREN

Although many aromatherapists advocate the use of essential oils for babies and young children, I feel it is safer to use only almond or olive oil for massage, and/or to vaporise low concentrations of recommended essences. In my opinion essential oils should never be used on the skin until the baby is over 12 months – and even then in very low dilutions (see page 201).

GENERAL PRECAUTIONS AT-A-GLANCE

- Keep bottles out of reach of children.
- Keep essential oils away from varnished surfaces as they may dissolve the coating. Despite this alarming fact, when correctly diluted as advocated in this book, essential oils are harmless to human tissue.
- Generally, do not apply neat oils to the skin. One exception is the occasional use of neat lavender, for example, on minor burns and cuts (see page 63).
- Keep essential oils away from the eyes, and do not rub your eyes after handling them. Should any essential oil get into the eyes, rinse it out at once with plenty of cool water.
- Never take essential oils by mouth, rectum or vagina, unless under medical instructions.
- Citrus oils, especially bergamot, increase the skin's sensitivity to sunlight, so do not use on the skin shortly before exposure to sunlight (or a sunbed) as they may cause unsightly pigmentation.
- Avoid citrus essences on the skin if you have symptoms or a history of melanoma, pre-melanoma, senile patches, large moles, warts, extensive dark freckles or skin cancer. There is a remote chance that citrus oils may promote the advance of these conditions.
- Never use an essential oil about which you can find little or no information.
- Avoid prolonged use of the same essential oil (i.e. daily for more than three months) as there is a slight risk of developing a sensitivity to the oil. Take a two month break before using it again.
- If you suffer from sensitive skin or allergies, it is advisable to carry out a simple skin test or a patch test before using an essential oil for the first time (see page 22).
- If you suffer from epilepsy, it is advisable to avoid the essential oils of rosemary, fennel and sage, as there is a remote chance that these essences may trigger an attack.
- If you suffer from asthma, avoid steam inhalations. With or without essential oils, concentrated steam may trigger an attack.
- Some homoeopaths believe that all essential oils (and other strong odours) weaken or cancel out the effects of homoeopathic remedies. Other practitioners believe that only the camphoraceous oils are contra-indicated. Always tell your homoeopath that you are using essential oils.

5
APPRENTICED TO AROMATHERAPY

Nature's aromatic essences can be used in many different ways to promote health of body and serenity of mind. Whether you wish to harness their powers to treat a specific ailment, to buffer the adverse effects of stress, or simply to enhance mood, this chapter is devoted to the basics of preparing and applying essential oils for healing purposes. While the mixing of massage oils is explained, the art of massage itself is explored in Part 4.

BUYING ESSENTIAL OILS

It is vital to obtain only the purest aromatherapy grade essential oils. Most aromatherapists buy their oils from specialist mail order suppliers, not from shops concerned with beauty and perfumery. The advantages offered by mail order suppliers include a wider range of oils and lower prices on larger quantities. However, if you are new to aromatherapy, it may be best to buy your oils from a health shop or other retail outlet specialising in natural remedies. This will give you the opportunity to smell the essences before buying.

But do check that an essential oil labelled as such is in fact 100 per cent essential oil. You may come across a bottle labelled 'Aromatherapy Oil', which often means it is a mixture of about 2–3 per cent essential oil in a carrier such as grapeseed or almond oil. These are fine as ready-mixed massage oils, albeit an expensive way to enjoy aromatherapy. For instance, a 10 ml bottle (the average size) of a diluted essence is barely enough for a single face and neck massage, whereas a 10 ml bottle of concentrated essential oil, once correctly diluted, is enough for over 100 face and neck massages

Moreover, ready-mixed oils are not concentrated enough to be used by the drop to perfume the bath water; neither are they suitable for use in vaporisers for perfuming rooms. Indeed, the entire contents of a 10 ml bottle (approximately two teaspoonfuls) of ready-mixed oil added to a bath full of water would emanate a faint aroma, whereas just two drops of the concentrated essence would result in a stronger aroma. Diluted oils also have a limited shelf-life (see below).

CARING FOR YOUR OILS

Essential oils evaporate readily and are easily damaged by light, extremes of temperature and exposure to oxygen in the air. For this reason they are sold in well-stoppered, dark glass bottles. They must never be sold in bottles with a rubber pipette (as was common several years ago). A few essential oils, especially cedarwood, cause rubber to perish into a sticky mess.

In theory, most essential oils will keep for several years. However, with the exception of bergamot, citrus oils may deteriorate within six to nine months. A few oils improve with age, rather like some good wines. Examples of these are sandalwood, patchouli and frankincense. But the more often you open the bottle, the greater the chance of oxidation – a process whereby a substance is chemically combined with oxygen and its original structure altered or destroyed – as reflected in the deterioration of the aroma.

To prolong the life of your oils, store them in a dark place in normal to cool temperatures (65°F or below). If you have a large selection of oils, they could be stored in a fridge (perhaps a second-hand fridge used exclusively for this purpose), but not in the freezer compartment. Although many essences turn cloudy when kept cold, after an hour or two at room temperature they become clear again. Citrus essences, however, are the exception and may become irreversibly cloudy if stored in very cold conditions. Nevertheless, this will not affect their therapeutic properties.

Should you decide to store essential oils in the fridge, always take them out at least an hour before use. If too cold, essential oils do not flow freely. Certain essences need special treatment. Rose otto, for instance, is semi-solid in cool temperatures, but becomes liquid with the slightest warmth, so rub the bottle between your hands for a few seconds before use. Other oils such as vetiver, cedarwood, patchouli and myrrh become increasingly viscous as they age and therefore take much longer to become liquid. In fact, myrrh becomes quite solid as it ages. In this instance, you may have to steep the bottle in a cup of hand-hot water for about ten minutes. Although heat speeds up the oxidation process, with myrrh it seems there is no other choice.

Although concentrated essential oils have a long shelf-life, once diluted in a base oil such as cold-pressed sweet almond or sunflower seed, the aroma will quickly deteriorate – along with the oil's therapeutic properties. Massage oil blends should be stored in the same conditions as concentrated essences, but for no longer than about two months.

AROMATHERAPY STARTER SELECTION

With such a vast array of essential oils from which to choose, a great many of which are endowed with similar properties, you will need some guidance on selecting oils for a starter kit. In fact, you could get by on just two essences: lavender and eucalyptus. But if you intend to take the art of aromatherapy seriously, you will probably need a basic selection of about eight carefully chosen oils; enough to create a variety of fragrant compositions. Essential oils often smell better when two or three are carefully blended together. Since the therapy is meant to be enjoyable, appreciation of the aroma is a vital part of the treatment.

Even though your final choice will be influenced by personal preference, it is also important to be open-minded. Unless you are familiar with essential oils, they may smell rather strange at first. Remember, plant essences are highly concentrated substances. With a few exceptions, it is only when they are correctly diluted that they become pleasant. You may also discover that a previously disliked oil takes on an intriguing persona when carefully blended with other essences.

Take patchouli and vetiver, for instance. On first encounter with their heavy, earthy, overtly Eastern aromas you may feel overwhelmed. But blend either of these oils with larger quantities of fresher-smelling essences such as bergamot, lavender and geranium and the aroma takes on a more delicate quality. Then there is clary sage; despite its reputation as a 'euphoric', its sweet-herbaceous aroma can be disappointing. Yet clary has great potential; blend with a tiny amount of the deeply resonating vetiver and a tinge of cheery bergamot, and you create a relaxing aroma reminiscent of woods and dappled sunlight.

Ideally, any initial selection of essential oils will include a representative from the floral, woody, citrus, spicy, resinous, herbaceous, camphoraceous and earthy groups, as shown in the Aroma Families chart. As well as presenting a wide range of therapeutic possibilities, such a selection offers plenty of scope for creative blending.

AROMA FAMILIES

When choosing oils for your starter kit, you may wish to include a representative from each of the aroma families. Those listed are the most popular essences used in aromatherapy. Many others are profiled in Part Seven where you will also find information regarding the therapeutic properties of and safety data for individual oils. The asterisks offer a guide to the price range of the oil. One asterisk indicates the least expensive oil, and five asterisks the most expensive.

Citrus: bergamot FCF**, grapefruit*, lemon*, lime*, mandarin*, orange*.

Floral: geranium**, chamomile (Roman)***, rose otto (or rose phytol)*****, lavender*, ylang ylang**, neroli*****.

Herbaceous: chamomile (Roman)***, lavender*, peppermint*, rosemary*, marjoram**, clary sage***.

Camphoraceous: eucalyptus*, cajeput**, rosemary*, peppermint*, tea tree*.

Spicy: coriander*, black pepper**, ginger*, cardamom**.

Resinous: frankincense***, elemi*, myrrh**, galbanum**.

Woody: cedarwood (Virginian)*, sandalwood***, pine*, juniper berry**, cypress*.

Earthy: patchouli*, vetiver**.

As you can see, a few essences belong to more than one group – a reflection of their complex chemical make-up.

Suggested Starter Kit: bergamot FCF, geranium, lavender, eucalyptus (or tea tree), coriander, frankincense, juniper berry, patchouli.

CHOOSING OILS FOR THERAPY

Having created an aromatherapy starter kit, the next stage in your apprenticeship is to learn the basics of choosing the right essence(s) for therapy. Oils need to be chosen to suit your physical and emotional needs, or those of the person you wish to help.

It is fine to use aromatherapy as a symptomatic treatment for short-term problems such as coughs and colds, muscular aches and pains due to exertion, acute bronchitis, and reactive 'stress' (that which can be pinpointed to tangibles such as overwork, moving house, the ending of a relationship, and so on). But long-term problems, such as susceptibility to every passing infection, arthritis, chronic anxiety and depression, need to be treated within the context of an holistic healing regime (see Chapter 19). Otherwise the treatment will do little more than soothe the surface.

> **IMPORTANT** *Before embarking on a self-help regime for a long-term health problem, it is essential to seek the co-operation of a doctor (someone who is also sympathetic to complementary therapy), and perhaps to consult a qualified aromatherapist as well. If you are suffering from severe anxiety or depression, it would be advisable to seek the help of an accredited counsellor (your doctor may be able to recommend someone) and to use aromatherapy as a supportive measure.*

STEP 1

Consult the therapeutic reference charts in Part 2. You will find that there is always a choice of essential oils (and often more than one recommended method of application) to help any given ailment. Your final decision will depend upon price and availability as well as your aroma preference. If you wish to use two or three appropriate essences in a blend, refer to the creative blending guidelines given in Chapter 6 where you will also find some useful at-a-glance references.

STEP 2

Whatever health problem you intend to treat, decide whether you wish the aromatic formula to be relaxing, enlivening or simply 'balancing'. If you cannot judge this by smelling the diluted oil and assessing how it makes you feel, refer to the psycho-aromatherapy chart in Chapter 21. However, never let dogma override your own instincts. If you dislike a particular aroma, no matter what its 'mood-enhancing' properties may be, you are less likely to respond to its charms. Aroma preference is probably less important in the symptomatic treatment of problems such as athlete's foot, burns or sprains – though some aromatherapists would disagree.

STEP 3

Most Important Whether you are choosing an essential oil for health or pleasure, check that the essence is safe for you to use; for example, take extra care during pregnancy or where there is a history of allergies. Refer to the safety data in Chapter 4 and/or the at-a-glance CAUTION note included at the end of individual essential oil profiles given in Chapter 29.

Choosing oils for aromatherapy

METHODS OF USE

Having established which oil (or blend) would best suit your condition, you will need to apply the healing oil using one (or more) of the basic methods you are about to learn (e.g. aromatic bath, steam inhalation, massage). If you carry out the step-by-step instructions given above, Step 1 will lead you to the therapeutic charts in Part 2 where you will find the recommended applications for whatever condition you wish to treat.

AROMATIC BATHS

Essences can be added to the bath simply for pleasure, to aid restful sleep, to help skin problems, relieve muscular and other pains, or to subtly influence mood. If you are fortunate enough to live in a house where the water comes directly from an underground spring (as is the case in certain rural areas) the water itself will be health giving. While it may lack the miraculous powers attributed to the healing waters of Lourdes, certainly it will be much kinder to the skin than chlorinated tap water. Nevertheless, city water can be made more vibrant with the addition of essential oils.

Sprinkle four to eight drops of essential oil on to the water's surface after the bath has been drawn. Agitate the water to disperse the oil. If you add the essences whilst the water is running, much of the aromatic vapour will have evaporated before you get into the bath. If you have dry skin, you may wish to mix the essences with a few teaspoonfuls of a vegetable base oil, such as sweet almond, but only if you don't mind cleaning an oily bath afterwards. Neat essences never leave a greasy tide mark due to their tiny molecular structure.

> **CAUTION** *Certain essential oils can irritate if you use more than one or two drops in a bath, especially if you have sensitive skin (refer to Chapter 8).*

Bath Temperatures

Very hot baths (100°F or 38°C) increase the efficiency of the sweat glands, which is beneficial when you are suffering from a cold or flu and can go straight to bed afterwards to 'sweat it out'. However, hot baths can be draining, and if taken frequently have a loosening effect on the skin causing it to age rapidly.

The ideal temperature for the 'neutral' bath is around 85–94°F (29–34°C). The effect of such baths is to reduce tension in body and mind. Adding relaxing essences such as chamomile and lavender to the bath enhances the effect, making this an ideal treatment for insomnia, anxiety, nervous tension and other stress-related problems.

For a bracing bath, the water should be cooler (65–70°F or 18–21°C). Adding stimulating essences such as pine, rosemary and eucalyptus will enhance the effect. However, if these essences are added to a much warmer bath, their bracing properties will be reduced by the tranquillising effect of the warm water. Similarly, relaxing essences are made more stimulating by the enlivening effect of fast-moving water – as in the shower. So, if you need to be energised but dislike the idea of a cool bath, try using stimulating essences in a warm shower instead (see page 30). Thermometers suitable for testing bath water are available from good chemists; otherwise use your own judgement.

EPSOM SALTS BATH

By inducing copious perspiration, the old-fashioned Epsom salts bath is one of the most effective methods for eliminating metabolic wastes through the surface of the skin. Epsom salts (magnesium sulphate) are inexpensive and can be purchased from most chemists. Ask for a large bag of 'industrial' Epsom salts. Alarming as this may sound, it just means the grains are coarse and therefore more suitable for the bath. The more expensive finely powdered version is sold in small quantities for use as a proprietary laxative.

The Epsom salts bath eases muscular aches and pains, and can even ward off cold and flu symptoms. It is also a superb relaxant during periods of prolonged stress. Due to the alkalising effect of Epsom salts, the treatment is also highly beneficial to sufferers of rheumatism and arthritis. The salts relieve pain by drawing acidic wastes (mainly uric acid) from the muscles and joints through the pores of the skin.

As if this was not enough, according to a well-known health guru, the effects of the Epsom salts bath go far beyond chemical detoxification. From an energetic point of view, magnesium sulphate dissolved in a body of water creates a static, unified, electrical field. Immersing yourself in this field helps neutralise excess electrical charges in the body, thus creating a magnetic balance. In practice, this means that an Epsom salts bath can counter the effects of low-level radiation, such as that experienced as VDU stress or jet lag.

Best results are achieved by taking a warm Epsom salts bath (95°F or 35°C) once or twice a day as required. For arthritis or rheumatism, however, the bath should be taken once a day for a week and then on alternate days until there is marked improvement; thereafter, take an Epsom salts bath once a week. If possible, try to rest for at least two hours afterwards, and avoid becoming chilled.

The method is as follows: dissolve 450 g (1 lb) of Epsom salts in a few pints of boiling water and add to your bath. Relax for about fifteen minutes, but do not use soap as this interferes with the beneficial action of the salts.

Essential oils can be added to the water, but this is primarily for the psychotherapeutic effects of the aroma. True, the skin absorbs essential oils more efficiently when it is warm and moist, for example, during and after a 'neutral' bath. However, the skin cannot absorb essences very efficiently if it is busy throwing off toxic wastes through profuse sweating. An aromatherapy massage oil containing essences such as lavender, chamomile and cajuput can be massaged into the skin an hour or two after the Epsom salts bath. The oil will also counter the drying effects on the skin caused by the Epsom salts.

IMPORTANT *Always move arthritic joints as much as possible after an Epsom salts bath to prevent congestion which will cause further pain.*

CAUTION *Avoid the Epsom salts bath if you have high blood pressure or a heart condition. Elderly or very frail people should use 225 g ($\frac{1}{2}$ lb) of Epsom salts to start with, gradually increasing as the bath becomes better tolerated.*

FOOT AND HAND BATHS

These can be used to ward off chills as well as rheumatic aches and pains, excessive perspiration, athlete's foot and other skin disorders of the hands or feet – or just for the sheer joy of it! If you have not already tried it, a foot bath at the end of a tiring day can be as relaxing as a soak in a full-size bath and can even alleviate tension headaches. Foot and hand baths are also beneficial following reflexology treatment (pressure point massage to the feet or hands) or before ordinary foot or hand massage.

Sprinkle five to six drops of the appropriate essential oil in a bowl of hand-hot water. You could dilute the essential oil in a couple of teaspoonfuls of vegetable oil if you wish, or in one teaspoonful of honey, or in one dessertspoonful of cider vinegar. Soak feet, or hands, for about ten minutes. Dry thoroughly and massage a little vegetable oil containing a few drops of the same essence(s) into the skin.

HIP BATH

The hip bath is a simple way of treating vaginal thrush and healing the perineum after childbirth. Run a warm bath to hip level or use a bowl which is large enough for you to sit in. Add two or three drops of essential oil and swish around to disperse the fine droplets. Sit in the water for about five minutes. Carry out two or three times daily for several days as necessary.

ALTERNATE HOT AND COLD SITZ BATH

Although rather awkward to take, these are highly beneficial for relieving congestion in the female reproductive area, treating haemorrhoids and easing constipation. The alternate hot and cold sitz bath (employed by European nature cure practitioners) operates like a pump, stimulating venous and lymphatic drainage. When applied to congested areas the bath reduces pain and inflammation.

Ensure that the bathroom (or wherever) is very warm. You will need two bowls large enough to sit in (two plastic baby baths would work well). Fill one bowl with tolerably hot water, the other with cold water. Add two or three drops of an appropriate essential oil to each bowl, then agitate the water to disperse the oil. Sit in the hot bath, and put your feet in the cold bath. Stay there for three minutes, splashing the water over your abdomen, then change position. Sit in the cold bath with your feet in the hot water, and stay there for 30 to 60 seconds, again splashing the water over your abdomen. Repeat the cycle two or three times, *concluding with the pelvic area immersed in cold water.* Carry out twice daily for several days as necessary.

AROMATIC SHOWER

This method is basically a wake-up treatment, rather than a serious therapeutic measure. Running water is enlivening no matter which essential oils you use. Simply choose the aroma you love the best. After washing as usual, put two or three drops of essential oil on to a clean face-cloth or sponge; while standing under the shower rub it briskly all over your body. The softer skin of the face, however, responds best to less vigorous treatment (see Chapter 26).

SAUNA

The purpose of the sauna is to encourage the elimination of metabolic wastes and the pollutants the body accumulates through stress, faulty diet and unclean air. As well as being a wonderful treatment for congested skin, it can even inhibit the growth of viruses and bacteria in the body.

The most appropriate oils to use in the sauna are

highly volatile and refreshing and have an affinity with the lungs, for example eucalyptus, lemon, peppermint and pine. This means that much of the aromatic vapour enters the body by inhalation and leaves by exhalation, thus acting as an expectorant for catarrh. The skin cannot absorb essential oils very efficiently if it is busy eliminating toxic wastes (see Epsom salts bath).

Mix just two drops of essential oil into 600 ml of water and throw on to the heat source. Never use more than the recommended quantity of essential oil as the aroma will be overpowering.

> **CAUTION** *Avoid saunas if you suffer from heart disease or a serious respiratory ailment such as asthma or emphysema. Avoid using sweet-smelling essences such as rose, geranium and ylang ylang as they may cause nausea or headache when inhaled in the confines of a steamy sauna.*

Incidentally, over the years I have received a number of reports regarding the nauseating effects of using lavender oil in the sauna (the oil is often included as a free gift when a new sauna is installed). However, it may not be the oil itself which is at fault – at least not in every case. People who are unfamiliar with essential oils are often tempted to use far more than the recommended quantity. Indeed, one person of my acquaintance admitted to using a half teaspoonful of lavender oil in the sauna – nearly fifty times the recommended amount! Not surprisingly, she feels nauseous at the mere mention of the word 'lavender'.

There is another reason why lavender does not always receive a rapturous welcome from sauna users. Unfortunately, the market is flooded with synthetic aromatic oils. Since the majority of sauna manufacturers know nothing about essential oil purity, they could easily mistake a 'nature identical' product (normally half the price of authentic lavender oil) for the real thing. Synthetic oils are far more likely to cause symptoms such as nausea, skin irritation, sneezing and wheezing – especially in the jungle-like atmosphere of the sauna.

COMPRESSES

A compress is a valuable way of treating muscular pain, sprains and bruises as well as reducing pain and congestion in internal organs. However, it is important to know when to apply a cold compress and when to apply a hot compress.

Cold: These are for recent injuries such as sprains, bruises, swellings and inflammation, and for headaches and fever.

Hot: These are for old injuries, muscular pain, toothache, menstrual cramp, cystitis, boils and abscesses.

To make a hot compress, add about six drops of essential oil to a bowl containing about 500 ml of water, as hot as you can comfortably bear. Place a small towel, or a piece of lint or cotton fabric, on top of the water. Wring out the excess and place the fabric over the area to be treated. Cover this with a piece of clingfilm, then lightly bandage in place if necessary (for an ankle or knee, for example). Leave the compress on until it has cooled to body temperature; renew at intervals as required.

For a cold compress, use exactly the same method as above, but with very cold, preferably icy, water. Leave the compress in place until it warms to body heat, then renew at intervals as required.

Alternate Hot and Cold Compresses

While massage can be very helpful for sufferers of arthritis, it should be avoided at all costs whenever there is a 'flare up' of inflammation and swelling in the joints. Massage over inflamed or swollen areas will cause further pain and damage to body tissue. The most effective way to reduce pain and swelling is to alternate hot and cold essential oil compresses. Each compress should be applied for two or three minutes. Repeat the cycle of hot and cold applications two or three times, always ending with a cold compress to prevent the hot application from having an enervating effect upon the skin.

GARGLES AND MOUTHWASHES

Gargles containing essences such as sandalwood or lemon are helpful for sore throats and laryngitis. A mouthwash with essential oils such as peppermint, coriander and sweet fennel will sweeten the breath by killing off putrifying bacteria. The simplest method for making a gargle or mouthwash is to add one drop of essential oil to a small glass containing two teaspoonfuls of cider vinegar. Stir well to disperse the oil, then fill the glass with warm water. Use twice daily or as required.

Why cider vinegar? Essential oils dissolve a little better in vinegar than in water, and cider vinegar in particular because it has therapeutic properties of its own. For instance, it is a well-known folk remedy for sore throats and laryngitis. When mixed with essential oils its healing effect is greatly enhanced. In my own experience, adding cider vinegar to an essential oil mouthwash helps reduce the build-up of tartar (calcium deposits) on the backs of the teeth.

INHALATIONS

Inhalations can help relieve cold and flu symptoms, sinusitis, coughs, catarrh, hay fever and other respiratory ailments. They can also be used to bolster a flagging memory or to enhance mood. Essences of rosemary and peppermint, for example, are said to stimulate clarity of thought.

For acute distress, such as panic attack or fear of facing some ordeal, the simplest method is to put a single drop of an appropriate essential oil (e.g. lavender, ylang ylang or clary sage) into the palm of the hand. Rub your hands together to warm the oil, then cup them over your nose and inhale the aroma. Keep your nose covered as you breathe slowly and deeply, in and out, for at least four cycles – or until you experience calm.

To help clear the nasal passages when you have a cold or flu, put five to ten drops of an essential oil such as eucalyptus or peppermint on to a handkerchief and inhale as required. Essential oils can also be sprinkled on your pillow to ease nasal congestion and to aid restful sleep. If you do not wish to put essential oils directly on the pillow, put them on a clean handkerchief and leave nearby.

A more powerful decongestant is the steam inhalation. This can be employed to help respiratory problems such as those mentioned above, or as a deep-cleansing facial (see page 215).

Pour about 500 ml of near-boiling water into a bowl and then add two to four drops of essential oil. The quantity depends on the strength of the essence. Peppermint, for example, is extremely powerful and will make you catch your breath if you use too much. Inhale the vapours for about five minutes, but no longer than ten. In order to trap the aromatic steam more efficiently, drape a towel over your head and the bowl to form a 'tent'.

You can take steam inhalations two or three times a day over a short period, for example, if you are suffering from a cold or flu.

CAUTION *Avoid steam inhalations if you suffer from asthma; concentrated steam may trigger an attack.*

VAPORISATION

This method can be used to purify the air when infectious illness is around. It can also be used to rid the air of cooking smells, repel insects, subtly influence mood – or simply to create a delightful ambience in the home or workplace.

Although there are many ways to vaporise essential oils, the purpose-designed essential oil vaporiser or 'burner' is by far the most effective. The essential oil burner is usually earthenware (sometimes glass, porcelain or marble), with decorative openings cut out of the sides to afford a free flow of air for the nightlight candle which is placed inside. A small, sometimes detachable, reservoir fits over the nightlight and is filled with water with a few drops of essential oil floated on the surface. This is gently heated by the flame. As the water evaporates, the room becomes permeated with fragrance.

There is one drawback, however: if you forget to refill the reservoir after the water has evaporated (which can be quite soon with some vaporisers) you may be left with a sticky blackened residue of burnt oil. This can be difficult to remove unless you use an alcohol-based substance, such as surgical spirit. To reduce the possibility of the nightlight vaporiser running dry too quickly, ensure that the model you choose has a reservoir deep enough to accept at least two dessertspoonfuls of water.

There is a high-tech alternative to the humble nightlight vaporiser in the shape of the electric diffuser. Here, a few drops of undiluted essential oil are dropped on to the ceramic or filter surface which is kept at a constant warm temperature. Some electric fragrancers, like the classic nightlight vaporiser, are designed to accept water as well as essential oil. These are to be preferred, partly because they use less essential oil in the long run, and also because the oils smell much better in dilution. Electric diffusers are particularly suitable for the workplace (they do not pose a fire risk) and certainly much safer than nightlights for use in the bedrooms of children and elderly people.

The most recent innovation is the stream diffuser. A cold-air pump blows minute droplets of neat essential oil into the atmosphere. Although manufacturers extol the virtues of this method on the grounds that heat radically alters the chemical structure of essential oils, I am not convinced that this is a superior method. Indeed, *gentle* heat actually enhances the aroma of essential oils, and other aromatic materials. Stream diffusers are often exorbitantly priced, which says it all!

When using the vaporiser, you will need between four and ten drops of essential oil depending on the odour intensity of the individual oils used (let your nose be your guide) and the size of the room. As a rough guide, six drops of essential oil will be enough to perfume a room up to three metres square. For a larger room you may need up to 15 drops; and for a very large space, such as a community centre, you will need more than one vaporiser.

AROMATIC OINTMENT

You can make a healing ointment for all manner of problems, including cuts, grazes, insect bites and stings, athlete's foot, ringworm, cold sores and chilblains. Simply doctor 30 g of an unperfumed shop-bought cream (preferably a natural product) with up to 20 drops of essential oil. For example: ten drops of lavender, five drops of geranium, five drops of tea tree *or* five drops of eucalyptus. For a cooling foot balm (which also heals athlete's foot) add two drops of peppermint instead of the five drops of tea tree or eucalyptus.

Put the cream into a little sterilised glass pot, and stir in the essences with the handle of a teaspoon. Cover tightly and store in a cool dark place. The ointment will keep for at least three months, depending on how often the jar is opened (see also the ointment recipes in Chapter 8).

If you cannot find a suitable base for the ointment recipe, a bland purpose-designed cream can be obtained by mail order from most essential oil suppliers (see addresses in the appendix).

NEAT APPLICATION

Provided that the skin is cooled first under cold running water for at least five minutes, lavender, eucalyptus, tea tree or geranium can be applied neat to minor burns and scalds. Larger burns and scalds are best treated with a cold compress. While lavender is the most popular essence for treating burns, in my own experience geranium is even better. The only drawback is that neat geranium (also eucalyptus and tea tree) may irritate very sensitive skin. Lavender is much more benign in this respect.

CAUTION *Serious burns need urgent medical attention.*

ORAL DOSES

Although essential oils are employed as internal medicines by European aromatherapy doctors, the home user (and non-medical aromatherapist) is advised against this method of treatment. Essential oils are highly concentrated, and therefore potentially toxic if taken internally. Without a thorough knowledge of the condition for which the oil is being administered, combined with an incomplete understanding of the oil's mode of action, the consequences could be serious.

MASSAGE OILS

Essential oils intended for aromatherapy massage need to be diluted in a natural base oil such as olive, almond or sunflower seed – preferably labelled 'unrefined' or 'cold

pressed'. If a vegetable oil is not labelled as such, it is certain to be a highly refined product extracted by high pressure, intense heat and possibly petroleum derived solvents. Moreover, the oil will also have been bleached, deodorised and artificially coloured. The devitalised end-product may then receive a dose of synthetic vitamins to replace those which were destroyed during the refining process. To add insult to injury, it is quite legal to describe such a product as 'pure'.

While a refined base oil will not harm the skin (unless you have an allergy to the plant from which it derives), unrefined oils are far superior. Indeed, they are health treatments in themselves. The oils contain naturally occurring nutrients such as vitamins D and E, essential fatty acids and trace minerals such as calcium and magnesium, all of which are highly beneficial to the skin whether taken internally or used topically (see the Repertory of Base Oils at the end of this chapter).

For many years aromatherapists have promoted refined oils such as grapeseed and soya (unavailable in an unrefined state) on the grounds that they have almost no odour of their own and therefore do not interfere with the aromas of essential oils. Yet to my nose, essential oils do harmonise with unrefined oils. For instance, the fruity-peppery aroma of extra virgin olive oil blends especially well with citrus essences; and while unrefined almond oil is a good base for all essential oils, its dulcet aroma marries exceptionally well with rose and chamomile.

Aromatherapists are somewhat divided over the issue of refined base oils – some believe they are ideal for aromatherapy treatments, some would argue otherwise. Most choose to compromise by mixing a refined oil such as grapeseed with a smaller percentage of an unrefined oil such as avocado, olive or jojoba.

However, there is consensus of opinion regarding mineral oil: it should never be used as a base for essential oils. Mineral oil (often available as 'baby oil') is derived from petroleum. Not only does it lack the health-giving properties of unrefined vegetable oil, according to some health experts mineral oil applied to the skin (or taken by mouth) makes fat-soluble nutrients leach from the body. It also tends to clog the pores of the skin, contributing to the development of blackheads and pimples. Also, when used as a base for essential oils, it hinders their absorption through the skin. Above all, the use of synthetic oil of any nature runs counter to the philosophy of aromatherapy.

SHELF-LIFE OF BASE OILS

If kept in the fridge (or in a cool larder) most cold-pressed oils will keep for up to nine months (check the best before date). Extra virgin olive oil will probably keep for much longer, even at room temperature. Although unrefined oils will turn cloudy when kept refrigerated, this is a good sign indicating that the oil is of a high quality.

It is important to remember that once unrefined oil has oxidised, it will have a detrimental effect on the skin. During the oxidation process, oil molecules break down to produce what are known as free radicals. These substances, if left unchecked, can damage and destroy cells. They have also been implicated as a primary cause of the ageing process itself, so it is imperative to buy unrefined oils in small quantities and to use them up quickly.

MIXING MASSAGE OILS

Essential oils need to be diluted at a rate of 0.5–3 per cent (see Easy Measures below) depending on the odour intensity of the essential oil (see page 42) and the condition for which it is being applied. The lowest concentrations (0.5–1 per cent) are best for facial oils and for those with sensitive skin, including children under 12. In practice, I rarely use concentrations above 2 per cent for adults (even for those with 'normal' skin). However, 3 per cent concentrations of certain oils can be most helpful when there is a great deal of muscular tension.

SHELF-LIFE OF BLENDS

If kept in a cool dark place, a massage oil blend will remain potent for up to two months. Not that the base oil will 'go off' in such a short space of time, rather the essential oil will begin to shape-shift or oxidise as soon as it comes into contact with the base oil. In an attempt to slow down this process many aromatherapists add up to 15 per cent of wheatgerm oil to blends because it is high in vitamin E, which is a natural antioxidant.

However, I am not at all convinced that wheatgerm oil extends the life of massage blends. True, the oil is sometimes added to vitamin capsules as a natural preservative, but just because the oil works well in the relatively air-tight space of a gelatine capsule, it does not necessarily follow that it will be as effective in a glass bottle – especially once opened. Any amount of space left in the bottle will be enough to accelerate the oxidation process – despite the vitamin E.

For some reason, it is rarely acknowledged that unrefined wheatgerm oil is highly unstable. Unlike extra virgin olive oil, which remains stable at quite high temperatures, wheatgerm oil must be kept in a cool dark place to prevent it from turning rancid within a few months of opening the bottle. Yet it contains thirty times more vitamin E than the long-lived extra virgin olive oil. Clearly, vitamin E is not the wonder preservative many would have us believe – at least not when it is in its natural state.

Therefore, it would seem preferable to forget about trying to prolong the shelf-life of blends and to mix just enough oil for each treatment – or perhaps enough to last for up to a week. Nevertheless, despite my own misgivings about wheatgerm oil, it does have therapeutic properties of its own and is deserving of a little space in the aromatherapists's larder (see the Repertory of Base Oils at the end of this chapter).

EASY MEASURES

If you intend to mix enough oil for a single massage, use a 5 ml plastic medicine spoon (available from chemists) to measure the base oil, as ordinary teaspoons generally hold less than 5 ml. For a full body massage you will need about six teaspoonfuls of oil (a little more if the skin is very dry or hairy). For a facial massage, you will need as little as one or two teaspoonfuls (see the Skin Care chart in Chapter 26).

Blend Percentage	Essential Oil in Drops	Base Oil in Teaspoonfuls (1 tsp = 5 ml)
0.5	1	2
1	1	1
2	2	1
3	3	1

MIXING LARGER QUANTITIES OF MASSAGE OIL

Inexpensive dark glass bottles suitable for storing aromatherapy massage blends are obtainable from chemists. The capacity in mls is usually imprinted into the glass at the base of the bottle. In my own experience, the 50 ml and 100 ml sizes are the most useful. When filling the bottles with base oil, a small kitchen funnel will ease the process. Having filled the bottle almost to the top with the base oil, add the essential oil; replace the cap and shake well to disperse.

Quantities given in drops for a 50 ml bottle of base oil.

Blend Percentage	Essential Oil in Drops
0.5	5
1	10
1.5	15
2	20
2.5	25
3	30

REPERTORY OF BASE OILS

Most of the oils profiled here are good all-purpose products suitable for body massage. The speciality oils such as avocado, jojoba and apricot are used mainly in beauty care. Although such oils are introduced in this repertory, more detailed profiles are to be found in the Beauty Care section (see Chapter 26).

ALMOND OIL
(*Prunus amygdalis var. dulcis*)

The finest quality almond oil is warm-pressed from the kernels of the sweet almond tree. It is also possible to obtain both a fixed oil and an essential oil from bitter almonds (*Prunus dulcis var. amara*). However, the essential oil (not the fixed oil) is potentially toxic. During the extraction process prussic acid (better known as cyanide) is formed. Therefore, commercial bitter almond essence, which is used as a flavouring agent, must be rectified to remove the prussic acid.

Sweet almond oil is pale yellow with a delicate nutty odour and slightly sticky texture. Although not rich in nutrients, it does contain trace minerals, linoleic acid and appreciable quantities of vitamins D and E. The oil is a good treatment for itchy skin conditions; it is also a natural sunscreen, filtering out, on average, up to 25 per cent of the sun's rays. However, sweet almond oil, like others which share this property, should not be used as a sunscreen on its own.

Percentage in blends: Can be used as a base oil, 100 per cent.
Availability: Refined almond oil is available from most chemists. The warm pressed oil is more difficult to find, but can be obtained from health shops or by mail order from essential oil suppliers.

APRICOT KERNEL OIL
(*Prunus armenica*)

An expensive, light-textured oil used mainly in beauty care (see Chapter 26).

AVOCADO OIL
(*Persea americana*)

A very rich yet highly penetrative oil used mainly in beauty care (see Chapter 26).

CASTOR OIL
(*Ricinus communis*)

A thick, sticky oil which can be used as a conditioning treatment for dry or damaged hair (see Chapter 26).

COCONUT OIL
(*Cocus nucifera*)

A light, highly refined oil captured by solvent extraction of the dried flesh of the coconut. Most coconut oil is semi-solid at room temperature, though it is possible to obtain a fractionated coconut oil which remains liquid even in cool temperatures. This is obtained by heating solid coconut oil and mechanically separating out the liquid fraction. Aromatherapists who choose coconut oil as a base do so because the oil is virtually odourless, and therefore does not mask the aromas of essential oils. Although devoid of nutrients (due to the refining process), *solid* coconut oil is known to block up to 20 per cent of the sun's harmful rays.

Percentage in blends: Can be used as a base oil for aromatherapy massage, 100 per cent. However, it is more useful as a bland carrier for essential oil perfumes.
Availability: Solid coconut oil is widely available from chemists. The fractionated oil is more easily obtainable from essential oil suppliers.

> **CAUTION** *Coconut oil may irritate sensitive skin. If you have sensitive skin carry out a skin test before use (see page 22).*

CORN OIL (*Zea mays*)

The highest quality corn oil is warm-pressed from sweet-corn kernels. It is bright yellow in colour with a slightly sticky texture and a faint corn-on-the-cob odour. The oil contains useful quantities of vitamin E and essential fatty acids.

Percentage in blends: An excellent all-purpose base oil which can be used 100 per cent.
Availability: Most of the corn oil on the market is heavily refined for blended cooking oils. However, it is possible to obtain the warm-pressed version from health shops.

EVENING PRIMROSE OIL
(*Oenothera biennis*)

Evening primrose oil has an exceptionally fine texture and a faint musty odour. It is captured from the minute seeds of the bright yellow flowers which bloom only at night. The oil is especially vulnerable to heat, so most producers extract the substance by employing the petroleum-derived solvent, hexane. The resulting oil is golden yellow, and almost identical in chemical composition to that which is found within the seed. It is possible to obtain warm-pressed evening primrose oil (labelled 'cold-pressed'). Unfortunately, the warm-pressed oil must undergo a process of refining in order to remove the dust-like seed husks which saturate the product. Having been subjected to a certain amount of heat – albeit naturally generated – as well as the refining process itself, the end product is a pale shade of yellow and contains fewer nutrients. In this instance, it is difficult not to concede that solvent extracted evening primrose oil is superior to that which is labelled 'cold-pressed'.

Evening primrose oil contains vitamins, minerals and essential fatty acids, including the important gamma linolenic acid. The oil is used mainly as a nutritional supplement to help conditions such as eczema, multiple sclerosis, heart disease, arthritis, PMS (pre-menstrual syndrome) and benign breast disease. When applied externally, the oil is a superb moisturiser, hence its popularity in beauty care (see Chapter 26).

Much more remarkable, evening primrose oil rubbed into the skin seems to reduce hyperactivity in babies and young children. Anecdotal evidence suggests that the nutrients of evening primrose oil reach the bloodstream via skin absorption.

Percentage in blends: For body massage, add the contents of two x 500 mg capsules of evening primrose oil to 50 ml (or less) of a relatively inexpensive base oil, such as sunflower seed. (Pierce the evening primrose oil capsule with a pin and squeeze out the oil.)
Availability: The oil is widely available in capsule form mainly from chemists and health shops. It is also possible to obtain bottles of evening primrose oil from a few chemists, essential oil suppliers and mail order vitamin companies. However, as well as being expensive (the tiny seeds produce very little oil), evening primrose oil is especially vulnerable to oxidation, which is why most suppliers prefer to encapsulate the product.

GRAPESEED OIL (*Vitis vinifera*)

The oil is heat extracted from the seeds of the fruit. Unfortunately it is unavailable in its natural state, for unrefined grapeseed oil is considered to be unpalatable – certainly it has an objectionable odour. The refined oil has an attractive green tint and an exceptionally fine texture. It is also virtually odourless, hence its popularity with those aromatherapists who prefer to use bland base oils.

Percentage in blends: Can be used as a base oil, 100 per cent, though many aromatherapists prefer to add at least 10 per cent of an unrefined oil, such as sunflower seed or hazelnut, to increase its vitamin content.
Availability: Widely available from supermarkets and health shops.

GROUNDNUT OIL
(*Arachis hypogaea*)

Groundnut oil (also known as peanut oil) has a pronounced nutty odour and sticky texture. Most groundnut oil is highly refined, though it is possible to obtain an unrefined version containing useful levels of vitamin E. Groundnut oil has a soothing effect on over-heated skin making it an excellent aftersun treatment.

Percentage in blends: Best used diluted 50/50 (or more) with a less viscous oil, such as almond or safflower.
Availability: Refined groundnut oil is available from many supermarkets, whereas the unrefined version can be found in a few health shops.

HAZELNUT (*Corylus avellana*)

The oil is warm-pressed from hazelnuts, also known as cobnuts or filberts. It contains useful levels of essential fatty acids, including the important linolenic acid. Hazelnut oil has a strong, sweet, nutty aroma and an exceptionally fine texture. It is also highly penetrative, exerting a slightly astringent effect on the skin. It is popular in beauty care (see Chapter 26).

Percentage in blends: A relatively expensive oil with a pronounced aroma. You may prefer to dilute it 50/50 (or more) with a cheaper less odorous base oil, such as corn or almond.
Availability: Available from good supermarkets, health shops or essential oil suppliers.

JOJOBA (*Simmondsia chinensis*)

A light, highly penetrative oil which is actually a liquid wax. Used mainly in beauty care (see Chapter 26).

MACADAMIA OIL (*Macadamia integrifolia* and *M. ternifolia*)

A nourishing, vitamin-rich oil popular in beauty care (see Chapter 26).

OLIVE OIL (*Olea europaea*)

The oil is usually extracted from hard, unripe olives. There are three grades of olive oil: extra virgin, virgin and 'pure'. Extra virgin olive oil is collected from the first pressing of the fruit. It is heavy and rich with a darkish yellow-green colour and fruity-peppery aroma. Virgin olive oil comes from the second pressing; it has a lighter yellow-green hue and a less pungent aroma. The so-called pure grade is usually a blend of highly refined olive oils from more than one country. It bears little resemblance to its cold-pressed relatives, being pale yellow with a relatively faint odour.

Both extra virgin and virgin olive oil contain useful levels of the essential fatty acid, alpha linolenic acid. Taken internally, the oil is said to be a preventative of heart disease. It is also a gentle laxative. Applied externally, olive oil is useful for dehydrated, sore or inflamed skin, for the prevention of stretch marks during pregnancy and for reducing the itchiness of pruritus. The oil is also a natural sun filter, screening out, on average, up to 20 per cent of the sun's rays. Of great interest from an aromatherapy perspective, for centuries olive oil has been used as an inunction (a substance which is absorbed through the skin) to alleviate rheumatic pain, and as a tonic for delicate babies whose bodies cannot utilise the oil's nutrients when taken by mouth.

Percentage in blends: Can be used as a base, 100 per cent. However, you may prefer to dilute it 50/50 (or more) with a less odorous oil, such as grapeseed or almond.
Availability: All three grades of olive oil are available from supermarkets.

PASSIONFLOWER OIL (*Passiflora incarnata*)

This oil is extracted from the seeds of the exotic passionflower and is used mainly in beauty care (see Chapter 26).

SAFFLOWER OIL (*Carthamus tinctorius*)

The safflower plant, which is related to the thistle, is thought to be native of Egypt and the Far East. The highest quality oil is warm-pressed from the seeds; it has a deep, golden-yellow hue and a faint, nutty odour. Unrefined safflower oil is rich in essential fatty acids and contains useful levels of vitamin E. It is also a natural sun filter, screening out, on average, up to 20 per cent of the sun's rays. However, the unrefined oil is especially vulnerable to oxidation and should be stored in the fridge.

Percentage in blends: Can be used as a base oil, 100 per cent.
Availability: The refined version is available from some supermarkets. The unrefined oil is more easily obtainable from health shops or from essential oil suppliers. It is also possible to obtain organic safflower oil from a few outlets.

SESAME OIL (*Sesamum indicum*)

The highest quality oil is warm-pressed from the tiny seeds. It is golden-yellow with a slightly bitter, yet pleasantly nutty aroma. There is also a dark brown, strongly flavoured sesame oil which is extracted from the toasted seeds. However, this pungent oil is not at all suitable for aromatherapy – unless you relish smelling like a Chinese stir-fry! Light sesame oil is rich in vitamins and minerals. It is also a natural sunscreen, filtering out, on average, up to 25 per cent of the sun's rays.

Percentage in blends: Can be used as a base oil, 100 per cent.
Availability: Available from most supermarkets and health shops.

SOYA OIL (*Glycine soja*)

It is extremely difficult to obtain warm-pressed soya oil. The beans contain very little oil, so producers favour solvent extraction because it gives a higher yield. If you can find an unrefined soya oil, it will contain appreciable quantities of vitamin E and lecithin.

Percentage in blends: Can be used as a base oil, 100 per cent.
Availability: Refined soya oil is widely available from supermarkets. The unrefined oil may be obtainable from a few health shops.

> **CAUTION** *Soya oil can be a sensitiser in highly allergic individuals.*

SUNFLOWER OIL (*Helianthus annus*)

Although most of the sunflower oil on the market is highly refined, the warm-pressed version is easy to obtain, and is usually labelled 'Sunflower Seed'. It is golden yellow with a slightly sweet, nutty odour and a fine texture. The unrefined oil contains useful amounts of essential fatty acids and a high level of vitamin E. Sunflower seed oil is popular in beauty care (see pages 218–27). In the past, it was taken internally as an expectorant to ease conditions such as bronchitis, laryngitis and even whooping cough.

Percentage in blends: Can be used as a base oil, 100 per cent.

Availability: While the refined oil is widely available from supermarkets, the unrefined sunflower seed oil is more easily available from health shops. It is also possible to obtain an organic sunflower seed oil.

WHEATGERM OIL
(*Triticum vulgare*)

The oil is either warm-pressed or solvent extracted from the 'germ' of the wheat. It is thick and sticky with an orangy-brown hue and a strong, earthy odour which is difficult to mask. However, the oil is extremely rich in vitamin E. Taken internally, wheatgerm oil is said to help eczema, prevent the development of varicose veins and to remove cholesterol deposits from the arteries. Applied topically, the oil is believed to penetrate deep into the skin, from where it acts to repair some of the damage caused by excessive exposure to sunlight. For this reason, wheatgerm oil is popular in beauty care (see page 219).

Percentage in blends: Wheatgerm oil is far too sticky to use on its own. Most aromatherapists add up to 15 per cent of wheatgerm oil to lighter base oils, such as almond or grapeseed. The oil is also thought to extend the shelf-life of blends because of its so-called antioxidant properties. However, I have grave doubts about the ability of wheatgerm oil to prolong the shelf-life of blends (see pages 26–27).

Availability: Widely available from health shops and essential oil suppliers.

> **CAUTION** *The oil may cause an allergic reaction in susceptible individuals, especially those with an allergy to wheat.*

INFUSED OILS

Aromatherapists sometimes use infused or macerated oils. By macerating fresh plant material (e.g. lavender or marigold flowers) in a high quality vegetable oil such as almond or virgin olive, it is possible to obtain a solution of the essential oil in the vegetable oil base. This can be used undiluted as a massage oil, or mixed 50/50 with a further quantity of vegetable oil. The diluted version is best for children and those with sensitive skin. A few drops of essential oil can also be added to infused oils at the rate of about 0.5 to 1 per cent (refer to the Easy Measures chart on page 34).

Several infused oils can be obtained from essential oil suppliers or from retail outlets specialising in natural remedies. However, it is much more fun to make your own, and this will also ensure the quality of the product, especially if you gather wild plants or use organically grown herbs from your own garden.

You can use almost any aromatic herb, for example, chamomile, lavender, lemon balm (also known as melissa), mint or rosemary, all of which can be used externally for the same conditions as their respective essential oils. Two of the most useful herbal oils are pot marigold (*calendula officinalis*) and St John's wort (*hypericum perforatum*). Marigold oil is soothing for all inflamed or itchy skin conditions, whereas St John's wort oil can be used as a rub to ease fibrositis and rheumatic pain (see the Profiles of Infused Oils below).

MAKING AN INFUSED OIL

Pick the healthiest looking flowers and/or leaves on a warm sunny day, after the dew has evaporated. This is the time when the essential oil is at its 'highest' (with the exception of night-scented flowers such as jasmine and honeysuckle). You will need about 4 oz (60 g) of plant material to 1 pint (600 ml) of oil. Bruise the herbs by placing on a wooden chopping board and crushing with a rolling pin or a wooden mallet. Half fill a large glass jar with the plant material, then cover with oil – preferably virgin olive (to avoid rancidity), but not the 'extra' grade as its pungent aroma may over-power that of the herb. Ensure that the jar is equipped with a tight-fitting lid, then give it a really good shake. Place the jar outside in the sun (or in a sunny window) for two to four weeks – weather permitting – but bring indoors at night. Remember to shake the jar hard whenever you pass by. The ability to judge when the infused oil is ready comes with experience, but intensity of colour and aroma are good indicators. When ready, press the mixture through muslin or a fine nylon sieve, then bottle the oil. If there is a separation of oil and herbal liquid (the oil will float on top), simply decant the oil into another bottle. If stored in a cool dark place, your herbal oils will keep for about one year – from one harvest to the next.

> **IMPORTANT** *Unrefined olive oil is one of the few natural oils capable of withstanding high temperatures. Most other natural oils, such as sunflower seed, safflower or hazelnut, are especially vulnerable to oxidation and must never be subjected to hot sun. If you would prefer to use a cheaper base oil, choose a refined oil, such as sunflower or corn.*

PROFILES OF INFUSED OILS

The two oils profiled here are commonly used by herbalists as well as aromatherapists. If you cannot make your own using the method just described, they can be obtained from essential oil suppliers and retail outlets specialising in natural remedies. Carrot oil is another popular infused oil used mainly as a skin care agent. Unfortunately, it cannot be successfully infused at home, but is obtainable from essential oil suppliers.

CALENDULA OR MARIGOLD OIL
(*Calendula officinalis*)

The pot marigold is a member of the daisy family, a popular garden plant indigenous to southern Europe.

Cultivation: Marigolds will grow in almost any soil, but they do require a sunny position. Sow the seeds directly in the ground in late spring, or sow under glass in ordinary potting compost during early spring. Plant out the seedlings when all danger of frost has passed. The large orange flowers are freely produced throughout the summer months. The joy of growing marigolds is that the more often the flowers are picked, the more prolific the flowering. Although the plants will not survive the winter, usually they will seed themselves the following spring.

Parts used: Flowers

Collection: Pick the healthiest flowers when they are in full bloom from early to late summer.

Actions of the oil: Anti-inflammatory, astringent, vulnerary (heals wounds), anti-fungal.

Therapeutic uses: Calendula reigns supreme in the soothing of sore, inflamed and itchy skin conditions, including burns (use in the later stages when the pain has passed), eczema, nappy rash, sore and cracked nipples. The oil can also be massaged into the perineum during labour to soften the area and to help make an episiotomy unnecessary. In skin care, the oil can be massaged into the hands after heavy outdoor work when there may be little cuts and abrasions in the skin. It can also be used to treat broken capillaries (also known as thread veins or spider veins) and varicose veins.

Combinations: To increase the oil's anti-inflammatory properties, mix 50/50 with St John's wort oil, or add 0.5 per cent concentration (refer to the Easy Measures chart on page 34) of any of the following essences: chamomile (Roman or German), lavender or yarrow. To enhance the anti-fungal properties of the oil, add 0.5–1 per cent of myrrh or tea tree. To enhance its astringent effect, add 0.5–1 per cent of geranium or cypress.

HYPERICUM or
St JOHN'S WORT OIL
(*Hypericum perforatum*)

St John's wort is a perennial weed found all over Britain and throughout Europe, on grassland, hedgerow and woodland clearings. The small, bright-yellow flowers open from midsummer onwards. The ovate leaves are dotted with tiny, reddish oil glands, which look like perforations when held up to the light, as reflected in the second part of the plant's botanical name. The essential oil found within the glandular dots is ruby red, and thus the infused oil takes on the same wonderful colour.

Cultivation: Although the plant is usually collected from the wild, you may be able to encourage it to grow in the garden. Collect the seed capsules in the autumn; put them in a paper envelope and store in a cool dry place until required. In early spring, shake out the small black seeds from the capsules and sow them under glass in ordinary potting compost. Plant out the seedlings in a sunny position when all danger of frost has passed. The plants will die in the winter, but they will appear again from the rootstock the following spring.

Parts used: Flowers and leaves.

Collection: In midsummer pinch out the flowering tops, including the leaves, preferably just before all the blooms are fully open.

Actions of the oil: Anti-inflammatory, astringent, vulnerary, anti-rheumatic.

Therapeutic uses: The oil can be used to heal wounds, sunburn, bruises, haemorrhoids, and to ease the pain of sciatica, fibrositis and rheumatism.

Combinations: To increase the oil's anti-inflammatory properties, mix 50/50 with calendula oil. To enhance the anti-rheumatic and pain-relieving properties of the oil, add a 1 per cent concentration (refer to the Easy Measures chart on page 34) of any of the following essences: cajeput, lavender, marjoram or rosemary.

> **CAUTION** *Excessive use of St John's wort oil causes a skin allergy in hypersensitive individuals, which becomes aggravated by exposure to sunlight.*

TINCTURES

A tincture is prepared by macerating plant material in an alcohol solution. Even though pharmaceutical grade alcohol is unobtainable in some countries without a practitioner's licence, you can obtain herbal tinctures from homeopathic pharmacies and from retail outlets specialising in natural remedies.

Herbal tinctures are not commonly used in aromatherapy, but they are an invaluable addition to the aromatherapist's and beauty therapist's store cupboard. They can be incorporated into aromatic ointments or diluted in water and used to treat a number of common ailments (see Chapter 7). The following tinctures are especially useful: calendula, hypericum, echinacea, euphrasia and myrrh.

6
CREATIVE THERAPEUTIC BLENDING

Having learned the basic methods of preparing and using essential oils, the next stage of your apprenticeship is the study of creative therapeutic blending. Should you wish to explore the related art of natural perfumery, the secrets of the craft are revealed in Chapter 27.

AROMATIC HARMONY

Aromatherapists rarely use single essences, but prefer to blend two, three or more oils to create a multifaceted aroma, thus reflecting the complex nature of the person for whom the blend is intended. A carefully composed blend often works better than a single essence due to the phenomenon of synergy – that is to say, when certain oils are blended together they have a mutually enhancing effect upon one another, so that the effect of the whole is greater than the sum of its individual parts. However, there is no reason why you should not use a single essential oil if it is indicated for your particular needs – and if the aroma appeals to your senses.

True, a disliked aroma can work well as a basic antiseptic, for example, but in order to embrace the all-important emotional aspect of our being, the scent must be perceived as agreeable. Aromatherapists have noticed that we tend to be instinctively drawn to the essential oil (or blend of essences) which best suits our physical and emotional needs at a given time. For the same reason, we can also 'go off' certain essences when we no longer need their particular properties. The healing power of a compatible aromatic blend, especially when combined with massage given by someone with 'good hands', lies in its ability to evoke pleasant feelings and images and to transport us into a state of reverie or tranquillity.

But what if we *detest* the odour? If it is obnoxious enough to elicit a gut felt 'ugh!', common sense tells us that the aroma cannot possibly act as a healer of the psyche – whatever its reputed 'mood-enhancing' properties. Indeed, studies carried out at Warwick University have shown that if we dislike an aroma intensely enough we can block its effect on the central nervous system.

However, it may not be necessary to adore the fragrance for it to work its special magic; it is enough to be accepting of the aroma. In so doing, we become more receptive to its charms (see also the section on Psycho-aromatherapy, page 159).

Intriguingly, the practice of blending essences can be as therapeutic for the blender as it is for the recipient of the fragrant prescription. Just like any other artistic pursuit whose aim is to create that which is generally perceived as 'beautiful' or 'harmonious', concocting mood-enhancing fragrances embraces our sense of the aesthetic, an aspect of our nature which suffers deprivation when awareness is centred on everyday things. Another important point: the act of preparing a therapeutic mixture for someone else can be experienced as a kind of healing ritual which enables us to focus our attention away from ourselves and on to the person we wish to help.

On a more tangible level, by blending different essential oils, we not only improve the aroma of a single essence, we also control the psycho-physiological effect of the oil. For instance, you may be feeling somewhat depressed and lethargic, yet love the soft, lingering aroma of sandalwood. However, you may benefit from a more uplifting aroma which will make you feel more alert. Even so, there is no need to disregard the sandalwood essence, thus flouting the aroma preference 'rule'. Instead, try blending the sandalwood with a touch of lively coriander and geranium, or perhaps a hint of light-hearted lavender and bergamot.

To take another example, you may be suffering the kind of depression that results in anxiety and insomnia as well as aching muscles (as is most common). Having scanned the therapeutic charts in Chapter 15, you may decide upon a muscle relaxant, sedative, antidepressant blend, such as chamomile and lavender. To cheer this up a little, you could add a tinge of rose or neroli, or a hint of clary sage or petitgrain.

A GUIDING HAND FOR THE PERPLEXED

Although some exact recipes for specific conditions are given in Part Two, for the most part you are advised to allow your intuition to be your guide – a daunting prospect for the novice who craves clear-cut instructions. Yet aromatherapists continue to develop their blending skills through practical experience and by trusting their instincts. There are no rigid rules, only possibilities. For this reason, no two aromatherapists will offer the same prescription to a person suffering from a given set of symptoms. Even if they come up with the same essential oils, chances are that the proportions of each oil in the aromatic prescription will be different. Indeed, it seems that the possible blending permutations are limitless! Nevertheless, it is still possible to offer a few guidelines which, no doubt, you will eventually surpass.

Generally speaking, 'families' of essences tend to blend well together, albeit in a rather conservative way; for instance, herbs (clary sage, lavender, marjoram, rosemary), citrus (bergamot, orange, lemon, lime, mandarin), flowers (rose, ylang ylang, neroli), spices (coriander, ginger, cinnamon), resins (frankincense, elemi, galbanum), woods (sandalwood, cypress, cedarwood). Other compatible aromas are spices with citrus (coriander and bergamot), resins with flowers and citrus (frankincense with rose and lemon). Woods and resins are a good match too: frankincense and cedarwood is a classic.

You could also try marrying wildly differing personalities, such as pungent black pepper or ginger with rose otto; the ancient and mysterious frankincense with the common or garden lavender; the bitter-sweet neroli with a hint of earthy vetiver or patchouli; the sweet scent of ylang ylang with the sharp scent of lemon, or whatever combination your developing sense of smell may suggest. (See also the 'Blends well with' note in the Aromatic Profiles section in Chapter 29.)

ODOUR INTENSITY

Certain essences are highly odoriferous, which means they will predominate your blends unless used in tiny amounts. Take the piercing aroma of lemongrass, for example; the oil is categorised as a top to middle note (see Chapter 27). This means it is highly volatile and will evaporate much more speedily than oils which resonate further down the odour scale. Yet add just a fraction too much lemongrass to a blend containing the less volatile middle to base notes, say, cypress and sandalwood, and the lemongrass will take over. However, if the blend is

not used up immediately, the more tenacious sandalwood and cypress will eventually win through – even though their aromas are masked at the outset. So a highly odoriferous oil is not necessarily a base note, as is commonly believed; rather, it has an intense, though sometimes relatively short-lived, aroma.

If blended in the correct proportions, a mixture of lemongrass, cypress and sandalwood will become an harmonious scent with no single essence predominating. The more tenacious essences will intermingle with the lemongrass – rather than being swamped by it – and will slow down its evaporation rate. Aromatherapists describe such a perfectly balanced mixture as a 'synergistic blend'. Quite apart from the aesthetic element, a synergistic blend is generally believed to be more efficacious. In fact, this intuitive understanding has been partially vindicated by science (see page 8).

Generally, when blending highly odoriferous essences with less odour-intensive oils it is important to start with a tiny amount of the most powerful-smelling oil and to add other essences drop by drop until you achieve the desired fragrance. For example, when creating a massage oil blend, you could begin with just one drop of tagetes or galbanum to 25–30 ml of base oil (very much lower than a 0.5 per cent dilution!). The less odoriferous essences can be added afterwards, in concentrations of between 1 and 2 per cent (refer to the Easy Measures chart on page 34). But it is advisable to add just one drop at a time, mixing well and smelling as you go. You may then find, for example, that three drops of lavender and six drops of bergamot essence, together with the single drop of tagetes or galbanum, make an harmonious brew. If you disagree, adjust the ratio of essential oils according to your own aroma preference.

When using highly odoriferous oils in applications other than for massage, such as baths, steam inhalations and compresses, unless the essences are first diluted in a base oil (not always appropriate) it is impossible to give precise quantities. As a rule of thumb, it is advisable to use no more than a single drop, perhaps blended with a few drops of another compatible oil.

Until your nose has become familiar with the odours of different essential oils, the following Odour Intensity chart will serve as an invaluable source of reference.

ODOUR INTENSITY OF AROMATIC OILS

Extremely high: carnation absolute, galbanum, mimosa absolute, oak moss absolute, tagetes, valerian.

High: angelica, basil, black pepper, cardamom, chamomile (Roman and German), cinnamon* (bark and leaf)*, clove* (stem, bud and leaf), elemi, eucalyptus, fennel, frankincense, ginger, hops, jasmine absolute, lemongrass, lime, melissa, myrrh, nutmeg, patchouli, peppermint, rose otto, rose phytol, tea tree, thyme (sweet), vetiver, yarrow, ylang ylang.

Fairly high: cajeput, clary sage, coriander, geranium, marjoram, myrtle, neroli, palmarosa, rosemary.

Medium: grapefruit, juniper, lavandin, lavender, lemon, orange, petitgrain, pine, rose absolute, spike lavender.

Low: bergamot, cedarwood, mandarin, sandalwood.

*Use as a room scent only

A SELECTION OF 'POSSIBLES'

When choosing oils for yourself it is relatively easy to compose a therapeutic blend which also suits your aroma preference. When deciding upon oils for another person, however, the process can be a little more difficult – especially if you have a limited selection. Even so, it may be helpful to illustrate how an aromatherapist might approach the task.

Although every aromatherapist will have their own method for determining which oils to use, the initial consultation always involves taking a thorough case history, as well as establishing the current emotional and physical state of the client. The aromatherapist may then refer to a therapeutic cross-reference of essential oils and/or use their intuition and knowledge to pick out a selection of 'possibles' – usually between three and six oils. The client may then be given the opportunity to smell each of the chosen oils and to decide which they like best. If more than one essence is to be used for the treatment, the aromatherapist will then apply their skill and intuition in preparing a test blend (see Aroma Test Your Blends below). If the client is happy with the mixture, then the blend will be used for that particular treatment (different combinations of oils may be used in subsequent treatments to suit the ever-changing pattern of the mind/body). If the client dislikes the blend, a good aromatherapist will try one or two other permutations until they hit upon a blend which the client finds agreeable. Although this may sound rather hit-or-miss – or even 'client-dominated' – in my own experience, the method works extremely well.

AROMA TEST YOUR BLENDS

The following economical methods for smell-testing blends are especially helpful when concocting mixtures for other people. Clearer responses are achieved if the area in which you intend to work is well ventilated, moderately warm and free from cooking and other household smells. In order to experience the different nuances of aroma (as described earlier) when testing a single essential oil it is important to put a drop of the test oil on a piece of blotting paper or a purpose-designed smelling paper (available from essential oil suppliers). If smelled directly from the bottle, the aromatic molecules are denied full contact with the surrounding air, thus hindering their ability to 'fly' or shape-shift to the required degree.

Another point, you will have to limit yourself to testing no more than three or four blends, or six single essences, per session. The nose becomes 'fatigued' after that and therefore less discerning. It is also important to have a notebook in which to record your successful blends (and also your failures) accurately. There is nothing more frustrating than discovering that you cannot quite recapture a certain aromatic harmony.

THE TESTS

I This test is best for assessing single essential oils rather than blends. Put a drop of essential oil on a damp cotton bud (dry cotton wool seems to hinder vaporisation), a smelling paper or a piece of blotting paper. If you are using blotting paper or a smelling paper, write down the name of the oil (or blend of oils) on the sample, or enter the information into a notebook. Before smelling, waft the sample around for a moment to encourage vaporisation of the essence. If the aroma is disliked, you have wasted only a small amount of essential oil.

2 A highly reliable guide for testing massage oil blends is to mix the sample combination of oils (up to five drops in all) in two teaspoon-fuls of base oil and apply to the inside of your wrist before smelling. The oils will then have the chance to interact with your skin chemistry. If the aroma is agreeable, mix a larger quantity of the same blend, incorporating the test mixture.

3 For the testing of water-based blends (for the vaporiser), add up to four drops in two or three tea-spoonfuls of luke-warm water and mix well. If you dislike the aroma (but don't absolutely hate it), sprinkle the mixture over the carpet rather than down the sink. The oils will not damage the fabric and may well improve its odour.

(See also the Advanced Smelling Technique in Chapter 27.)

SYNERGISTIC BLENDING

The therapeutic blending suggestions shown on the Synergistic Blending Chart are some of my own ideas, just to get you started. It would take volumes to explore every conceivable permutation, if, indeed, it were actually possible to do so. Instead, I have chosen to feature twelve essential oils and to blend each of these essences with one or two aroma-compatible oils. The resulting blends are examples of synergistic formulas for mind and body. For reasons of clarity and space, only three or four 'principal actions' of individual essences are emphasised. Most essential oils are endowed with numerous therapeutic properties (refer to Aromatic Profiles, Chapter 29).

It should also be mentioned that the sample blends demonstrate the *basic principles* of therapeutic blending. In reality, aromatherapists rarely mix purely 'physical' blends, as the chart suggests. In fact, it is impossible to do so – whatever affects the body must also affect the mind – and vice versa. So the Individual Prescription, as advocated by Marguerite Maury, reflects the whole person – body, mind and soul. However, it is common in aromatherapy to mix purely 'mental' blends (usually for stress), for the mind is believed to be the source of almost all our ills. Generally, a 'mind' blend can be inhaled from a handkerchief, added to the bath water, vaporised into a room or used for aromatherapy massage. Most of the 'body' blends are suitable for massage. However, steam inhalations or compresses may be more appropriate for certain ailments (see Chapter 5).

SYNERGISTIC BLENDING CHART

Bergamot

Principal actions

Antidepressant, heals wounds, combats fever.

Blending guide: Mind

To enhance its uplifting, antidepressant properties, blend with lavender and geranium, e.g. three parts bergamot, two parts lavender, one part geranium.

To create a more sedative blend, mix with clary sage and vetiver, e.g. three parts bergamot, one part clary sage, one part vetiver.

Blending guide: Body

To reinforce its wound-healing and fever-reducing properties blend with lavender and eucalyptus, e.g. two parts bergamot, one part lavender, one part eucalyptus.

Black Pepper

Principal actions

Stimulates the nervous system, aphrodisiac, stimulates the circulation, eases cold and flu symptoms.

Blending guide: Mind

To enhance its mentally stimulating effect, mix with bergamot and grapefruit, e.g. one part black pepper, three parts bergamot, two parts grapefruit.

To enhance its aphrodisiac properties, mix with ylang ylang and sandalwood, e.g. one part black pepper, one part ylang ylang, two parts sandalwood.

Blending guide: Body

To reinforce its stimulating effect on the circulation, mix with rosemary and coriander, e.g. one part black pepper, two parts coriander, one part rosemary.

To support its warming, decongestant properties, mix with ginger, e.g. two parts black pepper, one part ginger.

Cedarwood

Principal actions

Nerve sedative, decongestant, helps rheumatism and arthritis.

Blending guide: Mind

To increase its stress-reducing properties, mix with rose otto and sandalwood, e.g. three parts cedarwood, one part rose otto, two parts sandalwood.

Blending guide: Body

To support its decongestant properties, mix with elemi, e.g. three parts cedarwood, one part elemi.

To support its ability to reduce rheumatic and arthritic pain, mix with juniper berry and lavender, e.g. two parts cedarwood, two parts juniper berry, one part lavender.

Chamomile (Roman)

Principal actions

Nerve sedative, anti-inflammatory, eases muscular aches and pains.

Blending guide: Mind

To enhance its calming effect, blend with clary sage and neroli, e.g. one part chamomile, one part clary sage, two parts neroli.

For a less expensive calming blend, mix with lavender and petitgrain, e.g. one part chamomile, two parts lavender, one part petitgrain.

Blending guide: Body

To reinforce its anti-inflammatory properties, mix with lavender, e.g. one part chamomile, two parts lavender.

To increase its muscle relaxant properties mix with lavender and marjoram, e.g. two parts chamomile, one part marjoram, two parts lavender.

Coriander

Principal actions

Enlivening, aphrodisiac, stimulates the circulation, anti-rheumatic.

Blending guide: Mind

To enhance its enlivening effect, mix with bergamot and rosemary, e.g. two parts coriander, three parts bergamot, one part rosemary.

To emphasise its sensual quality, blend with rose otto and sandalwood, e.g. three parts coriander, one part rose otto, two parts sandalwood.

Blending guide: Body

To reinforce its ability to stimulate the circulation and alleviate rheumatic pain, mix with marjoram and rosemary, e.g. two parts coriander, one part marjoram, one part rosemary.

Frankincense

Principal actions

A meditation aid (deepens the breathing), anti-inflammatory, heals wounds, eases painful menstruation.

Blending guide: Mind

To enhance its ability to focus the mind during meditation, blend with juniper berry and cedarwood, e.g. two parts frankincense, one part juniper berry, one part cedarwood.

Blending guide: Body

To increase its anti-inflammatory and wound-healing properties, mix with lavender and geranium, e.g. one part frankincense, two parts lavender, one part geranium.

To enhance its ability to ease painful menstruation, mix with clary sage and cypress, e.g. one part frankincense, two parts cypress, one part clary sage.

SYNERGISTIC BLENDING CHART

Geranium

Principal actions

Antidepressant, restorative, anti-inflammatory.

Blending guide: Mind

To enhance its uplifting, antidepressant properties, mix with bergamot and lavender, e.g. one part geranium, two parts bergamot, two parts lavender.

To increase its ability to restore vitality during periods of prolonged stress, mix with clary sage and neroli, e.g. one part geranium, two parts clary sage, one part neroli.

Blending guide: Body

To increase its anti-inflammatory properties, mix with lavender, e.g. one part geranium, two parts lavender.

Juniper Berry

Principal actions

Nerve sedative, anti-rheumatic, relieves painful or difficult menstruation, eases cold and flu symptoms.

Blending guide: Mind

To enhance its ability to reduce nervous tension and anxiety, mix with bergamot and sandalwood, e.g. two parts juniper berry, three parts bergamot, one part sandalwood.

Blending guide: Body

To enhance its ability to relieve painful or difficult menstruation, mix with clary sage and lavender, e.g. two parts juniper berry, one part clary sage, one part lavender.

To enhance its anti-rheumatic properties, mix with rosemary and cypress, e.g. two parts juniper berry, two parts cypress, one part rosemary.

To reinforce its ability to ease cold and flu symptoms, mix with lemon and pine, e.g. two parts juniper berry, two parts lemon, one part pine.

Lemongrass

Principal actions

Antidepressant, eases muscular aches and pains, combats fever.

Blending guide: Mind

To enhance its ability to uplift the emotions and restore vitality during periods of prolonged stress, mix with mandarin and neroli, e.g. one part lemongrass, four parts mandarin, two parts neroli.

Blending guide: Body

To reinforce its ability to reduce muscular aches and pains, mix with rosemary and coriander, e.g. one part lemongrass, two parts rosemary, three parts coriander.

To enhance its fever-reducing properties (especially for colds and flu), mix with mandarin or orange and ginger, e.g. one part lemongrass, three parts mandarin or orange, one part ginger.

Rosemary

Principal actions

Mental stimulant, anti-rheumatic, stimulates the circulation, fungicidal.

Blending guide: Mind

To enhance its ability to increase mental clarity, mix with peppermint and lemon, e.g. three parts rosemary, one part peppermint, three parts lemon.

Blending guide: Body

To reinforce its anti-rheumatic properties, mix with lavender and frankincense, e.g. two parts rosemary, one part lavender, one part frankincense.

To increase its fungicidal properties, mix with geranium, e.g. one part rosemary, one part geranium.

Rose Otto

Principal actions

Antidepressant, reduces nervous tension, decongestant, promotes regular menstruation.

Blending guide: Mind

To enhance its antidepressant, stress-reducing properties, mix with bergamot and neroli, e.g. one part rose otto, five parts bergamot, two parts neroli.

Blending guide: Body

To increase its decongestant properties, mix with lavender and frankincense, e.g. one part rose otto, two parts frankincense, two parts lavender.

To support its ability to promote regular menstruation, mix with chamomile (Roman) and clary sage, e.g. one part rose otto, two parts clary sage, one part chamomile.

Ylang Ylang

Principal actions

Aphrodisiac, antidepressant, nervine, helps palpitations.

Blending guide: Mind

To enhance its sensual properties, mix with patchouli and sandalwood, e.g. one part ylang ylang, one part patchouli, two parts sandalwood.

To support its antidepressant, stress-reducing properties, mix with bergamot and clary sage, e.g. one part ylang ylang, two parts clary sage, three parts bergamot.

Blending guide: Body

To enhance its ability to slow down rapid breathing and heartbeat (palpitations), mix with lavender and neroli, e.g. two parts ylang ylang, two parts neroli, one part lavender.

INCOMPATIBLE AROMAS

Certain essential oils when mixed together seem to 'fight' or refuse to merge into an harmonious whole. Examples of incompatible aromas (at least to my nose) include ylang ylang/tea tree, fennel/clove, peppermint/fennel, cinnamon leaf/sweet thyme, Roman or German chamomile/myrrh, peppermint/orange, patchouli/German chamomile. As an experiment, try mixing some of these sparring partners (or any other unlikely sounding blend you can think of) and judge for yourself. Should you actually enjoy any of the aforementioned mixtures, then do feel free to ignore my comments about their so-called incompatibility. Indeed, an individual's perception of what is 'good' or 'not good' is highly subjective, and should be respected as such. Although there may well be a biochemical explanation for the 'incompatibility' of certain essences, there is no need to hold a degree in chemistry to perfect the art of blending. It is enough to apply your own aromatic good taste.

AROMATIC SIGNATURES

Believe it or not, no two people can blend an identical-smelling fragrance, even though they may use exactly the same blend of oils in exactly the same quantities from the same bottles. Amazingly, the oil will always take on an aspect of the blender's personality – their aromatic signature. Moreover, a massage oil or aromatherapy perfume blended while you are feeling depressed, angry or distressed will not smell right, no matter how beautiful the ingredients. It may smell rather flat, murky or somewhat harsh. On the other hand, a blend mixed while you are feeling relaxed and optimistic will be much more vibrant.

If this sounds unlikely, get together with a group of three or four friends – preferably of widely differing personalities – then prepare an identical aromatherapy blend, say, five drops of lavender, two drops of geranium and two drops of patchouli, in a 30 ml bottle of base oil. Each person should label their own blend with their name, then keep the bottle on their person for several minutes in order for the oil to become imbibed with their personal 'vibes'. Once everyone has completed the task, compare aromas. I think you will be surprised!

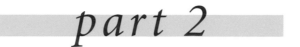

part 2

AROMATHERAPEUTICS

Forgotten and ignored for many years aromatic essences are coming back into their own, for many researchers and for a large section of public opinion, as the stars of medicine. Faced with a mounting toll of complications known to have been caused by aggressively synthesised chemical medications, many patients are now unwilling to be treated except by natural therapies, foremost among which plants and their essences have a rightful place.

THE PRACTICE OF AROMATHERAPY,
C.W. DANIEL, 1985
DR. JEAN VALNET

7

BEFORE YOU BEGIN HOME TREATMENTS

Aromatherapy can help a broad spectrum of physical and emotional problems but for lasting health and well-being it should form part of a healthy lifestyle and diet. Holistic healing is about cultivating a strong immune system by safe and natural means.

Where appropriate, included in the therapeutic charts are other supportive measures such as nutritional supplements, Bach flower remedies and herbal remedies. These can be used to complement aromatherapy treatments. Indeed, it is important to encourage a full and active participation in your own healing – the basic tenet of holistic therapy. Any of the suggested treatments shown on the charts can be used in conjunction with the basic deep breathing, relaxation and gentle stretching exercises given in Part 3.

The nutritional supplements mentioned are daily amounts which can be taken for as long as you feel necessary. However, they should never be regarded as an alternative to a healthy diet. A vitamin C tablet, for example, is not as welcome to the digestive system, nor as pleasing to the psyche, as a bowl of fruit salad. With the exception of evening primrose oil, supplements are best regarded as a short-term measure to help boost your immune system during periods of ill health or prolonged stress, and perhaps for a month or two afterwards to aid recovery. If you feel you need to take food supplements long term, it is advisable to seek the advice of a nutritionist who will devise a supplement programme to suit your specific needs. Pregnant women must obtain medical advice before taking nutritional supplements.

It is beyond the scope of this book to give a full account of the Bach flower remedy system of healing, suffice it to say that the remedies are prepared from non-poisonous wild flowers; they are benign in their action, non-addictive and can be taken by people of all ages. They help us transmute negative feelings such as anger, jealousy and fear into optimism and joy. The remedies are a wonderful adjunct to all other forms of treatment, be they orthodox medicine, herbalism or aromatherapy. Because they work on the mental/spiritual level, they will not interfere with any other means of healing the body; in fact they enhance other forms of treatment. If you

would like to know more about flower remedies, some useful books on the subject are included in the Suggested Reading section (page 288).

Internal doses of essential oils are best avoided by lay people. However, it can often be helpful to take an appropriate herbal remedy to complement external treatment with essential oils. In fact, French aromatherapy doctors usually employ herbs, dietetics and hydrotherapy to support treatment with plant essences.

The basic methods for preparing herbal remedies are to be found on page 51. Even though home treatment with simple herbal infusions is beneficial, a medical herbalist would in fact prescribe a synergistic mixture of herbs to suit individual needs. Similarly, a professional aromatherapist would create a personalised blend of essences to address both the physical and emotional state of the client. Advice on creating personalised aromatherapy blends can be found in Chapter 6.

IMPORTANT *If you are suffering from a long-term health problem such as eczema, asthma, arthritis, chronic anxiety or depression, it is advisable to seek the advice and co-operation of a qualified health practitioner before embarking on any of the self-help treatments advocated in this section of the book.*

It can be helpful to employ the conventional health service as a means of diagnosing any condition about which you may be concerned. You can then choose to embark on an holistic healing regime – incorporating dietetics, aromatherapy and other natural methods – should you so wish, perhaps under the guidance of a qualified holistic therapist. However, with certain conditions such as chronic high blood pressure and heart disease, natural treatments may have to be used in conjunction with prescribed medication, as a means of buffering the adverse effects of stress, thus promoting personal happiness and well-being.

PREPARING HERBAL MEDICINES

Although oral doses of essential oils are commonly prescribed by aromatherapy doctors, they are potentially harmful if unwisely administered. The herbal remedies suggested in the therapeutic charts are safe to use if you follow the correct procedure for preparing and administering the recommended dosage (see below).

Dried medicinal herbs are available from herbal suppliers and health shops. If you have a garden, however, you could grow a number of culinary and medicinal herbs. Some of the most useful and easiest to grow are mint, pot marigold, marjoram, lavender, thyme, lemon balm, common sage, rosemary and Roman chamomile.

Many herbal remedies are also available as tinctures (alcohol-based extractions) but these are only available from specialist herbal suppliers.

Alternatively, instead of preparing your own medicinal brews from home-grown or shop-bought herbs, many are also available in tablet or capsule form directly from health shops and herbal suppliers. However, with the possible exception of valerian (a foul-tasting medicine), I prefer to use fresh or dried herbs. Generally, smelling and tasting the herbal remedy feels like an important part of the treatment. Likewise, it is important to smell and taste our food in order to stimulate the flow of digestive juices. Indeed, as Hippocrates said 'Let food be your medicine and medicine your food'.

INFUSION (TEA)

Put 15 g dried herbs into a warmed china, enamel or pyrex vessel. Pour 600 ml boiling water over herbs and allow to steep for 10 to 15 minutes. If using fresh herbs, you will generally need three times as much. Seeds such as fennel and coriander should be bruised in a pestle and mortar to release the essential oils from the cells before being made into an infusion.

Dosage
The usual dosage is one wineglassful three times a day.

DECOCTION

This is used for hard woody plant material such as roots and woods, e.g. root ginger, cinnamon stick. Put 15 g dried plant material, or 45 g fresh, broken into small pieces, into an enamel saucepan or other heatproof vessel. Never use aluminium as poisonous seepage will react with the plant's chemistry, thus damaging the medicinal properties. Pour 300 ml water over the material and bring to boiling point; then turn down the heat and simmer with the lid on for 10 to 15 minutes.

Dosage
The usual dosage is one wineglassful three times a day.

HERBAL TINCTURES

Herbal tinctures (alcohol-based extractions) have the advantage of being quick and easy to administer.

Dosage
Ten to 15 drops in one wineglassful of water three times a day.

A WORD ABOUT THE BODY SYSTEMS

Even though the body systems outlined in the rest of Part 2 have been categorised as separate units, each system is an interrelated aspect of the mind/body complex. As we shall see, when one part of the organism manifests an imbalance, whether it be the nervous system, skin, respiratory system, or whatever, it is a reflection of disharmony within the whole. The holistic approach is explored further in Part 3.

8
THE SKIN

The skin is incredibly hard working, renewing and repairing itself ceaselessly. Apart from the obvious function of being a protective envelope which keeps blood and organs in and water out, it has numerous other vital functions. It protects from extremes of temperature through sweating, and invasion from micro-organisms by secreting anti-microbial substances. Indeed, the skin is an essential part of the immune system. It is laced with scavenging Langerhans cells whose function is to 'catch' micro-organisms and other antigens and present them to the T-cells (a type of white blood cell) which then produce an appropriate immune response.

Even though the skin protects against excessive loss of water, salts and organic substances, it is also responsible for excretion. For this reason, dysfunction in the other organs of elimination, the kidneys, lungs and colon, will manifest as spots, rashes, scaling, pallor, dark rings around the eyes, and puffiness, or perhaps the skin will take on an unhealthy waxy appearance. Of special importance to aromatherapists is the fact that the skin is a two-way street: as well as eliminating substances, it is also capable of absorption.

The skin also supports a network of underlying nerve endings whose function is to relay sensations to the brain, such as cold, heat and pain. Moreover, the blood vessels which lie just beneath the surface of the skin are especially responsive to emotion: when we are angry, excited or catch sight of someone we find attractive, blood rushes to the surface causing flushing of the face and neck (this is much more noticeable in fair-skinned northern Europeans). Fear, on the other hand, causes the blood vessels to contract, so we get cold feet:

A well-known function of the skin is the formation of vitamin D from the action of sunlight on the skin-resident substance known as *ergosterol*. But this is no excuse to expose your skin to the dangers of excessive suntanning. The skin of the face and hands of white people has become super-efficient at absorbing ultraviolet rays. As little as twenty minutes' exposure can supply the minimum level of the vitamin required for a whole day's quota. However, dark-skinned people require much

more light than this to maintain adequate levels of vitamin D. Any shortfall must be balanced by eating foods containing appreciable quantities of this important nutrient, such as eggs, oily fish, sunflower seeds, butter, whole milk or yoghurt.

The apocrine glands in the skin, found mainly in the armpits and pubic area, secrete hormone-like substances called *pheromones* which may have a role to play in human sexual attraction.

The skin is also an organ of respiration, a function which is often overlooked in medical text books. Indeed, Eastern healing philosophies often refer to the skin as the 'third lung'. A graphic example of this became apparent some years ago when the media reported the horrific story of the small boy who was painted all over with gold leaf for a carnival and who consequently died of respiratory failure. From this we can see why it is important to allow the skin to breathe by wearing natural fibres, at least directly against the skin (synthetics trap perspiration and hinder the free flow of air), and avoiding the use of chemical deodorants and antiperspirants (safe alternatives to these are discussed in Chapter 26).

PATTERNS OF SKIN DISORDERS

Unfortunately, the orthodox approach to treating skin ailments often overlooks the internal origin of the problem, concentrating instead on treating the skin locally as if it were a separate entity. The danger with this approach is that by suppressing the condition, the ailment may go deeper and perhaps manifest as a more serious complaint, a phenomenon which is widely recognised by homoeopathic physicians. For this reason it is important to be careful when attempting home treatment of chronic skin disorders such as psoriasis and atopic eczema. From my own experience, if the underlying cause of the problem is not dealt with (be it a food allergy or perhaps prolonged stress), treatment with essential oils can be little better than suppressive orthodox treatment.

The main reason for failure in natural methods of healing is that too few people are prepared to stick for long to the dietary and lifestyle disciplines which are an important part of holistic therapy. This is largely due to social pressures. Indeed, the stress of being a 'social outcast' can outweigh many of the benefits of a faultless diet and lifestyle. In such cases it may be worth consulting a qualified homoeopathic practitioner. Certainly a great many homoeopaths (though not all) are less concerned about diet; in fact homoeopathy is especially helpful for people suffering from food allergies. Instead of demanding that certain foodstuffs be removed from the diet, treatment is geared to promoting greater tolerance of the offending morsels.

Regular full-body massage can be used to complement homoeopathic treatment. This will help reduce stress levels and promote a sense of well-being, thus creating the ideal conditions for the mind/body's self-healing processes to come to the fore. However, do bear in mind that some homoeopaths believe that most essential oils antidote or weaken homoeopathic remedies. A view which was not, in fact, held by aromatherapy pioneer Marguerite Maury and her husband Dr E.A. Maury. They successfully combined the two therapies, believing that aromatherapy (in conjunction with dietetics) actually enhanced the efficacy of homoeopathic treatment.

The majority of homoeopaths, however, believe that it is only camphoraceous essences, such as camphor, eucalyptus and peppermint, which cancel out the effects of homoeopathic medicines. Whatever the truth may be, it is advisable to seek the advice of your homoeopath before combining the two therapies. Certainly, massage with plain vegetable oil will not interfere with homoeopathic medicine. In fact, by reducing stress levels, it should hasten the healing process.

ACTIONS OF ESSENTIAL OILS

The principal actions of essential oils used to treat skin problems are as follows:

Antiseptic: All essential oils are antiseptic to a greater or lesser degree, though good examples include eucalyptus, lavender, tea tree.

Anti-inflammatory: Helpful for skin rashes and wounds, for example chamomile, lavender, geranium.

Cicatrisant: (stimulates the growth of healthy skin cells): Helpful for burns, wounds and scars, for example chamomile, lavender, neroli.

Deodorant: Helpful for excessive perspiration and the cleansing of wounds, for example bergamot, cypress, lemongrass.

Fungicidal: Helpful for fungal conditions of the skin such as athlete's foot and ringworm, for example cedarwood, lemongrass, patchouli.

Insect repellent To repel insects such as midges and mosquitoes, for example lavender, eucalyptus, geranium.

Parasiticides: (prevents and destroys parasites): For treating conditions such as headlice and scabies, for example eucalyptus, rosemary, tea tree.

THERAPEUTIC CHARTS: SKIN PROBLEMS

ACNE VULGARIS

Description

Inflammatory disorder of the sebaceous glands of the skin, characterised by blackheads, whiteheads and clusters of pustules on the face, neck, chest and back.

Possible causes

Hormonal imbalance: the 'male' hormones androgen and testosterone are implicated; although a male hormone, females have it in small quantities too.
Food intolerance: the most common allergens being wheat or milk. A disturbance in carbohydrate metabolism may also be implicated.

Aggravated by

A diet high in fat and sugar, and by iodised salt, salt water fish, shellfish and kelp; oxalic acid in coffee; drugs containing iodides or bromides, e.g. cough syrups, sedatives and cold medications; excessive use of steam treatments (more than twice weekly); paint and industrial fumes; excessive sunlight; stress and PMS.

Recommended Essential Oils

Cajeput, chamomile (German and Roman), cedarwood, cypress, frankincense, garlic (see Nutritional Supplements), geranium, juniper berry, lavender, patchouli, rosemary, tea tree, vetiver.

Methods of use

Warm compress, moderate use of facial sauna (see page 215), baths, full-body massage (to balance nervous system), aromatic skin tonic (see pages 222–3 and other advice in the Beauty Care section, Chapter 26).

Suggested Herbal Remedies

A decoction of equal quantities of burdock and dandelion root, blended with an infusion of nettles. Other useful herbs are chamomile, peppermint and sage.

Nutritional supplements

Two × 500 mg evening primrose oil. If PMS exacerbates the condition, increase to four × 500 mg evening primrose oil during the pre-menstrual phase (or Efamol pre-menstrual formulation, available from chemists). One garlic capsule, 500 mg vitamin C, 30 mg beta carotene, six tablets brewer's yeast, two × 15 mg chelated zinc or zinc gluconate may be taken daily for as long as felt necessary.

Further suggestions

Moderate sunbathing (one hour a day maximum), plenty of fresh air and exercise, deep breathing and relaxation exercises. If feeling stressed, Bach flower remedies. If there is no significant improvement after three months, seek professional advice.

ATHLETE'S FOOT (*Tinea pedis*)

Description

A fungal infection between the toes, sometimes spreading over the whole foot. The skin may be cracked and sore.

Possible causes

Excessive perspiration in poorly ventilated footwear. Severe cases are indicative of a run-down state in general.

Aggravated by

Warm, moist conditions, poor hygiene.

Recommended Essential Oils

Lavender, garlic, patchouli, peppermint, pine, tagetes, tea tree.

Methods of use	Suggested Herbal Remedies	Nutritional supplements	Further suggestions
Aromatic vinegar, ointment (add the appropriate essences to the basic ointment recipe on pages 32–3), neat applications of lavender or tea tree, foot-baths, foot powder.	*To boost the immune system:* echinacea.	Four garlic capsules daily until infection has cleared. For severe cases, include a good multi-vitamin and mineral supplement.	Expose feet to sunshine and fresh air whenever possible and keep them scrupulously clean. Avoid hosiery made from synthetic fibres.

BOILS

Description	Possible causes	Aggravated by	Recommended Essential Oils
An abscess within infected hair follicles, having a livid appearance and extreme tenderness.	Physical neglect and/or emotional disharmony; also associated with acne and diabetes.	Squeezing, which spreads the infection.	Cajeput, chamomile (German or Roman), garlic, lavender, lemon, myrrh, thyme (sweet), tea tree.

Methods of use	Suggested Herbal Remedies	Nutritional supplements	Further suggestions
Warm compress, aromatic ointment, aromatic lotion.	*To boost the immune system:* infusions of echinacea. *External:* cabbage poultice (instructions are to be found on page 60).	A good multi-vitamin and mineral supplement, and four garlic capsules daily until skin has cleared.	Bach flower remedies for emotional disharmony.

CHILBLAINS

Description	Possible causes	Aggravated by	Recommended Essential Oils
An inflammatory condition of the skin, whereby the affected area (fingers, toes, ears or nose) becomes swollen and itchy, sometimes leading to ulceration.	Exposure to cold winds, coupled with poor circulation and sometimes calcium and silicon deficiency.	Rubbing, which can cause the skin to break.	Black pepper, chamomile (German and Roman), garlic, lavender, lemon, marjoram (sweet).

Methods of use	Suggested Herbal Remedies	Nutritional supplements	Further suggestions
Alternate hot and cold aromatic foot/hand baths, aromatic ointment.	Nettles, horsetail (rich in silicon).	A good multi-vitamin and mineral supplement, taken daily.	*As a preventative measure:* plenty of exercise and regular full-body massage to improve circulation. For broken chilblains, pierce a garlic capsule and paint the contents on to the affected area (if you can stand the smell!). Otherwise apply neat lavender oil.

COLD SORES (*Herpes Simplex*)

Description

Painful sores, occurring on the lips or around the mouth caused by the herpes simplex virus.

Possible causes

The virus lies dormant in many people, flaring up during periods of stress (including PMS), or when the body becomes weakened through infections, such as colds or flu. Sunlight on the skin can be a trigger in susceptible individuals.

Aggravated by

Poor nutrition and stress.

Recommended Essential Oils

Chamomile (Roman or German), melissa (true), myrrh, tea tree.

Methods of use

Aromatic lotion.
To reduce stress: full-body massage with any oil(s) of your choice.

Suggested Herbal Remedies

Internally: Echinacea, yarrow, lemon balm (melissa), chamomile.
Externally: Hypericum and calendula ointment.

Nutritional supplements

A good vitamin B-complex formula, and two x 500 mg vitamin C, taken daily.

Further suggestions

Food intolerances are often implicated, so it may be advisable to consult an holistic practitioner, preferably someone who can carry out allergy tests.

ECZEMA

Description

Itchy, scaly fissured inflammation of the skin, sometimes with a sticky fluid discharge. There are two main types: atopic (chronic) eczema or contact dermatitis.

> **CAUTION** *Always carry out a patch test before using oils and ointments (see page 23).*

Possible causes

Atopic eczema commonly occurs in those who have a family history of the disease and also asthma, hay fever or migraine. Food allergies are usually implicated, especially to dairy products. In contact dermatitis there may be a local reaction to household and industrial chemicals, cosmetics, nickle, etc. Contact allergy is also highly likely to occur in those with atopic eczema.

Aggravated by

Stress. In some cases, oils and ointments are not tolerated because they cause the skin to overheat. Often more itchy immediately after bathing.

Recommended Essential Oils

Calendula (infused oil), cedarwood, chamomile (German or Roman), geranium (weeping eczema), juniperberry (weeping eczema), lavender, rose otto.

Methods of use

Lukewarm or cold compress, hand and foot baths (for localised eruptions), bath, full-body massage if possible (to reduce stress) but not if eczema is widespread and/or weepy. Massage where skin is clear. Aromatic ointment if tolerated.

Suggested Herbal Remedies

An infusion of red clover and nettles (equal quantities). Other herbs: chamomile, chickweed.

Nutritional supplements

Six x 500 mg evening primrose oil. Also, a good B-complex supplement and two x 500 mg vitamin C. Both to be taken daily.

Further suggestions

Bach flower remedies. If you suffer from atopic eczema, it is advisable to seek the advice and co-operation of an holistic practitioner, preferably someone who can carry out allergy tests.

HEADLICE (*Pediculosis Capititis*)

Description

Due to the head louse which affects the scalp, although it may sometimes involve the eyebrows, eyelashes, armpit hair and beard. Common in children, especially girls. The eggs or 'nits' are firmly attached to the hair shafts.

Possible causes

Headlice feed on blood and are transmitted by direct contact of hair and by sharing combs, hair brushes and head gear.

Aggravated by

Bites causing severe itching, especially around the nape of the neck and behind the ears. Persistent scratching can cause lesions which may become infected.

Recommended Essential Oils

Eucalyptus, garlic (see Nutritional Supplements), geranium, lavender, pine, rosemary, spike lavender, thyme (sweet).

Methods of use

Hair oil (see instructions on page 224).

Nutritional supplements

An infestation of headlice can leave you feeling 'lousy' or run down. Take a good multi-vitamin and mineral supplement and two × 500 mg vitamin C daily. Also, one or two garlic capsules daily.

Further suggestions

If the eyelashes are affected, seek medical advice. Essential oils should **never** be used in or around the eyes.

PSORIASIS

Description

Characterised by red, raised patches topped by silvery scales. Affects any part of the body, including the scalp.

Possible causes

Usually a family history of the condition. Believed to result from a disturbance in skin enzymes. Sometimes associated with arthritis.

Aggravated by

Stress.

Suggested Essential Oils

Cajeput, chamomile (Roman or German), lavender.

Methods of use

Warm compress, baths, ointment, general body massage to reduce stress. For psoriasis of the scalp: scalp lotion (see recipes on page 61).

Suggested Herbal Remedies

Decoction: equal quantities of burdock, cleavers, sarsaparilla, yellow dock.

Nutritional supplements

Six × 500 mg evening primrose oil, daily. (Studies have shown that 60 per cent of sufferers experience a lessening of symptoms.)

Further suggestions

Sunlight and sea water usually give temporary relief. Bach flower remedies help during periods of stress. If there is no significant relief after three months of treatment with essential oils, do seek the advice of an holistic practitioner.

RINGWORM (*Tinea*)

Description

A red, itchy rash appearing in circular patches anywhere on the body.

Possible cause

A fungal infection closely related to athlete's foot. Can be picked up from pets and farm animals.

Aggravated by

Poor hygiene, synthetic fibres, profuse perspiration.

Recommended Essential Oils

Calendula (infused oil), eucalyptus, garlic (see Nutritional Supplements), geranium, lavender, lemon, myrrh, peppermint, tagetes.

Methods of use

Lukewarm or cold compress, strong aromatic ointment, bath.

Suggested Herbal Remedies

To boost the immune system: echinacea.

Nutritional supplements

Four garlic capsules daily until infection has cleared.

Further suggestions

Expose your body to fresh air and sunlight as often as possible. Clothing and linen must be washed thoroughly as the fungus can survive the wash and thus reinfect the skin.

SCABIES (*Sarcoptes Scabie*)

Description

A highly contagious skin disease associated with the parasitic 'itch mite'. The burrowing activites of the parasites cause intense itching and blister-like lesions.

Possible causes

Can be caught from farm animals, particularly sheep. Also associated with poor hygiene.

Aggravated by

Scratching.

Recommended Essential Oils

Bergamot, garlic (see Nutritional Supplements), lavender, lemongrass, peppermint, pine, rosemary, thyme (sweet).

Methods of use

Strong aromatic ointment (see recipe on page 61), warm compress, bath.

Nutritional supplements

Four to six garlic capsules daily until infection has cleared. The sulphurous garlic is eliminated through the skin as well as the breath and will literally gas the squatters out!

Further suggestions

Bed linen and underwear must be boiled, or put through the hottest wash cycle if machine washed.

WARTS AND VERRUCAE

Description

Small hard growths on the skin. Anal and genital warts are highly contagious and may contribute to the development of penile and cervical cancers. Warts on the larynx can also be dangerous. These three types require medical attention. Verrucae are painful in-growing warts in the ball of the foot.

Possible causes

The papillomavirus which enters the skin through tiny breaks. There is also an inherited tendency to develop warts. Can also be indicative of poor health in general. Most common among children and young adults.

Aggravated by

Never cut a wart as there is a risk of bleeding, infection and scarring.

Suggested Essential Oils

Garlic (see Nutritional Supplements), lemon, thyme (sweet).

Methods of use

Apply neat. Put one or two drops on the gauze portion of a very small round plaster; apply over the wart, avoiding the surrounding skin as far as possible. Repeat daily, but leave skin to breathe at night. It will take about a month for the wart to shrivel and fall away.

Suggested Herbal Remedies

Dandelion: Squeeze the 'milk' from the freshly picked stem and apply to the wart two or three times daily.

Nutritional supplements

If in poor health, a good multi-vitamin and mineral supplement and two garlic capsules daily.

Further suggestions

Once the wart has gone, apply wheatgerm oil to the area. Wheatgerm is high in vitamin E which has been found to inhibit the formation of warts. Regular aromatherapy masssage will help to boost your immune system.

AROMATIC PRESCRIPTIONS AND PROCEDURES

AROMATIC VINEGAR FOR ATHLETE'S FOOT

4 teaspoonfuls cider vinegar
30 ml distilled water or boiled water
10 drops lavender
6 drops tea tree

Funnel the cider vinegar into a dark glass bottle. Add the essential oils and shake well. Then add the water and shake again. You will need to shake well each time before use to disperse the oils. Using cotton wool, or a cotton bud if only a tiny area is affected, apply three times a day.

ATHLETE'S FOOT POWDER

2 tablespoonfuls unperfumed talc or cornflour
15 drops lavender
5 drops peppermint

Put the talc or cornflour into a plastic bag, then add the essential oils. Tie the bag securely and allow the oils to permeate the base for at least 24 hours. Shake well the first time before use.

CABBAGE POULTICE FOR BOILS

A marvellous alternative to the warm aromatic compress (the usual aromatherapy method for bringing boils to a head) is the old-fashioned cabbage poultice. Place a cabbage leaf in between two pieces of gauze dressing. Heat the leaf by pressing with a fairly hot clothes iron for a few seconds. Without removing the leaf from between the gauze, apply directly over the area to be treated. Hold in place for five minutes. Repeat two or three times, using a fresh leaf each time. Follow this up with aromatic lotion (see below).

AROMATIC VINEGAR FOR BOILS

4 teaspoonfuls cider vinegar
30 ml distilled or boiled water
4 drops Roman chamomile (or 2 drops German chamomile)

Mix in the same way as for the athlete's foot vinegar above. Apply with cotton wool swabs three times daily.

COLD SORE LOTION

Genuine melissa essence is used by aromatherapy doctors in Germany for the treatment of cold sores. However, the oil is incredibly expensive, prohibitively so for many people. The following mixture is a good alternative, at a fraction of the cost.

2 teaspoonfuls cider vinegar
4 teaspoonfuls distilled or boiled water
4 drops tincture of myrrh
3 drops tea tree

Mix as for the athlete's foot vinegar. However, the tincture of myrrh, should be mixed with the cider vinegar before adding the tea tree essence. Tincture of myrrh (available from herbal suppliers) will cause the blend to turn cloudy, but this does not affect the therapeutic properties. Apply with a cotton bud several times a day.

NB *Since I have no experience of using true melissa oil for the treatment of cold sores, I cannot comment on the efficacy of the remedy which is popular with German aromatherapy doctors.*

EASY-TO-MAKE COLD SORE OINTMENT

The following recipe is a partially home-made version of the popular hypericum and calendula ointment (available from most health shops). In my own experience, the synergy of hypericum and calendula is the best remedy available for the symptomatic treatment of cold sores, clearing them up far more quickly than any essential oil mixture I have tried.

Tinctures of hypericum and calendula are available from herbal suppliers. A bland base cream suitable as a carrier for aromatic essences can be obtained by mail order from most essential oil suppliers.

50 g unperfumed ointment/cream
1 teaspoonful hypericum tincture
1 teaspoonful calendula tincture

Put the base cream into a sterilised glass pot, then stir in the tinctures with the handle of a teaspoon. Apply several times daily. The ointment will remain potent for at least eight months if stored in a cool, dark place.

ECZEMA OINTMENTS

Creams and ointments will not cure eczema, rather they are meant to reduce inflammation and itching. Holistic treatment is essential for this complaint (refer to the advice given on the therapeutic chart).

Recipe 1
50 g unperfumed commercial cream or ointment
  (available from most stockists, see Useful Addresses).
5 drops Roman chamomile or 3 drops German chamomile

Put the cream into a spotlessly clean glass pot, then stir in the essential oils with the handle of a teaspoon and cover tightly. Apply two or three times a day.

Recipe 2
For weepy eczema, add three drops geranium, two drops Roman chamomile (or one drop German chamomile), one drop juniper berry to the unperfumed base cream.

Recipe 3
Beeswax ointment
15 g yellow beeswax
60 ml almond oil
8 drops Roman chamomile or 4 drops German chamomile

Heat the beeswax and almond oil in a heatproof dish over a pan of simmering water (the bain-marie method). Stir well, remove from the heat and allow to cool a little before stirring in the essential oils. Pour into a clean glass pot and cover tightly. Apply two or three times a day.

As an alternative to almond oil, use infused oil of calendula and reduce the essential oils to: four drops Roman chamomile or two drops German chamomile.

> **CAUTION** *Some eczema sufferers respond best to lukewarm aromatic compresses. This is because creams, ointments and vegetable oils can cause skin to overheat, thus exacerbating the condition. Moreover, some eczema sufferers are allergic to beeswax, so do carry out a patch test before using (see page 23). Instead of the unrefined yellow beeswax, you could try the refined white version. This may be better tolerated, but it is still important to patch test it first. Both types of beeswax can be obtained from herbal suppliers.*

TREATMENT FOR HEADLICE

75 ml vegetable oil (e.g. olive, sunflower)
25 drops eucalyptus
25 drops lavender
25 drops rosemary

Put the essential oil into a dark glass bottle, add the vegetable oil and shake well. Apply to wet hair (otherwise it will be difficult to shampoo out the oil) by massaging well into the scalp to reach the hair roots. Pay particular attention to the areas around the ears and nape of the neck where the lice breed. Leave on for at least one hour, then shampoo out throughly. Remove the eggs (nits) with a regulation fine-toothed comb (these can be bought from your local chemist). It is essential to repeat this treatment twice more at three-day intervals to ensure that the infestation has completely cleared.

PSORIASIS OINTMENTS

Holistic treatment is necessary for this condition (refer to the advice given on the therapeutic chart). Either of the following ointments will help to reduce inflammation and itching.

Recipe 1
Follow the same basic method as for eczema ointment Recipe 1, but use six drops lavender and three drops Roman chamomile.

Recipe 2
Follow the same basic method for eczema ointment Recipe 3, but use twelve drops lavender and four drops Roman chamomile.

AROMATIC LOTION FOR PSORIASIS OF THE SCALP

4 teaspoonfuls cider vinegar
50 ml distilled or boiled water
15 drops lavender
5 drops cajeput

Funnel the cider vinegar into a dark glass bottle, then add the essential oil and shake well. Add the water and shake well again. Rub into the scalp several times a week. You will need to shake the bottle each time before use to disperse the oils.

RINGWORM OINTMENT

Follow the directions for eczema ointment Recipe 1, but use seven drops lavender, six drops geranium, seven drops eucalyptus instead.

SCABIES OINTMENT

Follow the directions for eczema ointment Recipe 1, but make a powerfully aromatic formula using five drops peppermint, 17 drops lavender, 12 drops rosemary. Avoid getting the ointment on healthy skin as far as possible as it may cause irritation.

SKIN FIRST AID

The chart on page 63 will help you to select essential oils for minor burns, cuts and abrasions (i.e. injuries to the upper layer of the skin) and many other problems. Serious burns and wounds, however, need urgent medical attention. Although an aromatherapy doctor may treat such cases with essential oils, it is certainly not advisable for lay people to do so. But how can we tell when a wound or a burn is serious enough to warrant urgent medical attention?

BURNS AND SCALDS

Superficial or first-degree burns can be treated at home for they involve the outer skin layer. Although sometimes very painful, they are not dangerous to health. Usually they will leave a reddened, sometimes weepy, area of skin, which eventually heals without leaving a permanent scar. Superficial burns may be caused by grasping the handle of a hot saucepan, for instance, or scalding yourself with water or steam. Always cool the skin under running water, or immerse the burned area in a basin of cold water (preferably icy) for 5 to 10 minutes before applying neat essential oil (see Skin First Aid chart).

Deep or extensive burns fall into two categories: second-degree burns and third-degree burns. Second-degree burns are characterised by blistering, pain and swelling. The burn may also be weepy. Third-degree burns are characterised by lack of immediate pain (because the nerve endings have been destroyed), whiteness and/or charring.

Second- and third-degree burns are usually caused by contact with naked flame, boiling liquids, corrosive chemicals, electricity or excessive sunbathing. **Never immerse second- and third-degree burns in water**;. Home treatment should be limited to applying a clean, dry dressing (if a sterile dressing is unavailable, a torn up piece of clean cotton fabric will suffice), then seek urgent medical attention. Never in any circumstances attempt to burst blisters or peel damaged skin as this will only encourage infection.

WOUNDS

Most cuts and abrasions can be treated at home, but in any of the following situations, it is vital to seek urgent medical attention.

- Deep puncture wounds, especially if caused by a dirty or rusty object. The risk of infection is very high with this type of wound.
- If bleeding comes in spurts, this indicates that an artery may have been severed. This type of injury is life threatening, so it is important to take immediate action. Cover the wound with layers of clean cotton fabric (a torn-up sheet for instance). Press directly on the wound for at least 15 minutes to help staunch the bleeding. If possible you should also raise the injured part above heart level (for example, an arm or a leg) and support it in this position. This will slow down the flow of blood by lowering local blood pressure.
- If a cut looks very deep, or if the edges of the wound gape open. Also, if the cut was caused by a jagged object, such as broken glass or a bread knife. You may need stitches with this type of wound.
- If a graze is very large (for example, the whole length of an arm or leg) and there are foreign bodies in it (for example, gravel and soil particles).
- Animal bites, especially deep ones which cause extensive bruising and swelling.
- Allergic reactions to insect stings (anaphylactic shock). Symptoms may include vomiting, flushing, irregular heartbeat or breathing difficulties, which can lead to coma and even death. If you fall into this high-risk

category, your doctor can provide a life-saving shot of adrenalin which can be injected under the skin in an emergency situation.
- Venomous snake, fish or spider bites. Immediate applications of essential oils may save life if medical treatment is unduly delayed (see Skin First Aid chart).
- Frostbite: never rub the skin, nor apply oils and ointments. Warm the affected area slowly and naturally to prevent further tissue destruction (e.g. blowing on skin, warming hands in armpits, covering frostbitten ears, nose and face with warm hands). In serious cases, arrange removal of individual to hospital.

NATURAL ADDITIONS TO THE FIRST-AID KIT

A bottle of the Bach five-flower composite, known as Rescue Remedy will keep indefiniteiy due to the brandy preservatives. It can be administered in any emergency situation to address emotional shock (not to be confused with medical shock, which is a systemic reaction involving serious loss of vital body fluids) and for hysteria. While the remedy cannot replace medical attention, it can alleviate much of the person's distress whilst they await the arrival of medical aid, thus enabling the mind/body's healing processes to commence without delay.

The usual dosage is four drops of the undiluted remedy on the tongue every fifteen minutes or until distress abates. Alternatively, put the same number of drops in a small glass of water and sip at intervals. If the patient is unconscious, the drops can be applied externally, either diluted or directly from the bottle. Moisten the lips, gums, temples, back of the neck, behind the ears, or the wrists.

Always include a bottle of lavender essence in your first-aid kit, especially whilst travelling. Lavender can be used in just about any emergency situation. However, unlike Rescue Remedy, it does not have an indefinite shelf-life, which is why it is best kept in the aromatic store cupboard and replenished when necessary. It may lose its potency if left in the first-aid box for very long periods, especially if the bottle has been opened.

Include some cider vinegar for treating wasp stings. Funnel a small amount into a dark glass bottle of a suitable size for the first-aid box. For treating ant and bee stings, you will need a similar sized bottle of distilled water, and also some bicarbonate of soda.

SKIN
FIRST AID CHART

ANIMAL BITES

Recommended Essential Oils

Eucalyptus, lavender, tea tree.

Methods of Application

Rinse wound with cool water, then apply neat essential oil or a cold aromatic compress. Apply a dressing if required, adding a few drops of essential oil to the bandage or gauze portion of a plaster.

Further advice

Rabies can be contracted from the saliva of dogs (and other animals). Although Britain is free of rabies, if you are bitten by an animal whilst abroad, do seek urgent medical attention, no matter how minor the wound.

BURNS AND SCALDS (MINOR)

Recommended Essential Oils

Eucalyptus, geranium, lavender, tea tree.

Methods of Application

If possible, cool the affected area under cold running water for 10 minutes, or immerse in cold water for the same amount of time. Then apply *neat* essential oil to the burn or scald. Larger burns and scalds can be treated with cold aromatic compresses.

Further Advice

Never apply ointments, vegetable oils, including essential oils diluted in vegetable oil, for treating the early stages of a burn or scald, i.e. whilst still inflamed. Fatty substances (apart from neat essential oil) will 'fry' on hot skin, thus increasing the possibility of infection. Applications of diluted essential oils, wheatgerm oil or the infused oils of calendula and/or hypericum applied during the healing period will help prevent permanent scarring. **Serious burns need urgent medical attention.**

CUTS AND GRAZES

Recommended Essential Oils

Chamomile (German and Roman), elemi, eucalyptus, frankincense, galbanum, lavender, lemon, myrrh, pine, tea tree, thyme (sweet), vetiver.

Methods of Application

First cleanse by swabbing with wet cotton wool or holding injured part under running water. Apply neat lavender or tea tree, or an aromatic antiseptic ointment (see pages 32–3). For larger wounds, apply cold aromatic compresses. Cover with a bandage or plaster if necessary.

Further Advice

If soil particles are clinging to the wound, remove with spotlessly clean tweezers (wipe tweezers first with neat essential oil).

INSECT REPELLENT

Recommended Essential Oils

Eucalyptus, lavender, patchouli, rosemary, tea tree.

Methods of Application

Apply a 3 per cent dilution of essential oil to exposed parts (e.g. arms and legs), use a 1 or 2 per cent dilution for facial skin (see Easy Measures on page 34).

Further Advice

See also Aromatherapy for Home and Garden, Chapter 28.

INSECT BITES AND STINGS

Recommended Essential Oils

Cajeput, chamomile (German or Roman), eucalyptus, lavender, lemon, tea tree.

Methods of Application

Add neat lavender or tea tree to the affected area, or an aromatic ointment. If swollen, apply a cold chamomile and/or lavender compress.

Further Advice

For advice on treating wasp, bee and ant stings, see page 65.

JELLYFISH STINGS

Recommended Essential Oils

Eucalyptus, lavender, geranium.

Methods of Application

If you need to pull tentacles off, protect your hand with an article of clothing if possible. Wash with sea water, then apply neat essential oil.

Further Advice

Don't rub or rinse the affected area with fresh water as this can discharge unactivated stinging cells. Most jellyfish stings are harmless. But Portuguese Man-of-War stings may require medical attention.

SNAKE BITES

Recommended Essential Oils

Lavender.

Methods of Application

Apply plenty of neat lavender oil. Try to hold still the affected part and keep it below the level of the heart to prevent rapid absorption of the venom.

Further Advice

The only poisonous snake indigenous to the British Isles is the adder, though some people keep poisonous snakes as pets. Treatment with essential oils is meant as an emergency measure whilst awaiting medical attention. It is important to identify the snake so that appropriate antivenom serum can be administered.

SPIDER BITES

Recommended Essential Oils	Methods of Application	Further Advice
Chamomile (German or Roman), lavender, tea tree (see Further Advice).	Apply plenty of neat lavender oil and/or a cold chamomile or lavender compress.	There are no poisonous spiders in Britain, though some of the large hunter spiders can give a painful bite. Tea tree oil is said to neutralise the poison of the Australian funnel web spider, whereas lavender will neutralise the venom of the notorious black widow. Treatment with essential oils for venomous spider bites is meant as an emergency measure whilst awaiting medical attention.

SUNBURN

Recommended Essential Oils	Methods of Application	Further Advice
Chamomile (German or Roman), eucalyptus, geranium, lavender, rosemary, tea tree.	Take two or three cool (preferably cold) aromatic baths throughout the day, adding up to eight tablespoonfuls cider vinegar and eight drops essential oil. Afterwards, pat the skin dry and apply an appropriate oil (see Easy Measures Chart on page 34). For very sore patches, it is less painful to paint on the oil with a small soft, bristle brush.	Never apply oils, creams or ointments to the skin until it has been cooled by an aromatic bath (or cooled by sponging gently with cold water). Take frequent sips of water to prevent dehydration. Serious sunburn, with skin appearing lobster red, tender and swollen with possible blistering, requires urgent medical attention.

FIRST-AID PRESCRIPTIONS AND PROCEDURES

WASP STINGS

Since wasp venom is alkaline, the most effective treatment is vinegar (preferably cider vinegar), which neutralises the poison. Apply as often as required, until pain and swelling have subsided. To prevent infection, add a single drop of lavender or tea tree to each dessertspoonful of vinegar.

BEE STINGS

The bee is the only insect which leaves its stinger embedded in the skin. To remove, don't pull at the stinger with your fingers because you may squeeze the venom sac and thus pump the remaining poison into your system. Take a pair of tweezers and hold as near to the skin as possible (avoiding the venom sac), grasp the stinger and remove it.

Bee venom is acid, so to relieve pain and swelling, apply an alkaline solution of bicarbonate of soda (one teaspoonful in about one tablespoonful water), which will neutralise the poison. To help prevent infection, add a drop of chamomile or lavender essence to the solution. A cold compress containing chamomile and/or lavender will also help reduce pain and swelling.

ANT STINGS

Ant venom is acid. To neutralise the poison, apply an alkaline solution of bicarbonate of soda, adding a drop of chamomile or lavender to prevent infection. A cold compress containing lavender and/or chamomile will also help to reduce pain and swelling.

INSECT STINGS INSIDE THE MOUTH OR THROAT

To reduce swelling, give the sufferer an ice cube to suck. Alternatively, rinse the mouth out with cold water. If caused by a bee or ant, give a solution of water and bicarbonate of soda, if available (one teaspoonful to a tumbler). Most important: arrange removal of the individual to hospital.

9

THE RESPIRATORY SYSTEM

The air we breathe is shared by all life on our planet. By becoming aware of the breath as it flows in and out we begin to recognise the pattern of life itself; the ebb and flow of the tides; the waxing and waning of the moon; day and night; the vernal and autumnal equinoxes – cycles within cycles. Our oneness with the trees (often referred to as the planet's lungs) becomes manifest fact.

When sitting quietly we breathe in and out about 12 to 15 times a minute; during strenuous exercise we double or treble that rate. Most of the time our breathing is under the automatic control of the *medulla oblongata* – the bulge where the spinal cord joins the brain. However, we can also control the breath to a certain extent; for instance, when we practise deep breathing exercises, or when swimming under water.

Breathing is the movement of air in and out of the lungs by means of the diaphragm and intercostal muscles. *Respiration* is the chemical process occurring inside cells whereby food substances are oxidised to produce energy, and carbon dioxide and other tissue wastes are eliminated from the system. If these wastes were allowed to build up they would eventually cause the cells to die. So tiny blood vessels, which surround the alveoli (air sacs) in the lungs, carry the waste back to the lungs, where it is eliminated on the out breath and exchanged for fresh oxygen when we breathe in. This complex process is known as gaseous exchange.

The process of taking in oxygen and eliminating poisonous wastes is essential to life. Therefore, any problem with breathing will affect the organism as a whole – leading to susceptibility to every passing infection, premature ageing and diminished functioning of brain and nerve cells. According to many health experts, the mental changes usually associated with old age, such as senility and vagueness of thought, are the result of too little oxygen being available to the cells, either as a result of shallow breathing or blockages in the circulatory system or both.

Indeed, supplying the cells with life-giving oxygen is the shared responsibility of the respiratory and circulatory systems. Moreover, since the lungs share the role of eliminating waste with the skin, kidneys and colon (bowel), if a problem develops in any of these systems, the body compensates by increasing the burden on the others.

THE PATTERN OF RESPIRATORY DISORDERS

Respiratory ailments affect the mucus membranes. These include the linings of the nose, sinuses, mouth, throat, windpipe (trachea) and lungs. The fine coverings of the eyes and the linings of certain parts of the inner ears are also covered by mucus-producing membranes. The function of mucus is to protect these delicate surfaces, keeping them moist and trapping airborne particles.

When in good health, we are hardly aware of respiratory mucus, which is swept downwards into the sterilising stomach by the action of the beating cilia. These are microscopic hairs which grow from the cells lining the air passages which wave two and fro. Should we lose our natural resistance, perhaps through poor diet, emotional disharmony or cigarette smoking, we become more susceptible to airborne bacteria and viruses. The mucus then becomes more viscous and profuse as it attempts to rid the body of toxins. However, should the cause of the problem be ignored, this can lead to congestion or chronic catarrh. The aim of natural treatment is to change the consistency of the mucus by using decongestant herbs and essences; the cilia will do the rest.

Interestingly, researchers at Exeter University in Britain have given scientific validation to the old-fashioned steam inhalation as a treatment for colds and flu. These viruses are very sensitive to steam, which can actually kill them off. In my own experience, steam inhalations in conjunction with hot spicy lemon and honey drinks are especially effective if taken at the onset of symptoms. They can actually prevent the condition from developing further.

Polluted air is the biggest challenge to the lungs. When subjected to badly contaminated air or cigarette smoke, the cilia cease to sway. A temporary paralysis sets in. Should the irritation continue for long enough, cilia wither and die, never to be replaced.

It is important to remember that while most organs in the body can tolerate an enormous amount of abuse, the lungs cannot. The best preventative measures for the respiratory system – and indeed for the whole of your being – are fresh air, adequate exercise and good breathing. Should any problems arise, essential oils, herbs and other gentle remedies will then be able to work more speedily and efficiently.

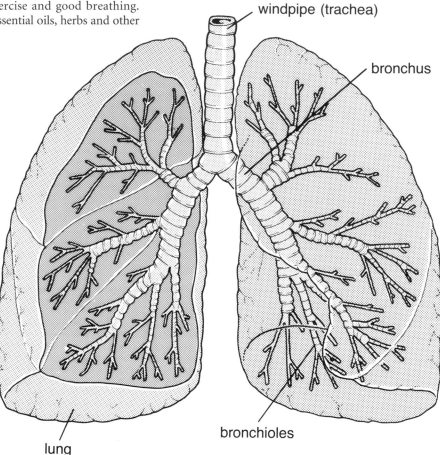

The respiratory system

windpipe (trachea)

bronchus

bronchioles

lung

ACTIONS OF ESSENTIAL OILS

Unlike herbal remedies, essential oils lack demulcent properties whose action is to soothe irritated and inflamed mucus membranes. Nonetheless, they are extremely helpful for a number of common respiratory ailments. The principal actions of essences having an affinity with the respiratory system are as follows:

Antispasmodics: (relax spasms in the bronchial tubes): For problems such as asthma and dry coughs, for example chamomile, cypress, thyme (sweet).
Antivirals: For colds and flu, for example clove, eucalyptus, tea tree.
Diaphoretics or Febrifuges: (induce sweating, and thus reduce fever): Helpful for feverish colds and flu, for example black pepper, ginger, thyme.
Expectorants: (promote the removal of mucus): For catarrhal problems such as bronchitis, sinusitis, coughs, colds, for example eucalyptus, peppermint, pine.

THERAPEUTIC CHARTS: RESPIRATORY PROBLEMS

Instructions for preparing essential oils for the various therapeutic applications are to be found in Chapter 6. Included in this chart are minor ear and eye ailments associated with respiratory infections and catarrh.

ASTHMA

Description

During an attack, breathing becomes difficult and audibly 'wheezy' with coughing, and expiration often being more affected than inspiration. There may also be agitation and confusion.

Possible causes

There is usually a family history of asthma, eczema and sometimes migraine. Allergies are often implicated, for example grass and tree pollen, animal fur, moulds, fungi, dairy products.

Aggravated by

Fear, nervous tension and anxiety, cigarette smoke. Also, avoid steam inhalations and saunas which may provoke an attack.

Recommended Essential Oils

Clary sage, cypress, eucalyptus, frankincense, galbanum, hyssop, lavender, melissa (true), marjoram, myrrh, peppermint, pine, rose otto, rosemary, tea tree, thyme (sweet).

Methods of use

Bath, regular massage (especially to chest, neck and shoulders), vaporiser, dry inhalation (drops on a handkerchief).

Suggested Herbal Remedies

Coltsfoot, echinacea, hyssop, lemon balm, peppermint.

Nutritional supplements

A good multi-vitamin and mineral supplement containing complete B-complex, plus 500 mg vitamin C, and one or two garlic capsules daily.

Further suggestions

Holistic treatment is essential. Serious cases may need to be treated in conjunction with prescribed medication. Breathing exercises, (see page 145), Alexander Technique (to correct poor posture), Bach flower remedies, allergy testing. A qualified homoeopath will prescribe constitutional treatment.

BRONCHITIS (ACUTE)

Description

An infection of the bronchial tubes that lead to the lungs. Symptoms are a chesty cough, high temperature, chest pain, aching muscles, irritation between the shoulder blades, depression.

Possible causes

Smoking, excessive consumption of dairy products and/or a junk food diet, incorrect breathing, air pollution, poor posture, stress and sometimes allergy. Often a complication of a cold or flu (bacterial infection is facilitated by viral inflammation).

Aggravated by

Cold damp air.

Recommended Essential Oils

Angelica, cajeput, cedarwood, cypress, elemi, eucalyptus, frankincense, galbanum, hyssop, lavender, lemon, marjoram, melissa (true), myrrh, orange, peppermint, rosemary, sandalwood, tea tree, thyme (sweet).

Methods of use	**Suggested Herbal Remedies**	**Nutritional supplements**	**Further suggestions**
Steam inhalations, vaporiser, bath, chest and back rub (see recipe, page 75).	Coltsfoot, hyssop, lungwort, thyme.	Four x 500 mg vitamin C, multi-vitamin and mineral supplement, two to four garlic capsules daily. Gradually reduce garlic and vitamin C as improvement takes place.	Bed rest, hot lemon and honey drinks. Chronic bronchitis is a much more serious disorder, often accompanied by emphysema. In this instance, seek the co-operation of your doctor as well as embarking on holistic treatment from a qualified practitioner, for example a medical herbalist, or a homoeopath.

CATARRH

Description	**Possible causes**	**Aggravated by**	**Recommended Essential Oils**
Excessive mucus as a result of a build-up of toxic matter that the body is forced to eliminate.	Infection, poor nutrition, stress and sometimes allergy.	Excessive consumption of dairy products and/or a junk food diet.	Cajeput, cedarwood, elemi, eucalyptus, frankincense, galbanum, garlic, ginger, jasmine, lavender, lemon, marjoram, myrrh, orange, peppermint, pine, rosemary, sandalwood, tea tree, thyme (sweet).

Methods of use	**Suggested Herbal Remedies**	**Nutritional supplements**	**Further suggestions**
Bath, regular massage (especially to chest), steam inhalation, vaporiser.	Chamomile, elderflower, lemon balm, peppermint.	Two x 500 mg vitamin C, six brewer's yeast tablets, multi-vitamin and mineral supplement, three to four garlic capsules daily (taper off to maintenance dose of one garlic capsule daily as improvement takes place).	Hot spicy lemon and honey drink (see page 76). Chronic catarrh should be investigated by an holistic practitioner, preferably someone who can carry out allergy testing.

COLDS

Description	**Possible causes**	**Aggravated by**	**Recommended Essential Oils**
A viral infection affecting the upper respiratory tract (nasal passages and throat).	We become more susceptible to colds during periods of prolonged stress and as a result of poor nutrition. Naturopaths regard the common cold as the body's attempt to cleanse the system, especially if they occur periodically during the spring and autumn.	A hot, stuffy or smoky atmosphere; symptoms often worse at night. Excessive amounts of mucus-forming foods such as dairy products, bread and potatoes.	Black pepper, cedarwood, cinnamon (bark or leaf), clove, eucalyptus, garlic ginger, lavender, lemon, melissa, orange, peppermint, pine, tea tree.

Methods of use	Suggested Herbal Remedies	Nutritional supplements	Further suggestions
Baths, steam inhalation, dry inhalation (drops on a handkerchief), vaporiser, massage oil (as a chest and throat rub, see page 75).	Chamomile, coltsfoot, elderflower, peppermint, yarrow.	As a preventative measure during the 'cold season', a good multi-vitamin and mineral supplement, one or two garlic capsules, two × 500 mg vitamin C daily.	Hot spicy lemon and honey drinks.

CAUTION *Cinnamon and clove essences should be used as fumigants only (see recipe, page 75).*

COUGHS

Description	Possible causes	Aggravated by	Recommended Essential Oils
The body's attempt to clear the air passages of irritating mucus, bacteria, dust, pollen or smoke.	Coughs often accompany other infections, such as colds and flu. Often the result of smoking, they can also be caused by an allergy.	As for Colds (see page 70) and Flu (see page 72).	Angelica, black pepper, cajeput, cedarwood, clary sage, cypress, eucalyptus, galbanum, garlic, ginger, hyssop, marjoram, melissa, myrrh, pine, rose otto, rosemary, sandalwood, tea tree.

Methods of use	Suggested Herbal Remedies	Nutritional supplements	Further suggestions
Gargle (one or two drops in warm water), dry inhalation (drops on a handkerchief), bath, vaporiser, massage oil (rub oil on chest and throat).	*Dry coughs:* coltsfoot, marshmallow. *Coughs producing phlegm:* hyssop, thyme.	As for Colds (see page 70) and Flu (see page 72).	Hot spicy lemon and honey drinks. For a persistent cough, seek medical advice and holistic treatment from a medical herbalist or homoeopath.

CAUTION *Garlic in any shape or form may be contra-indicated if you have a dry cough.*

EARACHE

Description	Possible causes	Aggravated by	Recommended Essential Oils
Often accompanies a cold or 'flu.	If associated with a cold or flu, it is brought on by the spread of infection from the throat to the Eustachian tube in the ear. Occasionally, an earache may be a symptom of middle-ear infection (see Further Suggestions).	Cold, damp and windy weather.	Chamomile (German or Roman), lavender, rosemary, peppermint.

Methods of use

Warm one eggcupful olive or sweet almond oil and add one drop essential oil. Using a medicine dropper (pipette), put a few drops into the ear and seal in with a small ball of cotton wool.

Suggested Herbal Remedies

As for Colds (see page 70), Coughs (see page 71) and Flu (see below).

Nutritional supplements

As for Colds (see page 70), Coughs (see page 71) and Flu (see below).

Further suggestions

Persistent or severe earache should be investigated by a medical practitioner, especially if there is pus or a bloody discharge.

EYES (STICKY OR IRRITATED)

Description

Often associated with upper respiratory infections such as colds and flu. However, styes are similar to boils (see Skin Disorders chart), but can be treated as suggested here.

Possible causes

As for Colds (see page 70), Coughs (see page 71) and Flu (see below).

Aggravated by

Overheated, dry atmosphere; bright fluorescent light.

Recommended Essential Oils

Essential oils should never be applied to the eyes as they can cause pain and irritation. If you can obtain genuine floral waters such as rosewater or cornflower water, these can be used to bathe the eyes.

Methods of use

Floral water: Cold compress for dry irritated eyes (soak cotton wool pads in floral water); warm compress for sticky eyes or stye (heat gently in an enamel or stainless steel vessel).

Suggested Herbal Remedies

Internally: Echinacea, eyebright (euphrasia).
Externally: For dry irritated eyes, bathe with *cold* infusion of eyebright, marigold or chamomile, or apply a cold compress. For sticky eyes, bathe with warm infusion of same herbs.

Nutritional supplements

As for Colds.

Further suggestions

Conjunctivitis is a more serious, contagious eye infection which may need medical attention. Various forms of the infection can often be relieved with herbal eye lotions. However, in chronic cases, especially where the subject has been feeling run down, holistic treatment (including nutritional advice) is essential. Nevertheless, the treatment suggested for dry irritated eyes will help if used as part of a holistic healing regime.

FLU

Description

A viral infection affecting the upper respiratory tract, causing fever, headache, general aches and pains and nasal congestion.

Possible causes

Factors such as prolonged stress, poor nutrition and overwork create the right conditions for viral infections to take root.

Aggravated by

Cold, damp weather, lack of sleep, physical exertion. Symptoms usually worse at night.

Recommended Essential Oils

As for Colds.

Methods of use	Suggested Herbal Remedies	Nutritional supplements	Further suggestions
Bath, steam inhalation, dry inhalation (drops of essential oil on a handkerchief), massage oil (rubbed on to chest and throat), vaporiser (see recipe, page 75).	As for Colds.	As for Colds.	Hot spicy lemon and honey drinks.

HAY FEVER

Description	Possible causes	Aggravated by	Recommended Essential Oils
A seasonal allergy to airborne pollens or mould spores. Symptoms manifest as excessive sneezing; itchy, blocked or runny nose; irritated watery eyes and sensitivity to light. Some people also develop a fever or suffer asthma-like symptoms, such as coughing and wheezing.	As for Asthma (see page 69).	Exposure to allergens, such as tree and grass pollens.	Chamomile (German or Roman), eucalyptus, rose otto.

Methods of use	Suggested Herbal Remedies	Nutritional supplements	Further suggestions
Bath, dry inhalation (drops of essential oil on a handkerchief), massage (especially to chest and back), vaporiser, hay fever balm (see page 75).	Elderflower, elecampane, eyebright (this can be used to bathe irritated eyes too), goldenseal.	As for Asthma (see page 69).	Deep breathing exercises (see page 145), Alexander Technique or yoga (to correct postural faults which may be hindering correct breathing), Bach flower remedies, allergy testing. If symptoms persist, consult a qualified homoeopath or medical herbalist who will offer constitutional treatment.

SINUSITIS

Description	Possible causes	Aggravated by	Recommended Essential Oils
An infection of the sinus cavities resulting in nasal congestion, pain around the eyes, headaches and sometimes bad breath as well.	Stress, food allergy and air pollution are contributing factors. May be triggered by a cold or 'flu.	Excessive amounts of mucus-forming foods such as dairy products, wheat and foods which are heavily laden with synthetic colourings and preservatives. Overheated, stuffy rooms.	Cajeput, eucalyptus, garlic (see Nutritional Supplements), lavender, lemon, peppermint, pine, tea tree.

Methods of use	**Suggested Herbal Remedies**	**Nutritional supplements**	**Further suggestions**
Steam inhalation, dry inhalation (drops of essential oil on a handkerchief), baths, vaporiser, facial massage oil, sinusitis balm (see page 75).	Elderflower, eucalyptus leaves, eyebright (use as a cold compress as well as by mouth), peppermint.	Two to three garlic capsules daily during acute stage, reducing to one a day as a preventative measure. A good multi-vitamin and mineral supplement and three x 500 mg vitamin C daily.	Seek the advice of an holistic practitioner if symptoms persist, preferably someone who can carry out food allergy tests.

THROAT INFECTIONS

Description	**Possible causes**	**Aggravated by**	**Recommended Essential Oils**
A sore throat is often the first symptom of a cold or 'flu virus or some other viral infection. Laryngitis is inflammation of the larynx (voice box), producing huskiness and weakness of voice and sometimes a harsh dry cough.	As with all respiratory infections, such factors as stress and poor nutrition invite passing bacteria and viruses to take root. Laryngitis often results from overuse or abuse of the voice and is common in public speakers, singers and actors.	Overheated, stuffy rooms; cigarette smoke; using the voice.	*Sore throat:* bergamot, cajeput, clary sage, eucalyptus, geranium, ginger, lavender, myrrh, peppermint, pine, sandalwood, tea tree, thyme (sweet) *Laryngitis/hoarseness:* clary sage, eucalyptus, frankincense, lavender, lemon, myrrh, sandalwood, thyme (sweet).

Methods of use	**Suggested Herbal Remedies**	**Nutritional supplements**	**Further suggestions**
Gargle (one or two drops in warm water).	Red sage or common sage. Make an infusion (see page 38). Add one teaspoonful cider vinegar and gargle often. Gently re-heat the infusion each time before use, but not the vinegar which should be added to the glass immediately before use.	As for Colds, Coughs and Flu.	Try to rest the voice.

AROMATIC PRESCRIPTIONS AND PROCEDURES

The following mixtures can be rubbed into the chest and throat as a decongestant for most minor respiratory ailments. The same combinations of essences can also be used in the bath, but you will need to adjust the quantities of essential oil accordingly.

RELAXING CHEST RUB (BEDTIME)

50 ml almond oil
5 drops frankincense
10 drops lavender
5 drops marjoram

Put the essential oil into a 50 ml dark glass bottle, top-up with the base oil and shake well.

STIMULATING CHEST RUB (DAYTIME)

50 ml almond oil
5 drops eucalyptus
10 drops spike lavender (or rosemary)
5 drops pine

Mix as for the previous recipe.

AROMATIC OINTMENT CHEST RUB

As an alternative to an oil-based chest rub, you could mix the same quantity of essential oil into 50g of an unperfumed shop-bought cream or ointment. Put the cream into a clean glass pot, add the essential oil and stir in with the handle of a teaspoon. In case of difficulty, suitable base-creams can be purchased by mail order from most essential oil suppliers.

FUMIGANTS

When infectious illness such as colds and flu are around, vaporise one of the following blends according to personal preference. Put the essential oil into a 50 ml dark glass bottle, fill the bottle with water and shake well. Add a small amount of the blend to the reservoir of a nightlight burner or electric vaporiser. Remember to shake the bottle each time before use to disperse the essential oil.

Recipe 1
50 ml water
5 drops eucalyptus
5 drops lavender
5 drops lemon

Recipe 2
50 ml water
2 drops clove
2 drops cinnamon (bark or leaf)
10 drops orange

Recipe 3
50 ml water
5 drops cypress
5 drops pine
5 drops juniper berry

HAY FEVER BALM

You may be surprised to discover that Vaseline is the main ingredient in this recipe. Although not an organic substance for it is derived from petroleum, Vaseline acts merely as a carrier for the essential oils, which can thus evaporate and enter the nasal cavities without being absorbed itself into the skin. The Vaseline will also trap dust and pollen particles which trigger attacks. Apply a very small amount to the nostrils two or three times daily.

1 dessertspoonful Vaseline
5 drops eucalyptus
5 drops pine

Melt the Vaseline in a small bowl placed over a saucepan of simmering water. Remove from the heat and stir in the essential oils. Pour the mixture into a little glass pot, cover tightly and label. Alternatively, and if you can afford it, use 5 drops of rose otto in the same quantity of Vaseline.

SINUSITIS BALM

1 dessertspoonful Vaseline
8 drops eucalyptus
2 drops peppermint

Make as for Hay Fever Balm and apply in the same way.

HOT SPICY LEMON AND HONEY DRINK

This is an excellent warming decongestant remedy for acute bronchitis, catarrhal coughs, colds and flu. If taken at the very first sign of cold or 'flu symptoms (sore throat, shivering and sneezing), I have known this spicy brew to stop the virus in its tracks.

1 pint (500 ml) still spring water
1 teaspoonful whole cloves
cinnamon stick, broken
1 level teaspoonful ground ginger
honey to taste
juice of one freshly squeezed lemon

Pour the water into a stainless steel or enamel saucepan, add the cloves and broken cinnamon stick and bring to boiling point. Turn down the heat and simmer in a covered pan for five minutes. Then turn off the heat, add the ground ginger and leave on the stove to infuse for about 30 minutes. Re-heat before use to just below simmering point. Pour some of the decoction through a tea strainer into a cup, then add one dessertspoonful lemon juice and as much honey as you wish to sweeten.

Drink a cupful two or three times a day, gently re-heating the spicy decoction (but not the lemon juice and honey) each time before use.

10

THE HEART AND
THE CIRCULATORY SYSTEM

To the romantic novelist, the heart is moody and fragile. While it is true that heartbeat is influenced by
emotion – speeding up when we are afraid or excited,
and slowing down when we feel calm – 'fragile' it certainly is not. In fact, the heart is incredibly hard working,
pumping blood around the body continuously. Indeed,
no muscles in the body are as strong as the heart – except
the uterine muscles during childbirth.

The average adult has six litres (10 pints) of blood cir-
culating in the body. The force (blood pressure) that
keeps this vital fluid moving comes from the heart itself.
However, a complex system of nerve signals, hormones,
and other elements, regulate the flow by widening or
constricting small muscular blood vessels called arteri-
oles, much like a tap controls the flow of water.

Blood pressure is normally defined in terms of the *sys-
tolic* pressure, which is the maximum pressure produced
in the larger arteries by each heartbeat, and the *diastolic*
pressure, the constant pressure maintained in the arteries
between heartbeats. The so-called normal figure for sys-
tolic pressure (as measured by means of a sphygmo-
manometer in millimetres of mercury) is 120 millimetres, and 80 millimetres for the diastolic, which is
expressed as 120/80 (one hundred and twenty over
eighty). The lower figure is the more important. The
higher that figure rises, the more the body is craving rest.
Without adequate rest the heart begins to weaken.

Yet many perfectly healthy people have a blood pressure reading which may be slightly below or above average. Moreover, there can be considerable fluctuations in
blood pressure from one moment to the next. The figure
may be affected by the time of day (it is lowest early in
the morning) and by your degree of physical exertion or
anxiety. In Western societies, blood pressure tends to
increase with age. Yet this is by no means the norm.
Population studies have found that in non-industrialised
countries, there is little increase in blood pressure with
age.

To cut an infinitely complex story short, the blood is
pumped by the right side of the heart through the pulmonary artery into the lungs, where it takes up oxygen. It
then returns via the pulmonary veins to the left side of

the heart to be pumped through the aorta and the arterial
system. Having given up its oxygen to every cell and
organ in the body, the deoxygenated blood returns
through the veins to enter the right side of the heart
again.

Because every cell in the body needs a constant supply
of blood to bring in oxygen and nutrients and to remove
metabolic wastes, should the supply be insufficient, the
vitality of the whole organism is lowered. The heart itself,
however, does not extract vital oxygen and nutrients
from the main circulation. It is nourished by the blood
which passes through its own coronary arteries – the
heart's main weak spot. Should they become narrowed
through cardiovascular disease, the amount of blood able
to pass through them to the heart is reduced. The more
heart muscle that is affected by this lack of blood, the less
efficient the heart becomes; the beat will become weak
and/or irregular. Coronary dysfunction is, in fact, the
greatest single cause of death.

PREVENTION IS EASIER
THAN CURE

The treatment of major heart and circulatory problems
are beyond the scope of home treatment. Nevertheless, so
long as you remain under medical supervision, there is a
great deal you can do to ease symptoms and perhaps even
halt the progress of problems such as high blood pressure
and angina pectoris. This can be achieved by giving up
smoking (or by not starting in the first place), taking adequate exercise, getting enough sleep, eating sensibly,
maintaining an average weight for your build, and by
seeking to reduce stress in your life.

Congenital defects apart, stress in its many guises is at
the root of a great many health problems, particularly
cardiovascular disorders. Aromatherapy, in tune with all
other systems of holistic healing, places great emphasis
upon preventative care. Of all the aromatherapeutic
treatments, massage with aromatic oils reigns supreme as

a means of reducing stress and engendering a sense of well-being. The only circulatory disorders which may not benefit from full-body massage are thrombosis or phlebitis, which means that blood clots are present and massage could dislodge them. However, gentle massage to the face, head, hands and feet are beneficial and will help to relax body and mind.

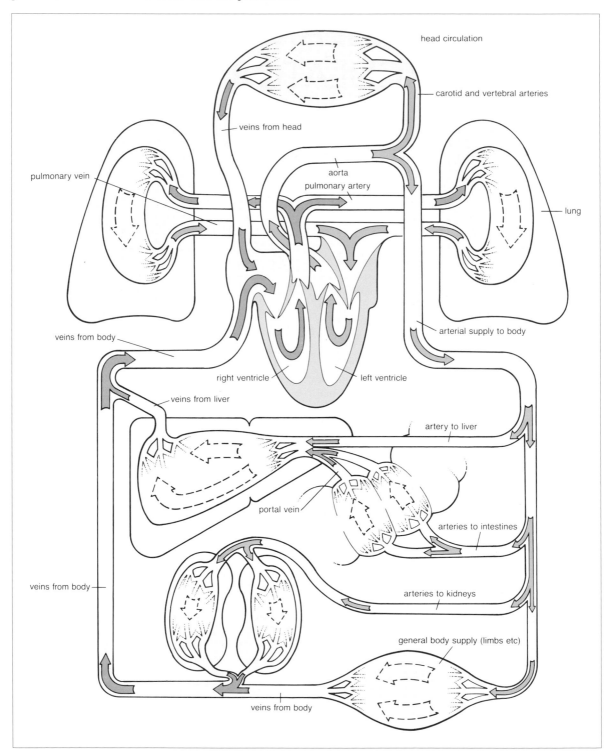

ACTIONS OF ESSENTIAL OILS

When circulatory problems arise there is often a need to deal with fluid retention. This is covered in the chapter on The Urinary System. However, regular massage (an essential part of aromatherapy) helps the body to eliminate excess fluid and toxic wastes, no matter which essences are applied.

The principal actions of essential oils used for circulatory problems are as follows:

Hypertensives (stimulate the circulation): Helpful for poor circulation and low blood pressure, for example black pepper, rosemary, thyme (sweet).

Hypotensives (lower high blood pressure), for example lavender, marjoram, ylang ylang.
Nervines (strengthen the nervous system): To reduce anxiety and stress which contribute to the development of cardiovascular disease, for example chamomile, lavender, neroli.
Tonics and Astringents (strengthen and tone the whole system): Especially helpful for varicose veins and haemorrhoids, for example cypress, geranium, lemon.

THERAPEUTIC CHARTS: CIRCULATORY PROBLEMS

Instructions for preparing essences for the various therapeutic applications are to be found in Chapter 6.

BLOOD PRESSURE, HIGH (HYPERTENSION)

Description	Possible causes	Aggravated by	Recommended Essential Oils
Although often symptomless in the early stages, signs include morning headache, dizziness on sudden change of position, palpitations, shortness of breath, blurred vision.	Heredity, prolonged stress, smoking, obesity, sedentary lifestyle, pregnancy. A diet high in animal fats, salt, chemical additives, alcohol and caffeine.	Stress.	Clary sage, lavender, lemon, marjoram, melissa (true), ylang, ylang.

Methods of use	Suggested Herbal Remedies	Nutritional supplements	Further suggestions
Baths, massage, personal perfume, vaporiser.	Hyssop, lime blossom, valerian (available in tablet or capsule form to disguise its unpleasant taste), yarrow.	Good multi-vitamin and mineral supplement containing calcium, magnesium and potassium. Plenty of fresh garlic in cooking or raw in salads.	Holistic treatment is essential, including deep-breathing and relaxation exercises (see Chapter 19) and regular aromatherapy massage. Persistent high blood pressure must be investigated by a medical practitioner.

BLOOD PRESSURE, LOW (HYPOTENSION)

Description

When blood pressure falls to a low level, the flow of blood to the brain is significantly reduced. Symptoms include debility and exhaustion, confusion, lightheadedness, unsteady gait and dizziness.

Possible causes

Nervous exhaustion, poor circulation, anaemia.

Aggravated by

Stress, getting up too quickly from a prone position.

Recommended Essential Oils

Black pepper, coriander, cypress, eucalyptus, galbanum, geranium, ginger, lemon, lemongrass, neroli, nutmeg, pine, rose otto, rosemary, thyme (sweet).

Methods of use

Bath, brisk massage.

Suggested Herbal Remedies

Ginseng (available in tablet or capsule form)

Nutritional supplements

Good multi-vitamin and mineral supplement, plenty of fresh garlic in cooking and raw in salads.

Further suggestions

Hypotension can be symptomatic of a more serious health problem, so do seek medical advice as well.

CIRCULATION, SLUGGISH

Description

Manifests as cold extremities, susceptibility to chilblains and exceptional intolerance to cold.

Possible causes

Heredity, advanced age, smoking, low blood pressure, anaemia.

Aggravated by

Sedentary lifestyle.

Recommended Essential Oils

Bergamot, black pepper, coriander, cypress, garlic (see Nutritional Supplements) eucalyptus, galbanum, geranium, ginger, lavender, lemon, lemongrass, marjoram, neroli, nutmeg, orange, pine, rose otto, rosemary, thyme (sweet).

Methods of use

Bath, foot/hand bath, massage.

Suggested Herbal Remedies

Lemon balm, lemon verbena, peppermint.

Nutritional supplements

A good multi-vitamin and mineral supplement, plenty of fresh garlic in cooking and raw in salads, or take one or two garlic capsules daily.

Further suggestions

Circulation is improved by regular full-body massage, dry skin brushing (see pages 213–4), fresh air and exercise, correct breathing, and good nutrition.

HAEMORRHOIDS

Description

Also known as piles. Swollen or varicose veins in the rectum or lining of the anus, causing pain, itching and sometimes bleeding.

Possible causes

Heredity, chronic constipation (causing straining during bowel movement), incorrect lifting of heavy loads, obesity, pregnancy.

Aggravated by

Low-fibre diet, stress, changing seasons (may worsen in the spring and/or autumn).

Recommended Essential Oils

Cypress, garlic (see Nutritional Supplements), geranium, juniper berry, myrrh.

Methods of use

Alternate hot and cold sitz baths, ointment (see page 33).

Suggested Herbal Remedies

Oral doses: Equal quantities of pilewort and marigold flowers.
Externally: Witch hazel applied on a gauze dressing.

Nutritional supplements

Plenty of fresh garlic in cooking or raw in salads, or take one to two garlic capsules daily (see also Varicose Veins).

Further suggestions

Where there is bleeding, seek medical advice as well as holistic treatment.

PALPITATIONS

Description

Pounding of the heart at times other than after exercise.

Possible causes

Stress, allergies, menopause, chronic high blood pressure, or when nicotine or caffeine have been taken. May be symptomatic of a serious heart problem.

Recommended Essential Oils

Lavender, melissa (true), neroli, rose otto, ylang ylang.

Methods of use

Dry inhalation (drops on a handkerchief or in palm of hand), vaporiser, personal perfume (see page 229). Regular full-body massage as a preventative measure.

Suggested Herbal Remedies

Chamomile, lemon balm, orange flower, valerian (tastes unpleasant, but can be obtained as tablets or capsules).

Nutritional supplements

Good multi-vitamin and mineral supplement containing the full range of B-complex vitamins. Otherwise, six brewer's yeast tablets daily to help reduce anxiety and stress.

Further suggestions

Deep-breathing and relaxation exercises (see Chapter 19). To alleviate 'panic attack'. Bach flower remedies, especially Rescue Remedy (see page 62). If chronic high blood pressure is suspected, seek medical attention.

VARICOSE VEINS

Description

Swollen, knotted superficial veins, causing pain and discomfort. Usually found in the legs, though can appear in other parts of the body.

Possible causes

Heredity, prolonged standing or sitting, heavy lifting, insufficient exercise, constipation, insufficient fluid intake, faulty diet, obesity, pregnancy.

Aggravated by

As for Possible Causes, including deep tissue massage over affected areas.

Recommended Essential Oils

Cypress, frankincense, lemon, rose otto.

Methods of use

Cold or luke-warm compress, ointment (see recipe, page 83), also *very gentle* application of appropriate essences diluted in vegetable oil.

Suggested Herbal Remedies

Oral doses: peppermint, vervain, yarrow.

Nutritional supplements

Good multi-vitamin and mineral supplements, plus 500 mg vitamin C and a rutin supplement (a riboflavonoid found in buckwheat and pith of citrus fruits). Together with vitamin C, rutin helps strengthen capillary walls and reduces swelling. One garlic capsule daily (or plenty of fresh garlic in cooking).

Further suggestions

Attention to diet and adequate exercise such as swimming and walking. Also yoga, especially the inverted positions. Alternatively, rest with feet higher than head for about 10 minutes every day.

AROMATIC PRESCRIPTIONS AND PROCEDURES

SLUGGISH CIRCULATION

Here are three massage oil blends to improve the circulation. They are also helpful for low blood pressure. Choose according to your aroma preference. The same blends of essences can be used in the bath, but remember to adjust the quantities accordingly (see page 29).

To mix a massage oil, put the essences into a 50 ml dark glass bottle, then top up with base oil. Give the bottle a good shake to disperse the essential oil. Apply after a bath or shower, or persuade someone with 'good hands' to give you an aromatherapy massage.

Recipe 1
50 ml almond oil
10 drops bergamot
5 drops geranium
5 drops lavender

Recipe 2
50 ml extra virgin olive oil
2 drops ginger
12 drops coriander
4 drops rose otto

Recipe 3
50 ml almond oil
10 drops cypress
5 drops rosemary
5 drops lemon (or 1 drop lemongrass)

HIGH BLOOD PRESSURE

The following three massage blends will induce relaxation and are therefore helpful if you suffer from high blood pressure. Choose according to personal preference. Mix as for the previous recipes.

Recipe 1
50 ml sunflower seed oil
5 drops clary sage
5 drops lavender
10 drops bergamot

Recipe 2
50 ml almond oil
5 drops lemon
5 drops petitgrain
8 drops ylang ylang

Recipe 3
25 ml almond oil
25 ml sunflower seed oil
5 drops marjoram
5 drops chamomile (Roman)
10 drops lavender

RELAXING ROOM SCENTS

Since stress in its many guises is a contributing factor in the development of cardiovascular disease, vaporise any of the following relaxing blends as your moods dictate. Put the essential oil into a 50 ml dark glass bottle, then fill with water and shake well. Pour a little of the mixture into the reservoir of a nightlight burner or electric vaporiser designed for water-based blends. Remember to shake the bottle each time before use to disperse the essential oil.

Recipe 1
50 ml water
3 drops neroli
8 drops mandarin
3 drops ylang ylang

Recipe 2
50 ml water
3 drops chamomile (Roman)
2 drops rose otto
10 drops bergamot

Recipe 3
50 ml water
3 drops frankincense
6 drops lemon
4 drops juniper

Recipe 4
50 ml water
1 drop galbanum
6 drops lavender
6 drops petitgrain

VARICOSE VEIN/HAEMORRHOID OINTMENT

The following ointment is made by 'doctoring' a shop-bought skin cream or bland ointment. Suitable base creams are available by mail order from most essential oil suppliers. Simply put the cream into a clean glass pot and stir in the essential oil with the handle of a teaspoon. For haemorrhoids, apply twice daily after alternate hot and cold shower or sitz bath (see page 30). For varicose veins, gently smooth into the affected areas twice daily or as required.

30 g unperfumed base cream
5 drops cypress
5 drops frankincense
5 drops geranium

11
THE DIGESTIVE SYSTEM

In the average size man, the digestive system is an amazing thirty-six feet long, beginning with the mouth and ending with the rectum. The purpose of digestion is to break down insoluble pieces of food into soluble molecules, thus enabling vital nutrients to be absorbed into the bloodstream. Even though the digestive system works as an integrated unit, for the sake of clarity, we shall take a brief look at the function of its various parts. This will give a clearer understanding of what is happening should things go wrong, and, most importantly, how to deal with such problems.

DIGESTION IN THE MOUTH

Digestion begins as soon as food enters the mouth, by the action of chewing and by the secretion of saliva.The food then begins its long journey, passing through the throat and into the *oesophagus* (food pipe). To prevent the food falling too quickly into the stomach and causing indigestion, *the epiglottis*, which is a valve-like muscle, sits perfectly over the *trachea* (windpipe). The epiglottis also prevents food from entering the airway and causing choking. However, choking may occur if pieces of food are inadequately chewed and hurriedly swallowed. When we eat slowly, the valve opens and closes where the oesophagus enters the stomach, passing along a little food at a time by the action of *peristalsis* (see below).

DIGESTION IN THE STOMACH

The stomach is tucked up in the abdomen at the lower rib line. While in the stomach, the food is churned by muscular contractions of the stomach wall, and converted into a semi-liquid state by being mixed with gastric juices –

mainly hydrochloric acid – secreted by numerous glands in the stomach lining. The liquid 'gruel' is then released from the stomach at regular intervals by the opening of the pyloric sphincter, from where it enters the *duodenum* – the foot-long first part of the small intestine.

DIGESTION IN THE SMALL INTESTINE

As the gruel passes through the duodenum, alkaline secretions from the *gall-bladder* and *pancreas* are also poured into it. Pancreatic juice – about two pints a day – pours into the duodenum, acting to neutralise the acid gruel. The gall-bladder acts as a storage for bile, which is produced in the liver. Bile is a green, alkaline liquid which breaks large fat globules into minute globules, thus enabling the pancreatic enzymes to process them.

Food is moved through the digestive system by means of muscular wave-like contractions known as peristalsis. When the digestive system is working normally, there are 10 to 15 of these movements a minute. It is by this action that the gruel is pushed into the *ileum*. The lining of the ileum is covered by millions of villi – microscopic finger-like projections. Their job is to convey nutrients from the liquid food into the bloodstream. The undigested material, chiefly cellulose from plant cell walls, dead bacteria, and dead cells, is passed out through a sphincter muscle into the *colon* or *large intestine*.

THE LARGE INTESTINE (COLON AND RECTUM)

It takes three to eight hours for the gut to process a meal. Once in the colon, water is extracted from the gruel and passed back to the blood. A semi-solid waste remains. Finally, this is expelled through the anus.

THE ROLE OF THE LIVER

The liver is the largest organ in the body. It is responsible for upwards of 500 vital functions. And in one way or another is involved with all the physiological processes. As well as governing the secretion of bile, the formation of blood, and the production of heat, it provides muscle fuel (glycogen), processes dietary fats, and manufactures vitamin A. The liver also deals with detoxification; so important is this process that if the caffeine and various drugs we might take were injected into exit vessels leading to the heart, we would be dead within minutes. Inject them into the entrance vessels of the liver, and the 'sting' is extracted within six to ten seconds – the time it takes for the blood to pass through the organ.

PATTERNS OF DIGESTIVE DISORDERS

Apart from the importance of eating a healthy diet and living a balanced lifestyle, the functioning and health of the digestive system is closely related to our emotional state. For instance, everyone at some time in their life has experienced a 'gut reaction' to powerful emotions such as anger, fear and anxiety. This may have simply resulted in a momentary tightening of the abdomen, or a fluttering sensation in the solar plexus area. However, prolonged stress can lead to disturbances, ranging from diminished appetite, constipation and heartburn, to diarrhoea and nausea. Or, more seriously, a gastric ulcer or irritable bowel syndrome.

Incidentally, just like the skin, the stomach flushes with anger and becomes pallid with fright! And when we get excited it reacts with vigorous contractions. One reason why some people lose their appetite and/or get constipated when they are depressed is because peristalsis all but stops, and so does secretion of gastric juice. If we ignore the signals and carry on eating, what we swallow just sits there, causing bloating and discomfort.

Worry and anxiety cause the stomach to produce excess acid. Such emotions may also cause acid from the stomach to regurgitate into the oesophagus, resulting in heartburn. Therefore, whenever you feel under stress, it would be wise to change your eating habits, as well as taking steps to reduce the stress through aromatherapy massage and/or relaxation exercises. Eating a number of small, light meals is the best way to control excess acid which, if left unchecked, may cause ulceration in the lining of the stomach or duodenum. However, even if acid has already begun to eat into the mucous membrane causing twinges of pain, this can be reversed in the early stages. As soon as you begin to relax, the stomach will pour out mucus to heal the wound. So as with almost every other condition mentioned in this book, holistic treatment (which takes into account the emotional state of the sufferer) is essential. Bearing this in mind, the following charts suggest natural treatments for a number of common ailments affecting the digestive system.

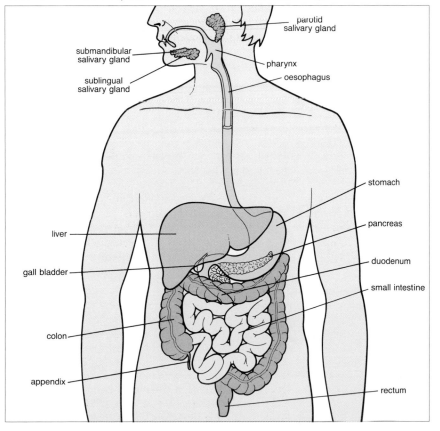

The digestive system

THE LIMITATIONS OF AROMATHERAPY

There are numerous herbal remedies that have a beneficial effect on the digestive system. However, because essential oils lack certain constituents such as bitters and demulcents, their action on the digestive system is somewhat curtailed. Taken internally, bitters promote the flow of saliva and gastric juices in a complex way via the taste buds and a reflex action in the brain, whereas demulcents soothe and protect an irritated or inflamed digestive tract. However, external treatment with essential oils in conjunction with herbal remedies becomes an effective healing tool for digestive ailments, but more especially for long-term problems such as chronic constipation, nervous indigestion and the prevention of gastric ulcers in prone subjects.

It is interesting to note that inhalation of certain essential oils can be helpful for digestive disturbances triggered by nervous tension. In fact, the aromatic molecules reach the bloodstream faster by inhalation than by oral administration. The problem is knowing how much to inhale. My own approach is to rely on internal doses of herbal remedies for an acute condition, such as an attack of heartburn or colicky indigestion, and to use aromatherapy (especially aromatherapy massage) as a preventative measure.

ACTIONS OF ESSENTIAL OILS

The principal actions of essences which have an affinity with the digestive system are as follows:

Antispasmodics: For spasm and pain, for example chamomile, fennel, peppermint.

Aperitifs: The aromas of most essential oils stimulate the appetite; good examples include bergamot, ginger, orange.

Carminatives and stomachics: For flatulence and nausea, for example cardamom, fennel, peppermint.

Cholagogues: For stimulating the gall-bladder, and thus the flow of bile, for example, lavender, peppermint.

Hepatics: For strengthening, toning and stimulating the secretive functions of the liver, for example, lemon, rosemary, peppermint.

THERAPEUTIC CHARTS: DIGESTIVE PROBLEMS

Instructions for preparing essential oils for the various therapeutic applications are to be found in Chapter 6.

CONSTIPATION

Description	Possible causes	Aggravated by	Recommended Essential Oils
Delayed emptying of the bowels so that stools become hard and dry and difficult to pass. Severe cases often lead to 'paradoxical diarrhoea' – fluid faeces from the large bowel being passed around the hardened mass of stool.	Lack of dietary fibre (especially fresh fruit and vegetables), inadequate fluid intake, sedentary lifestyle, nervous tension, depression, failure to adhere to a regular bowel opening habit, liver congestion.	Long-term use of chemical laxatives so that natural peristalsis is blocked.	Black pepper, fennel (sweet), garlic (see Nutritional Supplements), lemongrass, mandarin, marjoram, orange, palmarosa, rose otto, rosemary.

Methods of use

Dry skin brushing (see pages 213–14), followed by abdominal massage (see page 185). If stressed, regular aromatic baths and full-body massage with relaxing oils of your choice.

Suggested Herbal Remedies

Infusion of flax seed (linseed): pour 300 ml boiling water on two to three teaspoonfuls seed and leave to infuse for 10 to 15 minutes. Drink a cupful morning and evening.

Nutritional supplements

One garlic capsule daily, one dessertspoonful extra virgin olive oil (as a salad dressing).

Further suggestions

Drink two to three mugs of warm spring water immediately after breakfast to flush out toxins and stimulate bowels. Also, changes in diet and lifestyle may be appropriate. Chronic constipation should be investigated by a medical practitioner, and perhaps treated under the guidance of an holistic therapist.

DIARRHOEA

Description

Frequent loose bowel movements, with or without stomach cramp.

Possible causes

It is not, in itself, a disorder, but a symptom of an underlying problem such as stress, bacterial infection (e.g. holiday diarrhoea), gastric 'flu, side-effect of certain drugs, food poisoning, drastic and sudden change in diet.

Aggravated by

See Possible Causes.

Recommended Essential Oils

Chamomile (German or Roman), garlic (see Nutritional Supplements), ginger, marjoram, palmarosa, sandalwood, thyme (sweet).

Methods of use

Warm compress over abdomen

Suggested Herbal Remedies

Depends on cause, but generally peppermint and spearmint calm the digestive system. A decoction of ginger and cinnamon will wipe out most stomach bugs (sweeten with honey to taste).

Nutritional supplements

As a preventative of holiday diarrhoea, take one or two garlic capsules daily for a week or two before the holiday, and continue for the duration.

Further suggestions

Drink plenty of water and/or appropriate herb teas to prevent dehydration. For holiday diarrhoea, water must be boiled first. Persistent diarrhoea should be investigated by a medical practitioner.

GASTRIC ULCER (INCLUDING DUODENAL AND PEPTIC ULCERS)

Description

Ulceration of the lining of the stomach (or in the case of a peptic ulcer, the oesophagus and duodenum) as a result of excess gastric juices (i.e. hydrochloric acid and pepsin). Pain usually occurs within two hours of eating.

Possible causes

Faulty diet, smoking, prolonged stress.

Recommended Essential Oils

Any relaxing essential oils of your choice, for example chamomile (German or Roman), lavender, marjoram, neroli, rose otto, ylang ylang.

Methods of use	Suggested Herbal Remedies	Nutritional supplements	Further suggestions
The aim of aromatherapy is to reduce stress rather than to treat the ulcer directly. Regular, full body massage, aromatic bath, personal perfume (see Chapter 27), vaporiser.	Slippery Elm (available in tablet form).	Good multivitamin and mineral supplement.	Consult a medical practitioner for correct diagnosis. Regular and frequent light meals, avoiding foodstuffs which cause excessive secretion (such as bacon, egg white, tea, coffee, chocolate or alcohol). It would also be advisable to consult a holistic nutritionist. Seek to reduce stress (see Chapter 19).

GINGIVITIS

Description	Possible causes	Aggravated by	Recommended Essential Oils
Gums bleed when they are brushed or when hard, fibrous foods are eaten.	The result of invisible bacteria (plaque) which harden as a result of enzymes in saliva, forming calcium deposits (tartar). If left untreated, teeth may eventually drop out.	Poor dental hygiene, diets which are high in sugar and processed foods.	Bergamot, cypress, fennel, lemon, myrrh, tea tree, thyme (sweet).

Methods of use	Suggested Herbal Remedy	Nutritional supplements	Further suggestions
Mouthwash (see recipe on page 92).	Infusion of thyme or sage used as a mouth wash, two or three times a day.	A good multivitamin and mineral supplement (containing the entire B-complex group) together with 500 mg vitamin C.	If left untreated, gingivitis can lead to severe gum disease (pyorrhoea). Gentle, regular and effective brushing and flossing is essential. Visit your dentist regularly (preferably someone practising holistic dentistry).

HALITOSIS
(OFFENSIVE BREATH)

Description	Possible causes	Aggravated by	Recommended Essential Oils
Eating highly odorous foods such as garlic and onions. Otherwise, halitosis is the first sign of ill health.	Poor dental hygiene, periodontal disease, gastric disorders, respiratory infection or catarrh, smoking, excessive consumption of alcohol.	See Possible Causes.	Bergamot, cardamom, fennel (sweet), peppermint, thyme (sweet).

Methods of use	Suggested Herbal Remedies	Nutritional supplements	Further suggestions
Mouthwash (see recipe, page 92).	Chew a whole clove or the leaves of herbs such as peppermint, parsley and spearmint.	Best to avoid taking supplements until cause is clear.	Seek to remedy the cause. Chronic halitosis must be investigated by a medical practitioner, perhaps followed by holistic treatment under the guidance of a qualified practitioner.

INDIGESTION (DYSPEPSIA)

Description	Possible causes	Aggravated by	Recommended Essential Oils
Common forms are heartburn, flatulence and abdominal pain. Nausea may also be present.	Stress, eating too quickly, overeating, incompatible food combinations, for example bread with oranges, eating irregularly, food allergy. Indigestion, especially heartburn, is common during pregnancy and in cases of hiatus hernia. In a few cases, persistent indigestion is indicative of serious conditions such as peptic ulcers or gallstones.	See Possible Causes.	Angelica, black pepper, cardamom, chamomile (German or Roman), clary sage, coriander, fennel (sweet), ginger, lemongrass, marjoram, peppermint, spearmint.

Methods of use	Suggested Herbal Remedies	Nutritional supplements
Gentle abdominal massage in a clockwise direction, dry inhalation of peppermint (drops on a handkerchief).	Lemon balm, peppermint, spearmint.	Chamomile (German or Roman), lavender, marjoram, melissa (true), neroli, rose otto.

IRRITABLE BOWEL SYNDROME

Description	Possible causes	Aggravated by	Recommended Essential Oils
Symptoms include abdominal cramps, colic, flatulence and bloating, alternating bouts of constipation and diarrhoea.	Stress. Lack of dietary fibre, food allergies.	Although dietary fibre is an essential part of treatment, wheat bran is contra-indicated. Apart from not being a wholefood (having been separated from the rest of the wheat) it can irritate a sensitive digestive tract.	Chamomile (German or Roman), lavender, marjoram, peppermint, melissa (true), neroli and rose otto.

Methods of use

Warm compress (except for peppermint) over abdomen, very gentle abdominal massage in a clockwise direction. As a preventative measure to reduce stress; aromatic baths and full-body massage, *any* relaxing essences of your choice.

Suggested Herbal Remedies

Chamomile, lemon balm, marjoram, peppermint.

Nutritional supplements

Good multi-vitamin and mineral supplement. Peppermint oil capsules (available from health shops, follow directions on packet).

Further suggestions

Seek the advice of an holistic nutritionist, naturopath or medical herbalist, preferably someone who can carry out food allergy tests. Also, Bach flower remedies, stress reducing techniques (see Chapter 19).

MOUTH ULCER (APHTHOUS ULCER)

Description

An ulcerous sore inside the cheek, lips, gum, or underneath the tongue.

Possible causes

Inadvertently biting the inside of the mouth; irritation from a denture; a run down condition in general, perhaps through prolonged stress, faulty diet (especially deficient in vitamin C), or antibiotic treatment.

Aggravated by

See Possible Causes.

Recommended Essential Oils

Cypress, myrrh, tea tree.

Methods of use

Mouthwash (see recipe, page 92).

Suggested Herbal Remedies

Infusion: red sage (use as a mouthwash two or three times daily).

Nutritional supplements

If triggered by stress or antibiotics, take a good multi-vitamin and mineral supplement containing the entire B-complex group. Lacto bacillus supplements (yoghurt culture) may also be indicated, to restore the natural intestinal flora destroyed by antibiotics. Otherwise, eat lashings of live yoghurt. A 500 mg tablet of vitamin C is also recommended, twice a day, during the healing period.

Further suggestions

If necessary, seek to reduce stress in your life through regular aromatherapy massage and/or relaxation techniques. Bach flower remedies may also help in this respect.

NAUSEA (INCLUDING TRAVEL/SEA SICKNESS)

Description

The sensation of needing to vomit which can be brought on by virtually anything that affects gastrointestinal function, for example stress, constipation, faulty diet, overeating, mild food poisoning, indigestion, pregnancy, VDU stress.

Possible causes

Travel/sea sickness: Caused by movement of vehicle/boat affecting organ of balance in inner ear. Car sickness is often triggered by reading for any length of time whilst the vehicle is moving. May also be a conditioned reflex; if you expect to feel sick you are more likely to *be* sick.

Aggravated by

See Possible Causes.

Recommended Essential Oils

Cardomom, coriander, fennel, ginger, lavender, nutmeg, peppermint.

Methods of use

Dry inhalation (drops on a handkerchief).

Suggested Herbal Remedies

Peppermint, spearmint, ginger (it is possible to obtain herbal travel sickness tablets containing ginger).

Further suggestions

Fresh air tends to alleviate nausea, whatever the cause. Persistent nausea with no apparent cause should be investigated by a medical practitioner, then perhaps treated holistically with the help of a qualified practitioner.

TOOTH ABSCESS

Description

Extremely painful condition indicated by inflammation and swelling of gums (and often the face) around a decayed tooth. Infection can affect the whole system.

Possible causes

Faulty diet, poor health in general, stress and inadequate dental hygiene.

Aggravated by

Chewing on the affected area; usually sensitive to hot and cold drinks.

Recommended Essential Oils

Chamomile, garlic (see Nutritional Supplements), lavender.

Methods of use

First-aid measure whilst awaiting dental treatment: Mouthwash (see recipe, page 92), warm compress.

Nutritional supplements

To aid healing, especially for a month or two after antibiotic treatment: two garlic capsules daily, two × 500 mg vitamin C and a good multi-vitamin and mineral supplement containing the full B-complex group.

Further suggestions

Visit your dentist regularly, preferably someone practising holistic dentistry.

TOOTHACHE

Description	**Possible causes**	**Aggravated by**	**Recommended Essential Oils**
Severe and persistent pain.	Tooth decay (see Tooth Abscess, page 91).	See Tooth Abscess (page 91).	Clove, peppermint.

Method of use	**Nutritional supplements**	**Further suggestions**
First-aid measure whilst awaiting dental treatment: Apply one or two drops directly into tooth cavity. Repeat as often as necessary.	See Tooth Abscess (page 91).	As for Tooth Abscess (page 91).

CAUTION *Overuse of clove essence can cause gum damage, so use only as an emergency measure.*

AROMATIC PRESCRIPTIONS AND PROCEDURES

MOUTHWASHES

If used regularly, the following mixture will help to strengthen the gums. It can also be used to treat mouth ulcers and gingivitis. Tincture of myrrh (as used in the recipe) can be obtained from herbal suppliers. It will, however, cause the blend to turn cloudy, but this will not affect its therapeutic properties.

Recipe 1
30 ml tincture of myrrh
5 drops tea tree
10 drops cypress
20 drops peppermint

Add the essential oils to the tincture of myrrh and shake well. The mixture must be diluted before use. Add six to eight drops to a small glass or teacupful of warm water. Use two or three times daily. The mixture will keep for several months if stored in a cool dark place.

The following mixture can be used after meals to sweeten the breath. Floral waters can be obtained from some pharmacies, though do emphasise that you require a *distillate* rather than a synthetic substitute. In case of difficulty, genuine floral waters are available by mail order from a few essential oil suppliers.

Recipe 2
100 ml rosewater or orange flower water
200 ml distilled water
2 teaspoonfuls cider vinegar
1 drop cardamom
8 drops bergamot FCF
8 drops coriander

Put the cider vinegar into a dark glass bottle, then add the essential oils and shake well. Funnel the waters into the bottle. Remember to shake the bottle each time before use to disperse the essential oil. This mixture will keep for up to two months if kept in a cool, dark place.

MASSAGE OIL BLENDS

Either of the first two blends can be massaged into the whole body following a bath or shower, paying particular attention to abdomen and solar plexus area. The oils will help relax a stressed digestive system. Ideally, persuade someone with 'good hands' to give you a soothing aromatherapy massage.

The second two blends are more stimulating and will help a sluggish or congested digestive system. Again, massage into the skin (especially over the abdomen) immediately after a bath or shower, or get a skilled friend to give you an aromatherapy massage. In this instance, apply the oil with slightly faster strokes to enliven the whole system. (Aromatherapy massage is explained in Part 3.)

The same combinations of essences can be used in the bath to support aromatherapy massage. In this instance, you will need to adjust the quantities of essences accordingly (see page 29).

RELAXING MASSAGE BLENDS

Recipe 1
30 ml almond oil
2 drops chamomile (Roman)
8 drops lavender
2 drops marjoram

Recipe 2
30 ml almond oil
4 drops petitgrain
2 drops clary sage
4 drops lavender
1 drop geranium or rose otto

To mix the oils, put the essences into a dark glass bottle, add the almond oil and shake well.

STIMULATING MASSAGE BLENDS

Recipe 1
30 ml extra virgin olive oil
3 drops black pepper
8 drops coriander
1 drop palmarosa

Recipe 2
30 ml extra virgin olive oil
3 drops rosemary
5 drops mandarin
1 drop ginger

Mix as for the previous recipes.

12
THE URINARY SYSTEM

The kidneys form the body's main waste disposal system; the skin, lungs and colon following close behind. Yet the kidneys also work hard to conserve water, for much that passes through the kidneys is reabsorbed, with a comparatively small amount being excreted.

As well as controlling vital water balance, the kidneys are also involved with cleaning and filtering the blood, ridding this vital fluid of potentially deadly wastes. The kidneys also regulate the relative salt balance in the body, excreting excessive amounts of potassium salts and sodium chloride. Just a fraction too much or too little in the bloodstream and the consequences could be fatal.

Another important function of the kidneys is to maintain the optimum acid/alkaline content of the blood. In a healthy body the ratio between alkaline and acid is 4:1, that is, 80 per cent alkaline to 20 per cent acid. In fact, the acid/alkaline balance of the blood is also influenced by diet.

The most abundant waste product the kidneys have to deal with is urea, the end product of protein digestion. Of course, the kidneys also produce urine, two or three pints of it a day. Microscopic droplets of this waste-laden fluid continuously feed into a tiny reservoir (the ureter) in the centre of each kidney. Its exit (the urethra) reaches an opening in front of the vagina in women and the tip of the penis in men. In women, the urethra is shorter, which is why they are more susceptible to invasion by bacteria, resulting in problems such as cystitis (see pages 95–6).

THE PATTERNS OF URINARY DISORDERS

As with every other body system, problems arising within the urinary system reflect disharmony within the whole. Indeed, conventional medicine regards urine analysis as an extremely important diagnostic procedure, for the state of a person's urine can tell a great deal about what is happening elsewhere in the body. While pregnancy can be determined by the presence of certain hormones in the urine, disease states can also be detected. A high level of glucose in the urine, for example, indicates diabetes; whereas excessive uric acid points to kidney stones or gout. The presence of bile in the urine signifies jaundice. If the urine is persistently cloudy, malodorous or discoloured, this may indicate a kidney disorder. However, urine tends to cloud after heavy exercise, so it is important to differentiate. Should the urine contain high levels of protein this may indicate high blood pressure and/or serious dysfunction within the kidneys' filtering system. An immediately obvious danger signal, and one requiring urgent medical attention, is the presence of blood or pus in the urine. This reflects serious infection or disease within the urinary tract or the kidneys themselves.

In a healthy body, excess fluid is removed by the circulation of the blood (and also the circulation of lymph, see Chapter 16) and excreted via the kidneys. Oedema (fluid retention) or swelling occurring around the ankles is caused by excess fluid seeping out of the circulation. This usually results from poor drainage by the veins and is also seen in congestive heart failure and during pregnancy. Excessive facial oedema, manifesting as disfiguring puffiness around the eyes, cheeks and nose, may indicate kidney disease. The swelling is especially noticeable first thing in the morning after a night's sleep. This condition must be investigated by a medical practitioner. However, comparatively slight oedema around the eyes and elsewhere in the body is common in women during the premenstrual phase.

Before we go any further, it should be emphasised that the treatment of serious kidney and urinary disorders is way beyond the scope of home treatment – and indeed, beyond the training of the average aromatherapist. Nevertheless, there is still a great deal you can do to maintain the healthy functioning of the kidneys and urinary tract, and thus prevent the development of serious disorders.

As well as putting into practice the basics of a healthy diet and lifestyle, kidneys need to be flushed out. So drink copious amounts of water, preferably bottled or spring water. In fact, we need to drink about six or seven pints of fluid a day – but not in the form of excessive amounts of tea, coffee and alcohol, which put an enormous burden on the organs of elimination. Above all, never ignore the pressing demands of a full bladder. If urine is retained for too long, it is susceptible to chemical change which in turn can lead to infection. Moreover, a full bladder will press down on all the pelvic organs, especially the lower bowel and reproductive organs, and perhaps contribute to the development of prolapse.

DIURETIC HERBS

These are substances which increase the flow of urine. The problem with chemical diuretics, which are often administered to people suffering from high blood pressure, is that they leach potassium from the body. So potassium supplements need to be given as well.

Perhaps the most effective herbal diuretic is the root or leaf of the dandelion. Unlike a chemical diuretic, it contains a high percentage of potassium and other nutrients which act synergistically to maintain a healthy balance of mineral salts in the bloodstream. However, home-treatment should not step beyond certain limits. It is fine to take herbal diuretics for minor disorders, such as fluid retention associated with PMS or jet lag. But if you are suffering from a serious circulatory disorder or high blood pressure, on no account must you attempt to reduce or stop taking prescribed diuretics. In this instance, herbal remedies and aromatherapy massage must be regarded as complementary to conventional treatment. However, a good physician will monitor your progress and may even allow a slight reduction in medication should your condition improve enough to do so.

THE LIMITATIONS OF ESSENTIAL OILS

There are a number of essential oils such as fennel and juniper which are cited as diuretics. However, the diuretic effect of essential oils is generally thought to be negligible unless they are taken orally, for too little reaches the systemic circulation via skin absorption to stimulate the kidneys.

Nevertheless, massage therapy (with or without aromatic oils) is one of the finest treatments available for stimulating the circulatory and lymphatic systems, and thus the elimination of excess fluids (see Part 3).

TREATING URINARY INFECTIONS

Essential oils are very effective at wiping out the micro-organisms responsible for urinary infections. However, French aromatherapy doctors administer oral doses (sometimes suppositories) of essential oils for treating infections of this nature. Of course, internal administration of essential oils should never be carried out by the home user, nor prescribed by medically unqualified aromatherapists. With a few reservations, the only urinary infection which can be treated at home with herbs and essences is cystitis. And since it is the only condition in this chapter for which a suggested healing regime is given, it deserves a little more space than has been afforded to other ailments.

CYSTITIS

Description

Inflammation of the urinary bladder. If not treated properly it can damage the kidneys. Symptoms are burning pains when passing urine, as well as pain in the groin before, during and just after urination. Moreover, there is usually a frequent desire to urinate, even when the bladder is empty.

Possible causes

Many conditions predispose towards cystitis and only a medical examination and laboratory urine tests can ascertain the cause. Commonly, the condition is related to bacterial infection, inhalation of industrial chemicals or paint fumes, or by mechanical injury. Stress can also trigger an attack in prone individuals. Occasionally, food allergies are implicated.

Although cystitis mostly occurs in women, men are by no means immune. Those who have undergone surgery involving the urethra or who suffer from an enlarged prostate gland are more likely to suffer.

The prostate is the principal storage depot for seminal fluid. However, the small urinary tube that empties the bladder actually passes over the prostate; so anything that happens there to swell the prostate – infection, inflammation, cancer – can obstruct the flow of urine, and thus cause untold misery. The enlarged gland may press on the bladder causing a little urine to be trapped in a 'back pocket' where it soon becomes a breeding ground for bacteria.

In women, pressure from a back-tilting uterus may also

result in incomplete emptying. However, this can sometimes be corrected by osteopathic or chiropractic treatment. So-called 'honeymoon cystitis' may occur after a bout of prolonged sexual activity, in which case, the best preventative remedy is to drink a glass of water immediately after sex and to empty the bladder as soon as possible.

Aggravated by

Although douching with solutions of herbs or essences is often recommended by complementary practitioners, personally I would not promote this method – at least not without suggesting you seek professional advice beforehand. Medicated douches (and over-use of plain water douches) eventually disrupt the natural ecology of the vagina and allow the wrong kind of micro-organisms to thrive.

Recommended Essential Oils

Bergamot, cedarwood, chamomile (German and Roman), eucalyptus, frankincense, juniper, lavender, pine, sandalwood, tea tree.

Methods of use

Warm compresses over the lower back, sitz baths, ordinary baths. As a preventative measure, regular aromatherapy massage (paying particular attention to the lower back).

Suggested Herbal Remedies

Chamomile, dandelion, fennel, parsley, yarrow.

Further Suggestions

Flush out the kidneys with copious amounts of warm water to dilute the urine – at least 7 pints in 24 hours. Cranberry juice is an excellent alkalising remedy (helps to reduce the scalding effect of infected urine). Take one wineglassful three or four times a day at the onset of symptoms. If stress is a contributing factor, try Bach flower remedies. Also make appropriate changes in diet and lifestyle. If food allergy is suspected, do seek professional advice, preferably from a practitioner who can carry out allergy tests.

If you are especially prone to cystitis, it may be advisable to consult a homoeopathic practitioner who will prescribe constitutional treatment.

CAUTION *If there is blood or pus in the urine, seek urgent medical attention.*

AROMATIC PRESCRIPTIONS

Any of the following massage blends can be used as a preventative measure. The same combinations of essences can be used in the bath, though you will need to adjust the quantities accordingly (see page 29). However, it is important to take appropriate steps to improve your health as a whole, otherwise the oils will do little more than offer partial relief.

Recipe 1

50 ml almond oil
5 drops frankincense
8 drops cedarwood
5 drops juniper

Put the essential oils in a dark glass bottle, then add the almond oil and shake well.

Recipe 2

50 ml almond oil
5 drops Roman chamomile (or 2 drops German chamomile)
5 drops bergamot
10 drops lavender

Mix as for previous recipe.

Recipe 3

50 ml almond oil
5 drops eucalyptus
5 drops pine
8 drops lavender

Mix as for previous recipes.

Recipe 4

50 ml almond oil
8 drops juniper berry
6 drops bergamot
6 drops sandalwood

Mix as for previous recipes.

13
THE MUSCULAR AND SKELETAL SYSTEM

While the skeleton gives form, support and protection to the body, the muscles are concerned with movement. When our joints and muscles are supple and mobile, we radiate vitality and are much more resilient to the stresses and strains of life. Indeed, long-term tension in the musculature of the body saps energy simply because it is being used for maintaining the rigidity of the muscles. Massage therapy is perhaps the finest healing tool at our disposal for helping to release this pent-up energy. It is also one of the most accessible methods, for almost everyone can quickly master the basics (see Part 3).

In the meantime, we shall take a whistle-stop tour of the muscular and skeletal systems, the purpose of which is to instil a generalised understanding of how these systems work – and what happens when things go wrong. Armed with this knowledge, you will then have a better comprehension of the reasoning behind the various methods employed to alleviate specific problems.

THE BONES

The skeleton consists of about 206 bones. They are composed of two basic types of tissue: cancellous (also known as spongy bone) which is light and porous, and compact, which is dense and incredibly strong. Bones are bound together by ligaments. Tendons, on the other hand, connect bones to muscles, and thus make movement possible.

Far from being an inert framework for the living body, bones are a reservoir of the body's vital minerals such as calcium and phosphorus, and essential trace elements like copper and cobalt. The bones release minerals into the bloodstream, extracting any excess and storing this for future use. Some bones, like the tibia (shin-bone), also contain red bone marrow, where blood cells are formed.

The joints between bones are of three types: fibrous (allowing no movement), cartilaginous (limited movement) and synovial (freely moving). Free movement around synovial joints like the hip and shoulder is permitted by cartilage (a tough elastic material) coating the ends of the bones, and the lubricating substance, synovial fluid.

THE MUSCLES

Muscle is flexible tissue, which can initiate or maintain movement in the body. There are three types of muscle: skeletal or voluntary muscle, which moves the bones; smooth or involuntary muscle (found in the digestive tract, blood vessels, uterus and elsewhere); and cardiac muscle (found only in the heart). Voluntary muscles are so called because they are under the direct control of conscious thought. The textbook definition of involuntary muscle is that which is unaffected by conscious thought. For example, heartbeat cannot be slowed down or increased at will.

However, this is not strictly true. It is a well-documented fact that certain Indian adepts or yogis have been known to bury themselves alive for prolonged periods, having slowed down their heart and breathing rhythms to what can only be described as 'hibernation' mode. Of course, from what we have already learned about the mind/body complex, our thoughts and moods certainly do influence the so-called involuntary physiological processes, albeit unconsciously.

All muscles work in antagonistic pairs and groups. As one set of muscle fibres contracts, its opposite set relaxes. However, contrary to the popular notion that muscle bulk is a reflection of good muscle tone, nothing could be further from the truth. The elasticity of muscle tissue is the real measure of fitness. Excessive muscle size is a sign of chronic muscular tension.

The end products of muscle movement are tissue wastes such as carbon dioxide and lactic acid. A good flow of blood to the area acts to remove such wastes, which are eventually excreted via the organs of elimination, principally the skin and lungs. However, during prolonged physical activity, the muscle's main source of

energy (ATP and phosophocreatine) becomes depleted.
So the source of energy must be obtained from glucose.
This is derived from the breakdown of glycogen, which is
stored in the liver for this very purpose.

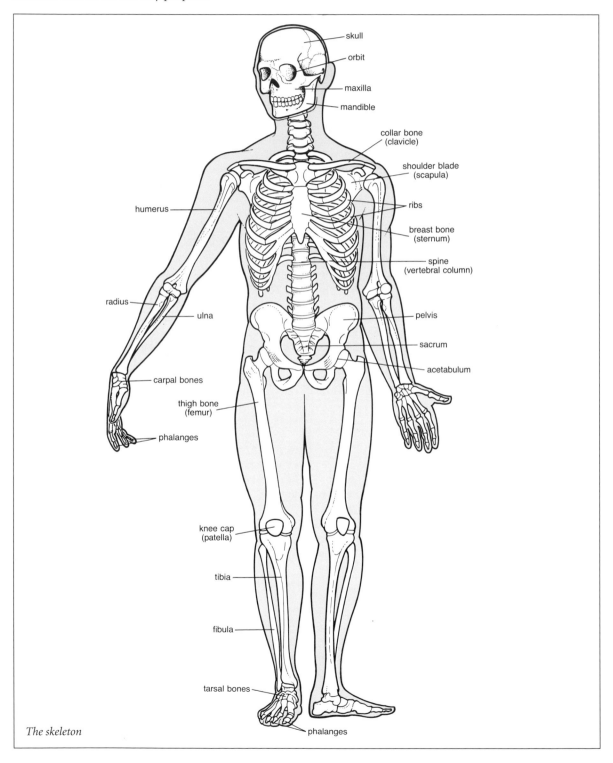

The skeleton

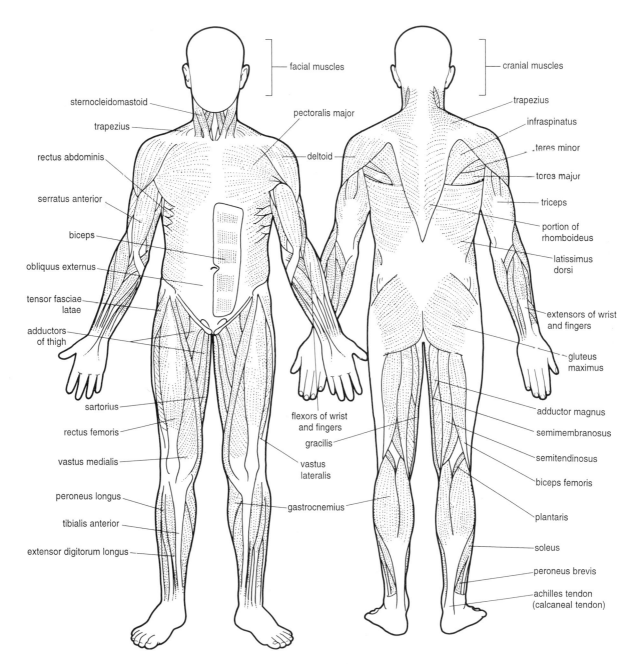

The superficial muscles

PATTERNS OF MUSCULAR AND SKELETAL DISORDERS

It is oft reported that more people take time off work as a result of back pain than for any other condition. This may be caused or aggravated by many factors, including poor posture, prolonged sitting, incorrect lifting of heavy loads, or psychological stress.

Another problem is the so-called slipped disc. Between each pair of vertebrae are cartilage discs containing a resilient, jelly-like substance. The purpose of these discs is to act as shock absorbers, thus preventing the vertebrae from grinding together whenever we move. However, discs are vulnerable to injury. A severe jolt caused by a fall, for example, can rupture the disc's tough envelope, permitting the enclosed jelly to ooze out. (The term 'slipped' disc is therefore a misnomer; *herniated* would be the precise definition.) The jelly-like material then presses on a nerve which results in excruciating pain. This is because the irritated nerve causes the surrounding muscles to go into spasm; a self-protective mechanism to prevent movement that might cause further damage. A slipped disc is best dealt with by an osteopath or chiropractor. However, regular aromatherapy massage can help during the recovery period.

Aromatherapy can also be of enormous benefit in dealing with activity injuries such as strains and sprains (see Muscles and Joints First Aid, page 104).

One bone disorder that afflicts almost everyone to some degree is osteoporosis or 'brittle bone' disease. This is an age-related problem characterised by decreased bone mass and increased susceptibility to fractures. Calcium and other essential minerals are leached into the bloodstream in greater quantities and are eventually excreted. Women (especially those of European or Asian descent) are especially vulnerable to osteoporosis after menopause, for the development of the disorder is believed to be related to decreased levels of oestrogens. But since elderly men are also in the high-risk category, oestrogen deficiency is not the sole cause.

Even though heredity plays an important role in the development of osteoporosis in both men and women, there is still a great deal we can do to lessen (perhaps even prevent) the development of this debilitating disorder. Once bone is lost, however, it cannot be restored with tissue of equal strength. Nevertheless, prevention lies in the area of diet and lifestyle. Studies have shown that regular weight-bearing exercise, such as walking, cycling and climbing, increase bone mass. But such activities need to be carried out regularly for at least twenty minutes, three to five times a week.

Of all the problems associated with the muscles and joints, arthritis and rheumatism are the best known, and perhaps the least understood by the medical profession.

Yet contrary to what the orthodox medics may tell you, it is possible to overcome these two potentially crippling diseases. Indeed, I have known several people (and have read about many others) who have used natural therapies such as acupuncture, massage, herbal medicine, homoeopathy and dietary reform to reduce pain greatly and increase mobility in affected parts of the body. However, there is no 'magic bullet'. Natural healing takes a great deal of time, patience and commitment. And it is for these reasons that comparatively few people give complementary healing a fair chance.

The main aim of treatment is to detoxify the system and to normalise the acid/alkaline composition of the blood (arthritis and rheumatism are associated with over-acidity). Treatment is also geared to reducing stress and increasing flexibility. This may be achieved by a combination of methods such as mineral salt baths, aromatherapy massage, aromatic compresses, gentle stretching, deep breathing and relaxation exercises, and by sticking to a predominantly alkaline diet. For example, by cutting out or reducing to a bare minimum acid-producing foods and beverages such as pork, tea, coffee and chocolate, and by eating plenty of fresh fruits, vegetables, sprouted seeds and grains.

However, no one diet is right for everyone. For instance, you may find that so-called 'goodies' such as apples or green grapes exacerbate your own particular symptoms. Therefore, it is advisable to consult an holistic nutritionist (see Useful Addresses, page 289) who will devise a personalised dietary plan.

ACTIONS OF ESSENTIAL OILS

Although essential oils cannot heal bone disorders like osteoporosis, they can help to alleviate the discomfort of arthritic and rheumatic conditions. The principal actions of essential oils which help in this way are as follows:

Anti-inflammatories: As well as helping to reduce pain and inflammation in arthritic joints, such essences also help reduce swelling around injuries, for example chamomile (German and Roman), galbanum, lavender.

Anti-rheumatics: Many essences have the reputation of preventing and relieving rheumatic problems, for example angelica, coriander, juniper.

Depuratives: These help to detoxify the system of metabolic wastes, for example juniper, lemon, rose otto.

Rubefacients: By stimulating the periphery circulation, such essences increase the blood supply to the affected area which in turn relieves congestion and inflammation, for example black pepper, ginger, rosemary.

THERAPEUTIC CHARTS: MUSCULAR AND SKELETAL PROBLEMS

Instructions for preparing essential oils for the various therapeutic applications are to be found in Chapter 6.

ARTHRITIS AND RHEUMATISM

Description

There are many forms, including bursitis, gout, sciatica, rheumatoid arthritis. All forms are painful and restrict movement. There may also be inflammation and swelling (this comes and goes), calcification of the joints, loss of synovial fluid which lubricates the joints.

Possible causes

Heredity, sedentary lifestyle, chronic emotional disharmony, advancing age, food allergy, injury, overuse of muscles and joints (dancers and sports people are especially prone).

Aggravated by

A cold, damp environment, stress, obesity.

Recommended Essential Oils

Cajeput, cedarwood, chamomile, coriander, cypress, eucalyptus, ginger, juniper berry, lavender, lemon, marjoram, rosemary, thyme (sweet), vetiver.

CAUTION *Never apply massage over inflamed and swollen joints. This state comes and goes, so massage over affected areas is fine in between flare-ups.*

Methods of use

Massage (but see Aggravated By), compresses, baths (including Epsom salts baths, page 29), aromatic ointment (see recipe, page 103).

Suggested Herbal Remedies

Internal: meadowsweet, celery seed or yarrow (or make an infusion using equal quantities of each), or devil's claw (available in tablet form).
External: hypericum oil (see page 39) rubbed into the affected areas.

Nutritional supplements

One tablespoonful cod liver oil daily (available in capsule form to disguise the foul taste), or three × 500 mg evening primrose oil daily.

Further suggestions

If there is little or no improvement after three months, seek the advice of an holistic practitioner, preferably someone who can carry out allergy tests. Also, Bach flower remedies (to address emotional disharmony). Other helpful therapies include acupuncture, homoeopathy, medical herbalism.

BURSITIS

Description

A painful inflammatory condition of a bursa (a fluid-filled sac which helps muscle and tendons move smoothly). It may affect the knee (housemaid's knee), elbow (tennis elbow), shoulders or hips.

Possible causes

Injury, infection, inflammatory arthritis, gout, rheumatoid arthritis, repeated friction.

Aggravated by

Use of the joint.

Recommended Essential Oils

Chamomile, lavender, peppermint.

CAUTION *Never massage inflamed or swollen joints as this will cause further pain and tissue damage.*

Methods of use

Cold compress, aromatic ointment (see recipe, page 103).

Further suggestions

If a recurring problem unrelated to injury, holistic treatment is essential (see Arthritis and Rheumatism).

GOUT

Description

An extremely painful form of arthritis causing swelling and inflammation around joints, especially the big toe. Common in middle-aged men.

Possible causes

Build-up of tissue wastes such as uric acid forming crystals in skin, joints and kidneys. Mainly caused by faulty diet and/or incomplete elimination of drug residues.

Aggravated by

Stress.

Recommended Essential Oils

Angelica, coriander, juniper, pine, rosemary, thyme (sweet).

> **CAUTION** *Never massage directly over the swollen joint as this will cause further pain.*

Methods of use

Footbath, bath, cold compress, ointment.

Suggested Herbal Remedies

Celery seed, nettles, yarrow.

Further advice

Holistic treatment is essential. Seek to reduce stress and improve diet and lifestyle.

MUSCULAR ACHES AND PAINS

Description

If caused by a recent injury or fibrositis, the pain will be sharp or searing. Old injuries and chronic muscular tension usually manifest as a dull ache. There may also be stiffness in the joints.

Possible causes

Over-exertion, poor posture, emotional trauma, or the condition may be related to an arthritic or rheumatic complaint.

Aggravated by

Stress.

Recommended Essential Oils

Black pepper, chamomile (Roman or German), coriander, cypress, eucalyptus, ginger, grapefruit, lavender, lemon, marjoram, pine, rosemary, thyme (sweet), vetiver.

> **CAUTION** *Never massage if the muscle is inflamed and swollen. Use cold compresses instead.*

Methods of use

Massage (see Aggravated By), baths, compresses.

Suggested Herbal Remedies

If stress is a contributing factor: chamomile, lemon balm, lime flowers, valerian (available in tablet form).

Nutritional supplements

If associated with arthritis and rheumatism, see relevant entry.

Further suggestions

Aromatherapy massage is the best treatment. If you are prone to muscular aches and pains, other useful therapies include: Bach flower remedies (for stress), Alexander Technique (to correct postural faults), yoga.

SCIATICA

Description

A form of neuralgia causing intense pain along the sciatic nerve extending from the buttocks to the foot.

Possible causes

Injury resulting in a slipped disc causing irritation to the spinal nerve roots and spasm in the surrounding muscles. Also, incorrect lifting of heavy loads, misalignment of the spine, constipation, childbirth, arthritic changes in bones and ligaments.

Aggravated by

Coughing, straining, bending, rising from a seated position, getting out of bed.

Recommended Essential Oils

Chamomile (German or Roman), coriander, eucalyptus, geranium, lavender, marjoram, peppermint, pine, rosemary.

Methods of use

Massage (especially to lower back, buttocks, hips and legs), bath.

Suggested Herbal Remedies

External: Massage with hypericum oil (see page 39).

Further suggestions

If aromatherapy massage does not help, consult an osteopath or chiropractor. Or try Alexander Technique to correct postural faults. If associated with chronic constipation and/or arthritis, seek to reduce stress and make appropriate changes in diet and lifestyle.

AROMATIC PRESCRIPTIONS AND PROCEDURES

ARTHRITIS AND RHEUMATISM OINTMENT

The following ointment will ease the discomfort of arthritis, rheumatism and fibrositis. It can also be applied to gouty joints, though apply very gently to prevent further pain. If you cannot obtain a suitable unperfumed shop-bought base cream/ointment, this can be obtained by mail order from essential oil suppliers.

50g unperfumed cream or ointment
10 drops marjoram
10 drops rosemary
5 drops juniper

Put the base cream into a little glass pot and stir in the essential oils with the handle of a teaspoon. Apply two or three times a day.

BURSITIS OINTMENT

The following ointment is best used immediately after an aromatic compress (see page 31). Apply to the affected joint two or three times a day, but do not rub too hard as this will cause further discomfort.

50 g unperfumed cream or ointment
20 drops lavender
5 drops peppermint

Mix as for the previous recipe.

MASSAGE OILS FOR ARTHRITIS AND RHEUMATISM

The following massage blends will help arthritis, rheumatism and fibrositis. The same combination of essential oils can also be used in the bath, but you will need to adjust the quantities accordingly (see page 29). Apply the oil after a bath or shower to facilitate absorption of the aromatic molecules. Ideally, persuade someone to give you a relaxing aromatherapy massage.

Recipe 1
25 ml sunflower seed oil
25 ml extra virgin olive oil
5 drops Roman chamomile (or 2 drops German chamomile)
10 drops lavender
5 drops lemon

Put the essences into a dark glass bottle, add the vegetable oils and mix well.

Recipe 2
30 ml hypericum oil
20 ml extra virgin olive oil
6 drops juniper berry
6 drops coriander

Mix as for previous recipe.

MASSAGE OIL FOR MUSCULAR ACHES AND PAINS

The following highly aromatic oil is best applied after a warm bath. As with all massage blends, it will be far more effective if you can find someone to give you a massage. If the aroma seems overpowering, dilute with a little more olive oil.
50 ml extra virgin olive oil
10 drops black pepper
12 drops coriander
6 drops grapefruit
2 drops ginger

Put the essences into a dark glass bottle, add the vegetable oils and shake well.

MASSAGE OILS FOR SCIATICA

The following blends will help ease the discomfort of sciatica and other aches and pains. Apply after a bath or shower. If you can persuade someone to give you an aromatherapy massage, all the better.

Recipe 1
30 ml hypericum oil
20 ml extra virgin olive oil
5 drops geranium
3 drops peppermint
10 drops lavender

Put the essences into a dark glass bottle, add the vegetable oils and mix well.

Recipe 2
50 ml extra virgin olive oil
5 drops pine
12 drops rosemary

Put the essences into a dark glass bottle, add the olive oil and mix well.

MUSCLE AND JOINT FIRST AID

Though sometimes referred to as sports injuries, problems such as strains and sprains, muscle cramps and knee injuries can also happen while walking in the countryside, climbing stairs, or when doing housework or gardening. The Muscles and Joints first-aid chart suggests treatments for such problems.

The chart does not cover serious conditions such as fractures and broken bones for such injuries need urgent medical attention.

MUSCLE AND JOINT FIRST-AID CHART

CRAMP

(See Massage for Sports Injuries, page 199).

SPRAIN

Description

This occurs at a joint when the ligaments and tissues around the joint are suddenly wrenched or torn, for example a sprained wrist or ankle.

Symptoms

Pain and tenderness around the joint, often followed by swelling and bruising.

Recommended Essential Oils

See Strain (below).

Methods of use

Cold or icy compress (see page 31), massage above and below the injury (*not* directly over the damaged tissue) to increase drainage of fluids. Aromatic ointment (see page 103).

Further Advice

Rest the injured part. Elevate the limb to prevent the accumulation of excess fluids (support with cushions or pillows).

STRAIN

Description

This occurs when a muscle or group of muscles is over-stretched and possibly torn by violent or sudden movement, for example back strain as a result of heavy lifting.

Symptoms

Sharp pain which may radiate outwards with subsequent stiffness and/or cramp. There may also be swelling at the site of injury.

Recommended Essential Oils

Chamomile (German or Roman), cypress, eucalyptus, geranium, lavender, marjoram, pine, rosemary, vetiver.

Methods of use

Cold or icy compress. Once swelling has subsided: hot aromatic bath (up to 8 drops essential oil and 3 tablespoonfuls sea salt) followed by massage (see Massage for Sports Injuries, page 199). An aromatic ointment will also aid healing.

Further Advice

Rest is a vital part of the healing process. If you have strained the muscles of an arm or leg, it is important to elevate the injured part above the level of the heart to prevent the accumulation of excess fluids (support with cushions or pillows).

KNEE INJURY

Description

This usually affects the cartilage in the knee. May be the result of a sporting incident, such as a missed kick, by slipping off a step or by twisting the body whilst the weight is balanced on one leg.

Symptoms

Pain around the knee, more commonly on the inner side. Difficulty in straightening the knee. Swelling may occur due to fluid collecting in the joint.

Recommended Essential Oils

As for Sprains and Strains.

Methods of use

Icy compress, massage above and below the site of injury (*not* directly over the swelling) to help drain off accumulated fluid (see Massage for Sports Injuries, page 199).

Further Advice

Having applied the icy compress, protect the knee by bandaging firmly enough to support the knee, but not so tight as to cause discomfort or affect circulation. Rest with knee elevated to prevent accumulation of excess fluid.

CAUTION *Never attempt to change the bent position of the knee or attempt to straighten it.*

14
THE ENDOCRINE SYSTEM

Classically, the endocrine system was defined as being responsible for secreting hormones into the bloodstream to provide a means of co-ordination of body functions, parallel to the nervous system. While hormones were said to travel in the circulation towards their target cells, neuro-chemicals merely passed on electrical signals which linked one nerve cell to another.

Nowadays, the separation of endocrine and nervous function is recognised as incredibly simplistic. Evidence is growing that the endocrine system, the nervous system and the immune system interact at many levels. For instance, insulin was once regarded as a classic hormone. But it has since turned up in nerve cells in the brain, just as brain chemicals such as transferon and CCK are now known to be produced in the stomach as well. Similarly, receptors for neuro-chemicals are to be found in the skin, and on cells in the immune system called monocytes. Moreover, endocrinologists have come to realise that the state of our body chemistry is closely related to physical activity (or lack of it) and to our thoughts and emotions.

Nevertheless, despite obvious pitfalls, we shall attempt to separate the parts that make up the whole, and thus glean a little insight into the functioning of the main glands which comprise the endocrine system.

THE PITUITARY AND HYPOTHALAMUS

The pituitary is a pea-sized knob of tissue connected to the underside of the brain by a short stalk. Despite being so tiny, it plays a major role in the functioning of the whole organism. Although once described as the master gland or the conductor of the endocrine orchestra, we now know that the pituitary takes its orders from the hypothalamus: a section of the brain to which the pituitary is attached. The hypothalamus in turn is influenced by a complexity of factors including the nervous system and the concentration of various substances in the blood.

The pituitary is divided into two sections: the posterior lobe and the anterior lobe. The posterior lobe is the storage site for two important hormones produced by the hypothalamus – oxytocin and anti-diuretic hormone (ADH), also known as vasopressin. The hormone oxytocin stimulates the onset of labour and helps with milk-production, while ADH acts on the kidneys to aid water conservation in the body. The larger anterior lobe produces a probable ten hormones (no one is quite sure) which direct the activity of other glands elsewhere in the body. For instance, thyroid stimulating hormone (TSH) increases the secretion of thyroxine (see The Thyroid), and adreno-corticotrophic hormone (ACTH) plays a part in the production of cortisone molecules in the adrenal glands.

The most plentiful of the pituitary's secretions is growth hormone (GH) which is necessary for growth of bone, cartilage and possibly other tissues. Deficiency of GH in childhood leads to dwarfism; excessive production, usually caused by a tumour of the pituitary, leads to gigantism. Even in adulthood, growth hormone may still have a role to play. If we break a bone, for instance, the hormone is believed to hasten the development of new bone tissue.

THE PINEAL

Attached to the base of the brain is the pineal body (so-called because it resembles a pine cone). Although many anatomical facts concerning the pineal have been known for years, its physiology is still somewhat obscure. Nevertheless, contrary to a once widely held belief, there is no evidence that the pineal atrophies with age. The presence of 'brain sand' (an accumulation of calcium which begins to surround the gland at the time of puberty) was thought to be a sign of the gland's diminishing activity. Recent studies indicate that the presence of 'brain sand' is actually a sign of increased secretory activity.

One hormone secreted by the pineal is melatonin – a light-sensitive substance produced during the hours of darkness. Melatonin is known to affect sleep, mood and the reproductive cycle. Usually levels of the hormone rise at night and subside at dawn. However, in recent years melatonin has also been associated with the depressive illness known as seasonal affective disorder (SAD). In this illness, melatonin production happens later at night than usual, resulting in a 'sleep hangover'. Symptoms include lethargy, irritability, loss of libido and self-esteem, mood changes, overeating and what can best be described as 'sleepaholism' (some sufferers can sleep upwards of fifteen hours at a stretch). The gloom begins to descend in the autumn, reaching an all-time low mid-winter, only to lift again magically with the first rays of the spring sunshine.

Treatment for SAD involves full-spectrum light treatment (phototherapy). The sufferer basks in front of a purpose-designed light-box first thing in the morning in order to kick-start the body for the rest of the day. Studies have shown that this treatment has an impressive 85 per cent success rate. Those who suffer a mild form of the condition (especially common in indoor workers) can be helped by installing full-spectrum light-bulbs which mimic natural daylight. These are widely available from electrical shops. The more sophisticated light-boxes (for those suffering from full-blown SAD) can be obtained by mail order.

THE ADRENALS

The adrenal glands lie on top of the kidneys. They are composed of two layers: the outer cortex and the inner medulla. Even though they are not much bigger than the tip of a man's finger, they synthesise over fifty hormones or hormone-like substances, most of which are essential to life. The best known is adrenalin.

When we experience any strong emotion like sudden rage or an overwhelming fear, or when we feel pressurised to meet a deadline, the medulla releases into the bloodstream the 'fight or flight' chemical, adrenalin. However, we have all the available energy to respond to the challenge. The body's systems are stimulated into increased activity. The liver immediately releases stored glucose, instant energy, into the bloodstream. There is also increased blood pressure, heart rate and oxygen intake. The digestive system comes to a halt, thus diverting blood to the muscles, which become tense in preparation for action.

The hormones produced by the cortex fall into three broad classifications: one batch (the cortisone family) is involved in a wide range of processes, including the metabolism of fats, carbohydrates and proteins; a second acts to stimulate the water and mineral balance in the body. The third group is the sex hormones. These are androgens (male hormones) and oestrogens (female hormones) which are produced in small amounts to supplement those produced by the gonads (sex glands).

While testosterone is generally regarded as an exclusively 'male' hormone, and oestrogen as 'female', in fact sex hormones are not the exclusive property of one sex or the other. Testosterone is produced in the female body too – albeit in comparatively miniscule amounts. Similarly, a tiny amount of oestrogen is produced in the male body, and is thought to have a role to play in cell growth and development. Interestingly, testosterone and its chemical relative androstenone (a pheromone) comprise the 'raw fuel' of the libido in both sexes. (For more on pheromones see page 232.)

THE THYROID

The thyroid gland is found in the neck, straddling the windpipe (trachea). Its principal job is to control the body's metabolic rate through the secretion of thyroxine. Lack of the hormone in childhood results in cretinism. Two outstanding clinical symptoms of this condition are dwarfism and mental retardation.

Adults who develop an under-active thyroid leading to thyroxine deficiency may become obese, slow and listless and feel cold. A common cause of thyroxine deficiency is lack of iodine in the diet, because iodine is an important constituent of thyroxine. On the other hand, an over-productive thyroid gland (sometimes triggered by prolonged stress and worry) causes the sufferer to develop a wolfish appetite. Yet the person remains extremely thin because food is burned up at an alarmingly rapid rate. If left untreated, the heart would race, possibly to the point of exhaustion and death.

A dysfunctioning thyroid (whether over-active or under-active) may become enlarged, causing swelling around the front of the neck, called a goitre. In England the so-called 'Derbyshire Neck' was due to a simple goitre caused by lack of iodine in the locally grown produce. The introduction of iodised salt caused this disease to die out. Other sources of iodine include fish, edible seaweed (especially bladderwrack) and vegetables grown in soil near the sea. A goitre caused by an over-active thyroid, however, will be made worse by eating iodine-rich foods. Treatment for this condition normally involves administration of anti-thyroid drugs that suppress the synthesis of thyroxine, or by surgical removal of part of the gland.

THE PANCREAS

The pancreas resides deep in the abdominal cavity, behind the stomach and between the duodenum and the spleen. It has two main functions, one of which is to produce various enzymes necessary for digestion. In its role as an endocrine gland, the pancreas produces insulin and glucagon which control several body functions, especially carbohydrate metabolism. Insulin helps the muscles and other tissues to obtain the sugar needed for their activity. A gross deficiency leads to diabetes, in which the blood sugar is not used by the body and increases to undesirable levels. Until substitute insulin from animals came along, many diabetics died of the disease. It is estimated that insulin has saved over 30 million lives since it was introduced as a therapy in the 1920s.

A change to a low-carbohydrate diet is often enough to control maturity onset diabetes. However, a growing number of nutritionists believe that a diet high in complex carbohydrates, such as wholemeal bread, brown rice, nuts and seeds, is better for the diabetic than the standard low-carbohydrate approach.

THE THYMUS

The thymus gland which is situated under the breastbone secretes thymosin, a recently discovered hormone believed to be related to the state of the endocrine system as a whole – it even appears to dictate how rapidly we age. However, the best-known function of the thymus gland is its role in helping us to develop a strong immune system (see Chapter 16).

THE ROLE OF AROMATHERAPY

The treatment and management of serious hormonal problems, such as juvenile-onset diabetes and thyroid dysfunction, is way beyond the scope of home treatment, and also beyond the skills of the average aromatherapist. So if you are suffering from such a complaint, it is essential to seek medical attention. However, aromatherapy can be used as a supplementary treatment, as a means of reducing stress.

Since prolonged stress and emotional disharmony can upset the delicate balance of the endocrine system, and indeed the functioning of any other body system or organ, this is where aromatherapy (especially aromatherapy massage) comes into its own. It is a wonderful preventative treatment which can be used to maintain the healthy functioning of the glands.

As a matter of interest, those essences known to influence the secretions of certain hormones are outlined in the chart opposite. Such essences (excepting garlic) can be used in any of the following recommended applications:

- Massage oil
- Aromatic baths
- Mood-enhancing room scents
- Personal perfumes

Instructions for preparing essences for the various therapeutic applications are to be found in Chapter 6. The art of perfume making is explored in Chapter 27.

There are also a number of essences which have a special affinity with the female reproductive system, such as chamomile, clary sage and rose (see Chapter 17). While many essences such as ylang ylang and sandalwood are reputed aphrodisiacs, a few like camphor and marjoram are said to have the opposite effect.

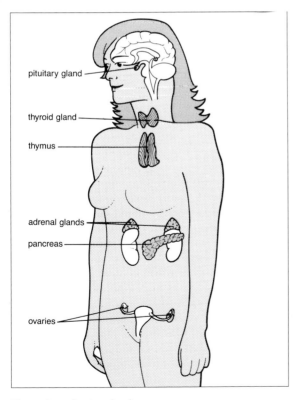

pituitary gland

thyroid gland

thymus

adrenal glands

pancreas

ovaries

The main endocrine glands

ACTIONS OF ESSENTIAL OILS

The principal actions of essences which have an affinity with the endocrine system are as follows:

Adrenal Stimulants: For stress-related exhaustion, for example basil, geranium, rosemary, pine.

Anti-diabetics or Hypoglycaemics: For helping to balance blood-sugar levels, for example geranium, juniper berry.

> **CAUTION** *These essences may need to be taken orally to exert their therapeutic effect – a potentially dangerous method for the home-user.*

Balance Thyroid Secretion: For balancing excessive secretions of thyroxine. Garlic is recommended by Valnet (the essence can be taken orally in the form of capsules). However, it may be that the juice and bulb of both garlic and onion are more effective for this particular disorder.

Contain oestrogen-like substances: Some plants contain phyto-oestrogens which have been shown to help menopausal symptoms, for example fennel, hops, sage. The essential oils of these plants may also contain the same substances (see also Chapter 2).

Contain Phyto-Steroids: These substances are said to resemble the male and female sex hormones and are found in frankincense and myrrh. Whether these essences exert a hormonal influence in humans has yet to be established.

AROMATIC PRESCRIPTIONS

Since direct treatment for disorders associated with endocrine dysfunction is beyond the scope of home treatment, the aromatic prescriptions suggested for the nervous system (see page 120) will help indirectly by reducing the adverse effects of stress on the mind/body complex.

15
THE NERVOUS SYSTEM

The nervous system is where the mind/body phenomenon can be observed as manifest fact, for every thought, emotion and action is reflected by a cascade of biochemical responses throughout the whole organism.

One major breakthrough came in the 1970s when a series of important discoveries centred on a new class of minute chemicals called neurotransmitters and neuropeptides. These chemicals were considered revolutionary at the time because they proved that the nerves did not work electrically like a telegraph system, as had been believed, but that nerve impulses were chemical in nature. As orthodox doctor and Ayurvedic practitioner, Dr Deepak Chopra, puts it:

> *The arrival of neuro-transmitters on the scene makes the interaction of mind and matter more mobile and flowing than ever before… They also fill the gap that apparently separates mind and body, one of the deepest mysteries man has faced since he began to consider what he is.*

Chopra comes to this conclusion because we now know that non-material thought can actually give rise to neuro-chemicals. 'To think,' says Chopra, 'is to practise brain chemistry.' But where does the guiding thought itself come from? A question that continues to baffle scientists and philosophers alike, and one that perhaps may never be satisfactorily answered.

On that enigmatic note, we shall continue with an overview of the nervous system and brain, and consider the role of aromatherapy as a healer of disease within the mind/body complex. (See also Chapter 21.)

ANATOMY OF THE NERVOUS SYSTEM

The central nervous system (CNS) is composed of the brain and spinal cord, to which a peripheral system of billions of neurones (nerve cells) are linked. The nervous system, as a whole, is concerned with the conduction of numerous electro-chemical messages received, every fraction of a second, from the sensory nerves, via the CNS, to the various muscles of the body. It is responsible for controlling movement and the reflexes, and for maintaining internal body functioning (the autonomic nervous system).

The brain is a soft, jelly-like structure, weighing about three pounds and looking like a giant walnut. No computer exists (nor ever will) that can begin to duplicate the brain's myriad functions. It contains a staggering ten thousand million neurones and eighty thousand million glial cells. The brain is the centre of our mental capacity, our actions, thoughts, feelings, senses – everything. Even when we are asleep, the brain's neurones continue to deal with thousands upon thousands of impulses stemming from our psyche and physiological processes.

But what of the neurones themselves? Each consists of a cell body, which gives rise to numerous branching processes called axons and dendrites. Axons conduct impulses away from the cell body, and dendrites pick up signals from adjacent neurones and conduct these towards the cell body. Yet the neurones never actually touch one another, for there are synapses (minute gaps) between the nerve cells. However, when an impulse reaches a synapse a chemical (neuro-transmitter) is produced in the ends of the nerve fibres. This diffuses rapidly across the gap between the cells and triggers off a fresh impulse in the cell on the other side.

The consensus of opinion is that for all their versatility, most types of nerve cells cannot reproduce themselves (the exception being olfactory nerve cells which are explored in Chapter 21). Skin, liver tissue, blood cells and bone tissue can be replaced after damage or loss, but lose a neurone and it is lost forever. But what causes the demise of neurones and is there anything that can be done to prevent this loss?

MIND OVER MATTER

It is known that the brain gradually loses weight as it ages. This is partly due to loss of protein and fats and to a lesser degree because it also loses water. However, from our mid-thirties onwards we also lose about 100,000 brain cells every day. This is hardly noticeable at first, but by the time we reach our sixties (or earlier), we may begin to notice our attention span diminishing and experience difficulty in remembering names, dates and telephone numbers.

Yet recent studies suggest that much of what used to be considered inevitable mental and emotional changes connected with ageing, such as senility and depression, and the belief that 'you can't teach an old dog new tricks' may not be as time-dependent as we may think. Such changes are at least partly determined by the negative expectations we may have about getting older. In other words, we become what we think.

Moreover, there is mounting evidence to suggest that science may be wrong in believing that neurones cannot reproduce themselves. Indeed, the mind/body's comeback powers can be miraculous. At the time of writing, the most remarkable example is that of Austrian-born David Verdegaal (now in his fifties) who lives in Lincolnshire (England). Eight years ago he 'died' when his heart stopped for 30 minutes after a massive coronary. Five minutes without oxygen is generally believed to be as much as the brain can stand without being irreversibly damaged. 'He had brain damage that was very severe,' explained one of his neurologists. 'We call it a pallic syndrome, where the whole cortex of the brain is damaged.' Indeed, his chances of survival were reckoned to be nil.

Yet Verdegaal made an astonishing comeback – though initially blind and paralysed. In eight years, at first his sight and then his limbs gradually responded to his superhuman determination. He has now completed two full marathons and one half-marathon for charity. And even though a lack of communication between eyes and brain leaves him unable to read or form letters, he can now write by pressing the keys of a word processor. Whatever caused Verdegaal to come back to life (he believes it was some kind of supernatural power) provided him with the will to make medical history.

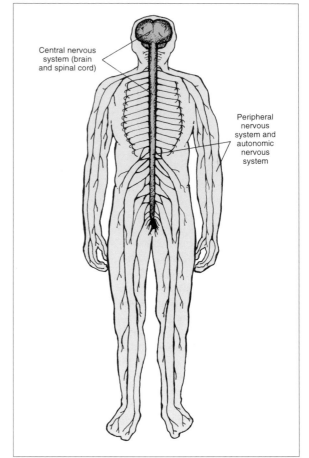

The nervous system

SELF-HELP MEASURES FOR NERVOUS DISORDERS

As mentioned in the previous chapter, prolonged stress can lead to serious health problems, though more often it will manifest as chronic muscle tension and fatigue. However, no matter how frenetic (or painfully monotonous) your life may be, there is usually an enormous amount you can do to prevent such a build-up of stress. You could perhaps use Bach flower remedies as a backup to aromatherapy; or maybe practise deep breathing, conscious relaxation or yoga; or you could opt for a relaxation tape; or maybe vigorous exercise is the answer. It is also important to mention that whatever form of activity or source of relaxation you decide upon, do ensure that it is something you actively enjoy. For, contrary to popular belief, holistic healing is biased towards the pursuit of pleasure!

THE ROLE OF AROMATHERAPY

Aromatherapy (especially aromatherapy massage) is one of the finest treatments available for problems associated with the nervous system – be it tension headaches, insomnia, mental fatigue, anxiety and stress, or mild depression. However, while you might simply choose a 'relaxing' or 'stimulating' oil, according to need, it is very important to ensure that the chosen oil (or blend) appeals to your senses (see Chapter 6). If the aroma is disliked, the treatment will be completely ruined.

As always, if you are suffering from a serious neurological problem, such as multiple sclerosis, it is important to seek the advice and co-operation of a medical practitioner, preferably someone prepared to let you use aromatherapy as a supportive measure. Likewise, if you are suffering from a serious psychological problem, such as deep depression and anxiety without apparent cause (i.e. that which cannot be pinpointed to obviously traumatic events like divorce, bereavement, financial difficulties, and so on), it is vital to seek professional support and guidance. Ideally, this would be given by a qualified psychotherapist or counsellor sympathetic to aromatherapy and holistic healing in general.

Bearing all this in mind, the following chart summarises the principal actions of essential oils used for problems associated with the nervous system.

ACTIONS OF ESSENTIAL OILS

The principal actions of essential oils used for problems associated with the nervous system are as follows:

Adrenal Stimulants: For stress-related exhaustion, for example basil, geranium, rosemary.
Sedatives: For calming a jangled nervous system, for example clary sage, lavender, marjoram, sandalwood, vetiver.
Hypnotics: Specifics for inducing sleep, for example chamomile (German and Roman), hops, neroli.
Stimulants: To help restore energy levels depleted through illness or nervous fatigue, for example black pepper, coriander, peppermint, rosemary.
'Normalising': For stimulating or relaxing, depending on the state of the individual, for example bergamot, geranium.
Nervines: For strengthening and toning the nervous system, for example clary sage, juniper, lavender, lemongrass, patchouli.
Antidepressants: For uplifting the spirits, for example bergamot, geranium, lemon, orange, rosemary, ylang ylang.

THERAPEUTIC CHARTS: ANXIETY AND STRESS-RELATED PROBLEMS

Instructions for preparing essences for the various therapeutic applications are to be found in Chapter 6.

ANXIETY

Description	Possible causes	Aggravated by	Recommended Essential Oils
A state of nervous apprehension and distress. Sufferers experience paralysing fear of an imminent, yet unspecified, danger and, in extreme cases, fall prey to unpredictable panic attacks. Anxiety is usually a response to stressful events, but can also occur apparently without provocation.	Chronic anxiety (sometimes accompanied by depression and/or insomnia), needs professional help, especially if an obvious cause cannot be pinpointed, though it may be linked to food allergy, excessive caffeine intake, or be the side-effect of certain drugs.	Lack of sleep and whatever the source may be.	Bergamot, chamomile, clary sage, frankincense, juniper berry, lavender, melissa (true), neroli, rose otto, ylang ylang.

Methods of use

Bath, massage, vaporiser, personal perfume.

Suggested Herbal Remedies

Chamomile, lemon balm, lime blossom, orange flower, valerian (also available in tablet form).

Nutritional supplements

If food allergies are suspected, seek professional advice. Otherwise use the same supplements recommended for Stress (page 119).

Further advice

Seek to reduce stress in your life. A professional aromatherapy massage now and again is a marvellous treatment, especially in conjunction with Bach flower remedies. You could also see a professional counsellor, or join a support group.

DEPRESSION

Description

Depression is characterised by excessive sadness, lethargy, a pronounced inability to concentrate and strong feelings of inadequacy. Regular sleeping patterns are often upset, with a sufferer having either too little, or too much sleep. It can be a perfectly normal response to a period of crisis, emotional upheaval or excessive level of pressure and stress.

Possible causes

Chronic depression is usually symptomatic of an underlying physical illness or a psychological disorder. Otherwise, treatment is similar to that recommended for Anxiety.

Aggravated by

Too much or too little sleep, or whatever has triggered the feeling.

Recommended Essential Oils

Specifics: basil (French), citrus essences, clary sage, lavender, neroli, sandalwood, vetiver, ylang ylang. *Others which may help:* black pepper, coriander, frankincense, juniper berry, lemongrass, pine, rose otto, rosemary.

Methods of use

Bath, massage, vaporiser, personal perfume.

Suggested Herbal Remedies

Lemon balm, lime blossom, ginseng (available in tablet form), rosemary, vervain.

Nutritional supplements

Depends on cause, but generally a good multi-vitamin and mineral supplement containing the full B-complex range of vitamins.

Further advice

Chronic depression needs professional help. Your GP may be able to put you in touch with a counsellor or psychotherapist. Mild or 'reactive' depression can be helped by aromatherapy (ideally, professional aromatherapy massage) and Bach flower remedies.

HEADACHE

Description

An extremely common ailment with numerous possible causes.

Possible causes

Nervous tension, low blood sugar, high blood pressure, food allergy, lack of sleep, muscle spasm at the base of the skull, structural misalignment, constipation, inhalation of toxic fumes, eye strain, and so on.

Aggravated by

See Possible Causes.

Recommended Essential Oils

Chamomile (German and Roman), clary sage, eucalyptus, lavender, lemongrass, marjoram, peppermint, rose otto, rosemary.

Methods of use

Icy compress, massage (especially to head, neck and shoulders), dry inhalation (a few drops on a handkerchief, or a single drop inhaled from the palm), headache balm (see recipe, page 121).

Suggested Herbal Remedies

Chamomile, marjoram, peppermint, rosemary, skullcap.

Nutritional supplements

Depends on causes.

Further suggestions

Seek to reduce stress in your life. Persistent headaches must be investigated by a medical practitioner.

INSOMNIA

Description

A frustrating problem which can leave you feeling drained, irritable and muddle-headed.

Possible causes

Excitement or anxiety, worry, overwork (especially mental work), lack of fresh air and exercise, eating a heavy meal late at night, caffeine, nervous tension, nutritional deficiencies, depression.

Aggravated by

A sleeping area that is either too hot or too cold.

Recommended Essential Oils

Chamomile (German and Roman), hops, lavender, mandarin, marjoram, melissa (true), neroli, petitgrain, rose otto, sandalwood, vetiver, ylang ylang.

Methods of use

Bath, massage (especially back massage), vaporiser, drops of essential oil on your pillow (or on a handkerchief placed nearby).

Suggested Herbal Remedies

Chamomile, hops, lime flower, orange flower, passion flower, valerian (also available in tablet form).

Nutritional supplements

Depends on cause. Seek professional advice.

Further advice

Seek to reduce stress in your life. Persistent insomnia, especially if it results in chronic fatigue, must be investigated by a medical practitioner. Usually, this can be followed up with holistic therapy (aromatherapy massage is excellent) in preference to long-term drug treatment.

JETLAG

Description

Symptoms may include fatigue, insomnia, swollen ankles, menstrual disturbances, general malaise.

Possible causes

A disruption in the body's biological clock, exacerbated by the aeroplane itself, i.e. compressurised cabin, dry atmosphere. Altitude is a problem for many people too, sometimes causing headaches and nausea.

Aggravated by

Alcohol contributes to dehydration, so drink plenty of bottled water instead.

Recommended Essential Oils

To calm: chamomile (Roman), cypress, geranium (lowest recommended quantity), juniper, lavender, neroli, petitgrain.
To enliven: bergamot, eucalyptus, geranium (maximum recommended quantity), grapefruit, lemon, peppermint, rosemary.

Methods of use

Massage (for puffy ankles, gently massage beneath and above the swelling, always towards the heart), aromatic bath. Epsom salts bath, dry inhalation (drops on a handkerchief).

Suggested Herbal Remedies

To help you sleep: chamomile, orange flower, passion flower, valerian (available in tablet form).
To wake you up: fennel, peppermint, rosemary, sage.

Nutritional supplements

To reduce stress levels short-term: 2 x 500 mg vitamin C, good multi-vitamin and mineral formula containing the full range of B-complex vitamins.

Further advice

During the flight, elevate your feet by resting them on a holdall or small suitcase to help prevent swollen ankles.

MENTAL FATIGUE

Description

Although common in young adults studying for their exams, it may also affect harrassed parents and office workers too.

Possible causes

Excessive mental work, tiredness, stress.

Aggravated by

Continuing to work without a break; boring work.

Recommended Essential Oils

Specifics (to clear the head): basil, eucalyptus, peppermint, pine, rosemary.
General: angelica, coriander, cypress, elemi, grapefruit, geranium, lavender, lemon, palmarosa, pine, rose otto.

Methods of use

Specifics: vaporiser, dry inhalation (drops on a handkerchief).
General: massage (especially head, face, neck and shoulders), baths.

Suggested Herbal Remedies

Peppermint, rose petal, rosemary.

Further suggestions

Deep-breathing exercises (see page 145), preferably in the fresh air or near an open window.

MIGRAINE

Description

Migraine occurs when blood vessels in the brain contract then dilate, causing searing pain. It may be accompanied by altered vision (bright spots before the eyes), nausea, numbness, a sensation of pins and needles and sometimes vomiting. Often regarded as a form of neuralgia.

Possible causes

Could be triggered by one or several factors, for example, stress, structural misalignment, muscle spasm at the base of the skull, depression, shock, hormonal disturbance (menopause, the pill), food allergy, extremes of temperature, personality (often anxious, hardworking, restless, perfectionists), heredity.

Aggravated by

Possibly by foods containing tyramine: chocolate, citrus fruits, cured meats, herring, cheese, caffeine, alcohol, yeast products, onions, peanut butter, pork, vinegar, yoghurt.

Recommended Essential Oils

Angelica, chamomile (German and Roman), coriander, clary sage, lavender, marjoram, melissa (true), peppermint.

Methods of use

As a preventative: regular aromatherapy massage, especially to head, neck and shoulders (see page 174).
During an attack: warm or icy compress (whichever gives the most relief).

Suggested Herbal Remedies

Feverfew, passion flower, valerian (also available in tablet form).

Further suggestions

Seek to reduce stress. If you cannot track down the cause, or if there is no improvement after a couple of months of home treatment, seek professional advice. Other helpful treatments include food allergy test, Bach flower remedies, osteopathy or chiropractic (to correct misalignment of spine), homoeopathy.

MULTIPLE SCLEROSIS (MS)

Description

A disease of the central nervous system (brain and spinal cord) where the myelin sheath, which insulates the nerve fibres, is destroyed. Symptoms vary dramatically from individual to individual, ranging from weakness in the limbs, numbness and tingling, to, in some cases, paralysis and incontinence.

Possible causes

There is no known cause.

Aggravated by

Symptoms relapse and remit over time, apparently without reason.

Recommended Essential Oils

Generally, choose according to aroma preference (to uplift the spirits), though you could also try rosemary in a base of hypericum oil (see page 39).

Methods of use

Massage (especially back, buttocks and legs), luke-warm bath.

Nutritional supplements

Evening primrose oil is the most popular supplement at present. Dosage: 6 x 430 mg daily. Many sufferers feel that the oil makes an incredible difference.

Further advice

There is no known 'cure' for MS, but aromatherapy can help to nurture the spirit, and alleviate depression and exhaustion (a common symptom during low phases of the illness). Also, do seek the advice of a holistic nutritionist as many sufferers have found that diet can have a beneficial effect on their symptoms. (See Useful Addresses, page 289.)

NEURALGIA

Description

Pain arising along the course of a nerve, which may be severe, dull, or stabbing.

Possible causes

A symptom occurring when a nerve is irritated or compressed or where there is inflammation and infection. Facial neuralgia can be triggered by cold wind.

Aggravated by

Stress.

Recommended Essential Oils

Chamomile (German or Roman), coriander, eucalyptus, geranium, hops, lavender, marjoram, nutmeg, peppermint, pine, rosemary.

Methods of use

Massage, bath.

Suggested Herbal Remedies

Internal: hops, passion flower, valerian (available in tablet form).
External: hypericum oil (see page 39).

Nutritional supplements

Good multi-vitamin and mineral supplement, including the full range of B-complex vitamins.

Further suggestions

Seek to reduce stress in your life. If symptoms continue, consult an osteopath or chiropractor who will be able to correct any structural misalignment.

STRESS

Description

Stress occurs when the natural equilibrium of the body and mind is upset, often as a result of disease, physical injury, emotional troubles and excessive demands made on an individual's mental and physical resources. Prolonged stress weakens the body's immune system and can be the source of many health problems, ranging from general aches and pains, to heart attacks and stomach ulcers.

Possible causes

The body's reaction to situations of potential stress is the classic 'fight or flight' response, triggered by the production of adrenalin. This hormone prepares the individual to resist ('fight') or avoid ('flight') attack. In modern life, however, it is rarely possible to deal with stress in this way and, as a result, there is no direct outlet for the physical and emotional effects of adrenalin production.

Aggravated by

The longer the 'stressed out' feeling remains, especially if there is no outlet for pent-up emotions, the more harmful it can be.

Recommended Essential Oils

Almost any, but especially citrus essences, cedarwood, chamomile (German and Roman), clary sage, cypress, frankincense, geranium, lavender, juniper berry, marjoram, patchouli, peppermint, pine, rose otto, rosemary, sandalwood, ylang ylang.

Methods of use

Massage, bath, vaporiser, personal perfume.

Suggested Herbal Remedies

As for Anxiety, though Siberian Ginseng may also help (available in tablet form).

Nutritional supplements

During acute stage: A good multi-vitamin and mineral supplement containing the full range of B-complex vitamins, and extra vitamin C amounting to 1 g per day, gradually tapering off as improvement takes place.

Further suggestions

Beat the hell out of a cushion! Other stress-releasing ideas are given on page 149.

VDU STRESS

Description

A wide range of symptoms, including headache, eye-strain, irritability, insomnia, nausea, muscular aches and pains, or a general feeling of malaise.

Possible causes

The effects of low-level radiation as a result of spending many hours each day in front of a computer screen.

Aggravated by

Spending more than two hours at a time in front of the VDU without a break. Symptoms are worse in those who dislike the work they are doing.

Recommended Essential Oils

As for Jetlag (see page 116).

Methods of use

Massage, bath, vaporiser, personal perfume (see Chapter 27).

Suggested Herbal Remedies

See Stress (above).

Nutritional supplements

See Stress.

Further suggestions

Take regular breaks, preferably in the fresh air, and do simple stretching exercises.

AROMATIC PRESCRIPTIONS

The following massage oil blends are best massaged into the skin after a bath or shower. If you have a friend or partner available to give you a nurturing massage, all the better. The same blends of essences can be used in the bath or vaporiser, but you will need to adjust the amount of essential oil accordingly (see pages 29 and 32).

TO HELP ANXIETY AND STRESS

Recipe 1

50 ml of light base oil such as almond or sunflower seed
8 drops bergamot
3 drops clary sage
3 drops neroli
5 drops frankincense

Put the essential oils into a dark glass bottle, add the base oil and shake well to disperse the essences.

Recipe 2

50 ml of light base oil such as almond or sunflower seed
6 drops juniper
3 drops rose otto
5 drops cedarwood
5 drops sandalwood

Mix as for the previous recipe.

TO HELP MILD DEPRESSION

Recipe 1

50 ml of light base oil such as almond or sunflower seed
9 drops bergamot
5 drops petitgrain
3 drops clary sage
3 drops vetiver

Put the essential oils into a dark glass jar, add the base oil and shake well to disperse the essences.

Recipe 2

50 ml of light base oil such as almond or sunflower seed
4 drops lemon
8 drops coriander
4 drops neroli
3 drops ylang ylang

Mix as for previous recipe.

TO HELP JETLAG AND VDU STRESS

For jetlag: As soon as possible after arriving at your destination, take an Epsom salts bath (see page 29). Afterwards, allow at least fifteen minutes 'sweating it off' time before massaging your whole body (or as much as you can reach!) with one of the blends suggested below. The first recipe is for when you need to calm down at night, the other is to pep you up in the daytime. Similarly, the treatment can be used to help combat VDU stress.

Recipe 1 (calming)

50 ml almond oil
4 drops cypress
5 drops petitgrain
10 drops lavender

Put the essential oils into a dark glass bottle, add the base oil and shake well to disperse the essences.

Recipe 2 (enlivening)

50 ml almond oil
4 drops peppermint
4 drops geranium
10 drops rosemary

Mix as for previous recipe.

TO HELP NEURALGIA

Recipe 1

25 ml extra virgin olive oil
25 ml hypericum oil
6 drops geranium
8 drops coriander
1 drop nutmeg

Put the essential oils in a dark glass bottle, add the base oil and shake well to disperse the essences.

Recipe 2

25 ml calendula oil
25 ml hypericum oil
4 drops peppermint
4 drops eucalyptus
4 drops pine

Mix as for previous recipe.

HEADACHE BALM

Rub a small amount into the temples and back of the
neck. If you cannot obtain an unperfumed base cream,
this can be purchased by mail order from most essential
oil suppliers.

30 g unperfumed base cream
2 drops peppermint
5 drops lavender
5 drops eucalyptus

Put the cream into a clean glass pot, add the essential oils
and stir well with the handle of a teaspoon.

VAPORISING BLENDS FOR MENTAL FATIGUE

Diffuse the essences into the room where you work. If
this is difficult, say, if you share a work space with others
who may object, put the drops on a handkerchief and
inhale at intervals throughout the day, in which case you
should adjust the number of drops to roughly half that
suggested in the following recipes, for example two drops
each of cypress and pine, and four drops of rosemary.

Recipe 1
100 ml water
5 drops cypress
5 drops pine
10 drops rosemary

Funnel the water into a dark glass bottle, add the essential
oils and shake well. Fill the oil burner reservoir with some
of the aromatic blend. Do remember to shake the bottle
each time before use to disperse the essences.

Recipe 2
100 ml water
5 drops grapefruit
5 drops coriander
10 drops pine

Mix as for the previous recipe.

16
THE IMMUNE SYSTEM

The immune system enables us to survive in an ecosystem swarming with invaders threatening us from within and without. It is the body's defence system, its fortress against an astounding variety of things that have the potential to make us ill. These include viruses, fungi, dust, pollen, harmful chemicals, transplanted tissue, blood transfusions, proteins from improperly digested food, just about anything. The most insidious are those that originate within our own bodies. According to Dr Michael A. Weiner, author of *Maximum Immunity* (Gateway Books, 1986) it is probable that cancer cells are produced spontaneously in everyone's body, but in most people the immune system is able to identify and eliminate these cells before they grow out of control.

How exactly does the immune system deal with all these enemies, and why do things sometimes go wrong? In order to answer these questions, we shall take a simplistic overview of the hottest medical subject to date. Then we shall consider the role aromatherapy can play in helping to build up immunity.

THE THYMUS AND OTHER LYMPHATIC ORGANS

Our internal defence force is supported by the spleen, lymph nodes, bone marrow, tonsils, adenoids and also possibly the appendix and portions of the intestine – but primarily by the thymus gland. Until recently, the thymus was largely ignored because it was thought that it was only involved in the growth process and the development of immunity in childhood. After that, it was simply redundant to the body. Today, this mysterious organ has moved into the limelight of medical research and has even been dubbed 'the throne of immunity'.

The thymus is located deep beneath the breastbone: a small blob of pinkish-grey tissue. However, the gland reaches its maximum size, relative to body weight, during early childhood, and begins to shrink as we reach maturity, hence the 'thymus redundancy theory'. Nevertheless, the thymus continues to be functional in adulthood, producing the hormone thymosin, which appears to be related both to the state of the endocrine system and to many brain chemicals, as well as to how rapidly we age.

Its role in immunity is to help produce T cells (thymus-derived), which act in concert with B cells (bone marrow-derived) to destroy invading microbes. Both types of cells are collectively known as *lymphocytes*. They are amazingly skilful warriors, instantly recognising a potential enemy – a flu virus, a pus-forming staphylococcus, a splinter that has penetrated a finger. They produce antibodies and call upon other cells to do the same. Each antibody is specific against a single invader – one for mumps, one for whooping cough, and so on. The body actually produces as many as a million different kinds of antibody.

There is another group of white blood cells collectively known as *phagocytes*. Should a foreign body actually penetrate the skin and mucus membranes or bypass the antimicrobial substances in the blood (as is most common with serious wounds), the T cells can call upon a certain type of phagocyte, the *macrophages* (meaning 'big eaters') to destroy bacteria or malignancies. Amoeba fashion, the macrophages surround the bacterial debris and digest it.

T cell lymphocytes also produce a group of hormone-like substances called lymphokines which are considered the immune system's natural drugs – the cancer-fighting substance interferon is a notable example. There are others with cryptic titles like SIRS and IL-2.

LYMPHATIC DRAINAGE

The immune system is also responsible for draining excess fluid and wastes from the system. It is therefore equipped with a vast network of vessels throughout the body (similar to the blood vessels) which transport a watery fluid known as lymph. This network of vessels is called the lymphatic system. Lymph itself is formed from the fluid that bathes all tissues of the body and contains material which is too large to enter the blood capillaries. It also carries lymphocytes and other substances concerned with immunity.

Unlike the circulatory system, which is controlled by the pumping of the heart, the lymphatic system has no such pump. The normal contractions and relaxation of the muscles through everyday movement, and the force of gravity, keep the lymph flowing. The wastes are eventually eliminated via the excretory organs – the skin, lungs, kidneys and colon.

The lymphatic system is interrupted at intervals by groups of glands known as *lymph nodes*. These have a role to play in immunity, producing both lymphocytes and antibodies. When a lymph node is stimulated into activity, for example by infection, it swells and becomes painful. This swelling may be noticeable even before the

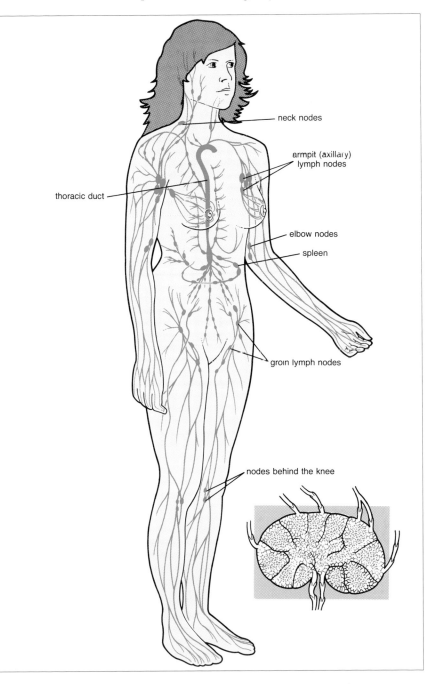

neck nodes

armpit (axillary) lymph nodes

thoracic duct

elbow nodes

spleen

groin lymph nodes

nodes behind the knee

The lymphatic system

infection itself is apparent (swelling of the glands in the neck during a throat infection is most common). Apart from those in the neck, the main groups of lymph nodes are to be found in the armpits and groin and the centre of the torso. Important secondary concentrations are found near the elbows and knees.

Interestingly, complaints such as arthritis, cellulite, high blood pressure and even depression have been linked to poor lymphatic drainage. Therefore it is important to keep this system in good health by taking adequate exercise. If this is difficult, perhaps because you are wheel-chair bound, elderly, or have a sedentary job, regular massage and/or dry skin brushing will help enormously with lymphatic drainage (see Part 3 for massage instruction, and Chapter 26 for the dry skin brushing technique).

WHEN IMMUNITY FAILS

With such an amazing system of immune defences, you may be wondering why we ever succumb to illness. This can be partially explained by the fact that there is a time lapse between the moment an invader enters the body and when the immune system finally destroys it. In the interim, the disease-producing organism, such as a virus or pathogenic microbe, is wreaking havoc – killing cells, producing toxins, devouring nutrients and sapping the body's vitality. Even when the immune system has the intruder under control, it still takes a while for the body to repair itself. The severity and duration of the attack is dependent upon many interrelated factors. These include the person's innate constitution (some people are born healthier than others), their age (the immune system begins to weaken as we grow older), and on how well nourished we are. Our standard of hygiene is important too. Immunity is also influenced by our mental and emotional state.

Sometimes the lymphocytes over-react to foreign invaders, responding too aggressively and producing an array of annoying symptoms. For instance, should the body over-respond to pollen grains, we get hay fever. In fact, all allergies are the result of an over-responsive immune system. Just why the body should behave in this way remains a mystery, though emotional disharmony combined with a faulty diet and lifestyle are regarded as contributing factors.

Perhaps the most alarming diseases associated with a dysfunctioning immune system (usually an underactive immune response) are those which are broadly categorised as auto-immune diseases; illnesses such as rheumatoid arthritis, lupus erythematosus, multiple sclerosis and AIDS. In such cases, the B cells and T cells go haywire. They fail to distinguish between 'self' and 'nonself' and start to attack the body's own tissue.

There are several theories to account for this, though they are far too complex to go into here. Suffice it to say, although there may be a genetic link, other possible triggers cited by researchers include environmental pollution in its many guises (e.g. toxic chemicals, radiation, noise, electromagnetism), over-zealous use of antibiotics, vaccination (a sensitive issue which is of concern to a growing number of medical researchers), poor nutrition, stress and other psychological factors.

MIND OVER IMMUNITY

For some considerable time scientists thought of the immune system as a self-contained unit which responded automatically to the stimulus of antigens. The nervous and endocrine systems were regarded as separate entities, having no part to play whatsoever in the intricacies of immunity.

In recent years a new understanding has arisen, a trailblazing realisation grounded in the field of psychoneuroimmunology. In tune with the beliefs of ancient healers, mystics and philosophers, disease is now defined as 'any persistent harmful disturbance of the mind/body's equilibrium'. And this equilibrium is maintained by the interrelatedness of the nervous, endocrine and immune systems.

According to the American psychoneuroimmunologist Dr Michael A. Weiner:

> It is now evident that our attitudes, beliefs and emotions can influence immunity, and that the immune system can even be conditioned – tricked into responding by psychological devices.

The 'psychological devices' he proposes include relaxation and deep-breathing exercises – methods which we shall explore in Part 3 along with several other paths to mind/body harmony.

THE ROLE OF AROMATHERAPY

Just about every essential oil used in aromatherapy has a beneficial action on the immune system, and this includes the indirect psychotherapeutic route to enhanced immunity. The exceptions, of course, are those essences which in some people trigger an allergic reaction.

Psychotherapeutic actions apart (individual responses cannot always be predicted), *the direct* actions of essential oils on the body's immune defences are shown in the following chart. Treatments for individual ailments ranging from colds and flu, stress and depression can be found in the therapeutic charts throughout this part of the book.

The psycho-physiological benefits of massage and its immuno-stimulant effects cannot be praised enough, so do try to incorporate this as part of your lifestyle. Not everyone, of course, can afford the services of a professional aromatherapist. However, you could try getting together with a group of like-minded friends with whom you can exchange aromatherapy massage on a regular basis. Everything you need to know about giving skilful, yet sensitive and nurturing massage is to be found in Part 3.

ACTIONS OF ESSENTIAL OILS

The principal actions of essential oils on the immune system are as follows:

Antibiotics and bactericidals: For fighting bacterial infection, good examples being lavender, lemongrass, rosemary, tea tree.

Antivirals: For protecting against and helping to reduce serious complications of viral infections such as coughs, colds and flu, for example garlic, eucalyptus, marjoram, tea tree.

Cytophylactics: For increasing the activity of white blood cells which help in our defence against infection, for example frankincense, lavender, rosemary.

Depuratives or detoxifying agents: For helping to combat impurities in the blood and organs, for example angelica, fennel, juniper, rose otto.

Fungicidals: For combating fungal infections such as candida, for example lavender, myrrh, tea tree.

Parasiticides: For destroying fleas and lice, for example eucalyptus, lavender, rosemary, tea tree.

Vermifuges*: For expelling intestinal worms, for example bergamot, lavender, lemon, peppermint, thyme.

Vulneraries: For helping to heal wounds, for example frankincense, lavender, marjoram, rosemary.

* Since oral doses would be required for this purpose, unsupervised home treatment is not recommended.

17
THE FEMALE REPRODUCTIVE SYSTEM

Aromatherapy is especially helpful for easing problems associated with the female life-cycle. Nevertheless, men have not been totally ignored. Indeed, aromatherapy can be helpful for problems such as emotionally induced impotency or 'performance pressure' (see Chapter 25).

Rather than following the pattern of previous chapters, which give brief physiological surveys of the various organs and body systems, here we shall concentrate on natural ways to manage the ebb and flow of the female life-cycle.

A WORD ABOUT TREATING 'WOMEN'S PROBLEMS'

Although the therapeutic charts in this chapter outline treatments for a number of common ailments, certain conditions need to be considered a little more closely; for example, pre-menstrual syndrome (PMS) and menopause. Mention is also made of anorexia nervosa and bulimia nervosa. Even though men occasionally succumb to eating disorders, young women are by far the most likely victims. However, treatments for these are not included on the therapeutic chart, because it would be ludicrously simplistic to suggest oils to increase the appetite (for anorexia nervosa) and oils to balance the appetite (for bulimia nervosa), for these two related illnesses are far more complex and require specialist psychotherapeutic intervention.

PRE-MENSTRUAL SYNDROME (PMS)

PMS can begin at any time from two days to two weeks before menstruation. Physical symptoms can include fluid retention, weight gain, constipation, breast tenderness, headaches, nausea, skin eruptions and nervous tension. As if this were not enough, there may also be other psychological symptoms such as lethargy, depression, low self-esteem, food cravings, tearfulness and irritability. Thankfully, it is unusual to suffer more than a handful of these symptoms at any one time. Nevertheless, all women experience some degree of pre-menstrual change, even if very slight and therefore requiring no treatment.

Interestingly, some women experience the pre-menstrual phase as a time of heightened creativity and deeper insight. There are also those women who experience a surge of energy at this time, the kind of energy that enables them to take on projects that would normally tax several workers. After the gush of energy, however, they usually feel totally drained.

But what causes PMS? Although it is fashionable in some quarters to consider PMS to be entirely psychosomatic, a 'rejection of the feminine processes', such a view is incredibly simplistic. On the other hand, it seems equally unbalanced to cite wayward hormones as the sole cause. Even worse, ardent feminists are now denying the very existence of PMS, believing that the condition is 'all in the mind', an obstacle to women's freedom and equality. For all those women who suffer from PMS, the condition is real enough.

Enlightened researchers support the multi-factorial model, and thus allow different factors to interact – physical, psychological, social and cultural.

It is my own opinion that a certain degree of PMS – and I do not include suicidal or murderous tendencies here – is a perfectly reasonable response by a healthy reproductive system to the unnatural state of non-pregnancy. Before you gasp in horror, I am not for one moment suggesting that women should give in to biology; rather I am saying that PMS is at least partly physical in origin. Interestingly, tribal women rarely get pre-menstrual because during their fertile years they are usually pregnant or breastfeeding (breastfeeding can delay the onset of menstruation for up to three years). So having a healthy attitude to femininity makes little difference in this instance. On the contrary, since menstruation is taboo in many primitive, patriarchal societies, it may be just as well that the women do not experience it very often. Such negative conditioning is hardly conducive to care-free bleeding!

It would seem that the real culprit is fluid retention (even though this is barely noticeable in some women) triggered by subtle changes in body chemistry. PMS is also exacerbated by stress and poor diet which is why it can, to a great extent, be remedied – as so many women have discovered.

MENOPAUSE AND BEYOND

The menopause marks the end of a woman's reproductive years and can begin at any time between the ages of 40 and 55 years of age (although the onset is commonly between the ages of 47 and 50). Symptoms may include the 'hot flush' and night sweats (caused by a rush of hormones into the bloodstream), mood swings, weight gain, palpitations, vaginal dryness, headaches and many other minor ailments. Understandably, there may also be irritability, poor concentration and insomnia. However, it should be emphasised that few women experience *every* symptom associated with the menopause. In fact, it is not at all uncommon to sail through the phase with little or no discomfort. It helps in experiencing a smooth passage through menopause if a woman feels loved by her family and friends and has a fulfilling life in general.

And while many women continue to enjoy a loving sexual relationship, others experience a new-found freedom in celibacy. The problem with celibacy, of course, is that a woman's partner may not share her enthusiasm for that particular path. Even though this may cause unhappiness at the outset, if the relationship is bonded with love and based on true friendship the partner will adjust to the new situation. The relationship may even blossom into something deeper, albeit on a level that needs to be experienced to be believed.

Unfortunately, this is not a view that is popular at present. Indeed, popular health and psychotherapy books are full of helpful suggestions about making yourself look more attractive for your man and seeking psychosexual counselling – and if all else fails, there is always the KY jelly!

Moreover, led by Hollywood and the glossy women's magazines, twentieth-century civilisation is obsessed with the cult of Youth Eternal.

Even those psychologists and health writers who try to present the positive features of menopause (and ageing in general) may, inadvertently, be guilty of ageism. Many times we read words to the effect that 'successful ageing' is about continuing to look and behave as we did when we were younger. This assumes that one age group's physical appearance and pattern of behaviour is inherently superior to that of another, and is, therefore, a value judgement which merely reinforces the idea of 'younger' being more desirable.

At risk of sounding trite, deep down we all know that *true* beauty emanates from the very essence of who we are. It cannot be found in the texture of our skin, the shape of our body or the colour of our hair, alluring as these things may be. Beauty is that which is enduring. Everyone has recognised it from time to time – when in the presence of a certain vibrant individual who may look like a crocodile but feel like an angel!

CULTURAL INFLUENCES

There is increasing evidence to suggest that cultural views on the nature of ageing profoundly influence a woman's psycho-physical experience of menopause. For instance, women in Mayan villages actually look forward to the menopause because it brings freedom from childbearing. Menopausal symptoms such as nervous anxiety and hot flushes are unknown. Similarly, peasant women on the Greek island of Evia who have few negative notions about menopause, suffer few of the symptoms linked to the change. Could this be at least partly attributable to the fact that their culture does not idealise youth?

Anthropologists Margaret Mead and Judith K. Brown have looked at the status of women in primitive patriarchal cultures throughout the world, and have found one constant: menopause marks the threshold of seniority and rank. Women at this time are 'crowned' Wise Women, midwives, healers and givers of initiation. Conversely, Western society views the menopause as an end, so it is not surprising that it should be a time of mourning for a great many women.

Nevertheless, it would be wrong to conclude that all menopausal symptoms are caused by our negative attitudes to life. As we have already seen with PMS, body and mind are inseparably linked, so natural hormonal changes are bound to cause a certain degree of emotional and physical discomfort – at least for a year or so until the body settles down. It is only when symptoms become extreme (not as common as you may think) that we need to consider taking drastic measures to control the menopause.

HORMONE REPLACEMENT THERAPY (HRT)

While it would be wrong to rule out HRT completely, far fewer women than the proponents of HRT would have us believe actually need medication to control their body chemistry. Despite tireless campaigns by doctors and drug companies, half of all women prescribed HRT stop within six months, according to a recent survey by the National Opinion Polls. So the 'feel good drug' is not living up to its expectations. Although women used to be given oestrogen-only versions of HRT, this was found to increase by twenty-fold the risk of endometrial cancer. To counteract this, women who still have a womb are now given the additional artificial hormone progestogen, which is supposed to mimic the naturally occurring female hormone progesterone.

It may be true that HRT offers some protection against osteoporosis (one of HRT's big selling points) but at what cost? Meticulous studies of almost all the scientific papers and research data regarding HRT have been carried out by researchers working for the British publication *What Doctors Don't Tell You*. Their findings are startling. Of the many facts they have unearthed, far too numerous to explore in this book, the following are especially interesting:

- Despite claims that the oestrogen/progestogen combined formulas of HRT are protective against breast cancer and cardiovascular disease, in fact the opposite is true (*The Lancet* 1991; 338: 274–7).
- Almost every study to date on HRT demonstrates a significant cancer risk (of the breast and womb). The only thing disputed is exactly how substantial the risk is. A Swedish study of 23,000 women on the oestrogen/progestogen combined drug showed that the risk quadrupled after six years of continuous use (*New England Journal of Medicine*, 3 August 1989).
- HRT preserves bone mass only when it is taken for upwards of seven years – far longer than most women stay on the drug. As soon as you stop taking it bone mineral density declines rapidly, and other menopausal symptoms like hot flushes and night sweats may return with a vengeance (*New England Journal of Medicine*, 14 October 1993).
- The Amarant Trust (a British pro-HRT campaigning organisation) asserts in its literature that HRT can stop you becoming 'seriously forgetful' in old age. 'Institutions are full of old women who have become virtual cabbages due to senile decay (Alzheimer's disease) which afflicts more women than men.' A scare tactic if there ever was one! This claim has, in fact, been disputed by American medical researchers (*Journal of the American Medicine Association*, 10 April 1991).
- Oestrogen implants (and transdermal patches) appear to create a 'tolerance' for oestrogen – in other words, the drug can be addictive. However, if we are to believe HRT protagonist John Studd, a leading gynaecologist at King's College Hospital, London, women who become dependent have psychiatric problems and therefore require larger than normal amounts. A wonderful example of blame-the-patient justification!

Of course, someone somewhere may well produce statistics to counter the above revelations. It should also be acknowledged that there are many women for whom HRT has indeed been a wonder drug, lifting them from the depths of despair. But are such women the exceptional few who perhaps suffer from uncommonly severe symptoms? In which case, is HRT prescribed too freely – even to those who might otherwise weather the passing storm? Since the experts cannot agree about the safety of HRT, my own approach is to err on the side of caution. This means promoting the use of natural treatments such as a well-balanced wholefood diet, sensible exercise like walking (to help develop strong bones), herbal remedies (especially Phytoestrol, see page 9) and aromatherapy as the first line of action – and should natural methods fail to control any distressing symptoms, HRT as a last resort.

As a final word on the HRT debate, it is of great concern to many people that some HRT formulas are based on hormones obtained from mares' urine. As well as being deprived of adequate amounts of water, the unfortunate animals are kept in appallingly cramped conditions and therefore suffer a great deal of distress. So if you really need to go on HRT, you may feel that it is preferable to opt for a totally synthetic formula.

EATING DISORDERS

One of the most pernicious maladies of our times, and one which claims young girls in particular (though boys are not immune), must surely be anorexia nervosa and the related eating disorder bulimia nervosa (binge eating followed by purging and vomiting). According to the Royal College of Psychiatrists, one in every 100 schoolgirls in Britain suffers from anorexia to a greater or lesser degree. Two in every 100 women aged between 15 and 45 have bulimia. There are high rates of both anorexia and bulimia among models, dancers and those in media-related jobs.

Whatever the underlying cause (and theories abound), the greatest pressure must surely come from modern society's obsession with the lean, muscular, almost androgynous body which few women could ever attain – at least not without indulging in an excessively time-consuming exercise programme. In fact, those responsible for promoting the 'ideal image' of women are often sick themselves. Jane Fonda, for instance, suffered from bulimia for many years, and Princess Diana, a paragon of modern feminine beauty, may still be struggling to overcome the bingeing vomiting cycle of self-starvation.

Even more disturbing, pre-adolescent dieting is on the increase. Born to compete, little girls, sometimes as young as six or seven, have been taught by their mother's example to associate femaleness with deprivation. Hunger is regarded as a prerequisite for entering into adult sexuality.

While aromatherapy massage given by a caring therapist may help during the early stages of an eating disorder, once the illness has taken a firm hold specialist care is essential. Moreover, it is unlikely that an anorexic woman would consult an aromatherapist or massage therapist, since being touched is almost certain to be abhorrent to the sufferer. In fact, massage would cause physical pain in the advanced stages of the illness. The problem is acknowledged here in the hope that it will open the eyes of those who may be caught up in such a nightmare. And that others may recognise the early signs in themselves or in their loved ones – and will seek help before it is too late (see Useful Addresses, page 289).

AROMATHERAPY FOR PREGNANCY AND CHILDBIRTH

Excepting the occasional aromatherapeutic treatment, I no longer advocate unsupervised daily use of essential oils on the skin during pregnancy and whilst breastfeeding (the reasons for this are outlined on pages 24–5). You can, however, enjoy gentle massage with plain vegetable oil throughout pregnancy and afterwards. But do seek the approval of your doctor or midwife first.

Moreover, certain essences can be vaporised in low concentrations during the massage to enhance the experience. Recommended oils include bergamot, chamomile (German or Roman), lavender, mandarin, neroli, sandalwood, rose otto and ylang ylang, depending on personal preferences and psycho-physical needs.

Essential oils can be of enormous help during labour. Indeed, a growing number of maternity units, are now offering aromatherapy to soothe both mother and baby during the birthing process. For instance, a drop or two of frankincense and rose, inhaled as required from the palm of the hand, has been successfully used to help women suffering from hyperventilation (over breathing) during labour. In addition, clary sage helps with the delivery of the placenta (afterbirth) when used as a warm compress over the abdomen.

If you would like to know more about aromatherapy and massage during maternity, including the joys of baby massage, see Part 4.

POST-NATAL DEPRESSION

After childbirth, progesterone and other hormones fall precipitously, which is the main reason why many women suffer from tearfulness or 'baby blues' a few days after delivery. But this normally passes within a week or so as the shock and/or elation of childbirth begins to abate.

However, some women may develop full-blown post natal depression lasting many weeks or months following childbirth (or as a result of miscarriage or abortion). Although the problem is related to hormone imbalance as a direct result of childbirth, the condition has also been linked to high levels of stress (especially sleep deprivation), poor health, change of lifestyle and social status, immediate separation from the baby after birth, an unexpected Caesarean, over-sedation during the birth and many other interrelated factors. As we have seen, emotional disharmony can affect our hormones, and just about any other physiological process.

Whatever the combination of factors, as well as employing aromatherapy (ideally, professional aromatherapy massage), it is advisable to seek guidance and support from your midwife, health visitor or health practitioner, and also from family and friends – especially women friends with babies or young children of their own. For it can be self-empowering to empathise with others in a similar situation – to know that you are not isolated in your feelings and experiences.

THE ACTIONS OF ESSENTIAL OILS

Apart from the indirect psychotherapeutic and stress-reducing benefits of aromatherapy, *the direct* actions of essential oils on the female reproductive system are shown in the chart opposite. It has also been confirmed by pharmacognosists (those who study the natural history, physical characteristics and chemical composition of plants) and pharmacologists (those who study the effects of substances on the human physiological processes) that a number of plants such as hops, fennel and sage contain oestrogen-like substances which have been shown to regulate the menstrual cycle and minimise menopausal symptoms like hot flushes and mood swings.

However, whether or not essential oils of the aforementioned plants (and others) contain the same phyto-oestrogens cannot be scientifically confirmed. As far as I am aware, there have been no official studies on the subject. Nevertheless, empirical evidence amongst aromatherapists and their clients confirms the efficacy of these and other 'hormonal influencing' essences.

ACTIONS OF ESSENTIAL OILS

The principal actions of essential oils having an affinity with the female reproductive system are as follows:

Antispasmodics: For preventing and easing menstrual pain and for easing labour, for example chamomile (German and Roman), clary sage, lavender, marjoram, rose otto.
Emmenagogues: For inducing menstruation and/or normalising menstrual flow, for example chamomile, clary sage, lavender, rose otto.
Galactogogues: For stimulating the flow of mother's milk, for example fennel, lemongrass.
Hormone Influencing: For a broad spectrum of problems associated with the female reproductive system, for example cypress, frankincense, geranium, hops, rose otto.

Anti-Galactogogues: For reducing milk flow, for example peppermint, sage*.
Uterine Tonics: For toning and regulating the female reproductive system, and for excessive menstruation, for example frankincense, melissa (true), rose otto.

NB Many essences are also reputed aphrodisiacs (see Chapter 27).

* Essential oil of common sage is very powerful and therefore not recommended for home use.

THERAPEUTIC CHARTS: WOMEN'S PROBLEMS

Instructions for preparing essential oils for the various therapeutic applications are to be found in Chapter 6.

AMENORRHOEA (LOSS OF PERIODS)

Description	Possible causes	Aggravated by	Recommended Essential Oils
Apart from cessation of periods outside pregnancy, the condition may manifest as irregular or scanty menstruation, perhaps leading to fertility problems.	Prolonged stress, emotional shock or excitement, obesity, anorexia nervosa, excessive exercise, sometimes symptomatic of an underlying serious health problem.	Depends on cause, though poor nutrition and/or emotional disharmony are nearly always implicated.	Clary sage, fennel (sweet), hops, juniper berry, marjoram, myrrh, rose otto.

Methods of use	Suggested Herbal Remedies	Nutritional supplements	Further suggestions
Bath, massage (especially to lower back and abdomen), warm compress (for scanty periods). Supplementary methods: vaporiser, dry inhalation (drops on a handkerchief).	Marigold (calendula), parsley, chaste tree, (available in tablet form under its botanical name *Vitex agnus-castus*.	Depends on cause.	Attention to diet and lifestyle. If there is no improvement after a few months, especially if you wish to conceive and are experiencing difficulties, do have a medical check-up.

DYSMENORRHOEA (PAINFUL PERIODS)

Description	Possible causes	Aggravated by	Recommended Essential Oils
In some women, the cramping pains experienced as the uterus contracts during menstruation can be incapacitating.	Heredity, lack of exercise, being fitted with an IUD, a fall in blood calcium levels (common prior to and during menstruation). Severe pain may be symptomatic of a gynaecological disorder such as endometriosis.	Stress, poor nutrition.	Chamomile (German or Roman), clary sage, cypress, frankincense, hops, juniper berry, lavender, marjoram, melissa (true), rose otto, rosemary.

Methods of use	Suggested Herbal Remedies	Nutritional supplements	Further suggestions
Bath, warm sitz baths, warm compress (abdomen), massage (featherlight stroking downwards over abdomen), also regular full-body massage as a preventative measure.	Cramp bark (decoction), chamomile, marigold (calendula), chaste tree (available in tablet form under its botanical name *Vitex agnus-castus*).	If caused by low calcium levels, a specially formulated vitamin and mineral supplement may help. 'Premenstrual' packs are widely available from chemists and health shops.	Attention to diet and lifestyle. Severe menstrual cramp must be investigated by a medical practitioner, perhaps followed up with holistic treatment from a qualified practitioner.

ENGORGEMENT OF BREASTS

Description		Aggravated by	Recommended Essential Oils
Too much milk, usually in the first few days of breast-feeding before milk production has settled down. Symptoms are hot, hard, swollen, lumpy and painful breasts.		By not feeding your baby, though if the breasts are too hard and congested, the baby will fail to get a proper hold on the nipple, thus preventing him/her from drawing milk. A little milk may need to be expressed manually (your midwife will show you how).	Geranium, peppermint.

Methods of use			**Further suggestions**
Cold compress.			Gentle breast massage (see page 201) after each feed will help prevent the development of mastitis (a painful inflammatory condition related to an infected or blocked milk duct).

MENOPAUSAL SYMPTOMS

Description	**Possible causes**	**Aggravated by**	**Recommended Essential Oils**
Including hot flushes and night sweats.	A drastic decrease in the output of oestrogen and progesterone.	Stress, poor nutrition, attitude/cultural conditioning.	*Specifics for hot flushes and night sweats:* cypress, clary sage. *General (supportive/balancing to mind/body complex):* bergamot, chamomile (Roman), clary sage, fennel, frankincense, geranium, hops, lavender, melissa (true), neroli, rose otto, sandalwood, ylang ylang.

Methods of use	**Suggested Herbal Remedies**	**Nutritional supplements**	**Further suggestions**
Specifics: bath, massage, dry inhalation (drops on a handkerchief). *General:* bath, massage, vaporiser, personal perfume.	*For hot flushes and night sweats:* sage. *As an alternative to HRT:* 'Phytesterol' (a herbal supplement containing plant-derived oestrogens) available from health shops.	A good multi-vitamin and mineral supplement. Specially formulated 'menopausal' packs are available from chemists and health shops.	Seek to reduce stress and improve your diet and lifestyle (see Chapter 19). If symptoms are still severe after a month or two of home treatment, do seek professional advice. Other helpful therapies: Bach flower remedies (for emotional disharmony), medical herbalism, homoeopathy.

MENORRHAGIA (HEAVY PERIODS)

Description	**Possible causes**	**Aggravated by**	**Recommended Essential Oils**
Although this condition can be helped with herbs and essences, it may be indicative of a serious gynaecological problem.	There are many possible causes, including endometriosis, fibroids and polyps.	Heavy lifting and sometimes even mildly strenuous activity.	Chamomile (German and Roman), cypress, rose otto.

Methods of use	**Suggested Herbal Remedies**	**Nutritional supplements**	**Further suggestions**
Bath, massage oil (gently massage into the abdomen and lower back), dry inhalation (drops on a handkerchief to supplement skin applications).	Cranesbill (decoction of the root), cypress (decoction of the crushed cones).	For short-term relief, try 4 × 500 mg vitamin C with added bioflavonoids (found naturally in the pith of citrus fruits).	If the excessive flow continues for more than a few cycles, do seek medical advice, perhaps followed up with holistic treatment from a qualified practitioner.

MILK FLOW (TO PROMOTE)

Description		**Aggravated by**	**Recommended Essential Oils**
There are many things you can do to improve the quantity and quality of breastmilk.		Low fluid intake, tiredness, inadequate diet, smoking, stress. Also, avoid excessive quantities of caffeine (stimulating to the baby) and avoid alcohol (which will end up in breastmilk).	Fennel, lemongrass.

Methods of use	**Suggested Herbal Remedies**	**Nutritional supplements**	**Further suggestions**
Massage (see Breast Massage, page 201), warm compress.	*Decoction*: fennel seeds, caraway seeds, fenugreek seeds. *Infusion*: goat's rue, vervain.	Seek the advice of a holistic nutritionist (see Useful Addresses, page 289).	Seek to reduce stress and improve your diet. Drink copious amounts of bottled spring water. Commence breastfeeding as soon as possible after birth to stimulate milk production. Wash off all traces of essential oil prior to feeding. Seek the advice of your midwife too.

MILK FLOW (TO DECREASE)

Description		**Aggravated by**	**Recommended Essential Oils**
If for some reason the milk flow needs to be stopped, there are ways to encourage this without resorting to drugs.		Regular feeding.	Peppermint.

Methods of use	**Suggested Herbal Remedies**		**Further suggestions**
Cold compress, massage oil (apply two or three times daily, but don't actually massage the breasts as this may stimulate milk flow).	*Infusion*: red sage or ordinary garden sage, three times daily until desired result.		Cut down on fluid intake, but do seek the advice of your midwife too.

PERINEUM (HEALING AFTER CHILDBIRTH)

Description

With or without stitches, the perineum is almost certain to feel uncomfortable after childbirth. There may also be bruising or swelling.

Possible causes

Episiotomy (small surgical incision to assist childbirth, especially forceps delivery) and also natural tears which may require stitches.

Aggravated by

Constipation, sitting on the sore area.

Recommended Essential Oils

Lavender, tea tree.

Methods of use

Alternate hot and cold sitz baths; full-size bath with two tablespoonfuls of sea salt added to aid healing.

Further suggestions

Massaging the perineum with extra virgin olive oil during the last few months of pregnancy will help prevent tearing during childbirth. Pelvic floor exercises before and after childbirth (see page 200).

PMS (PRE-MENSTRUAL SYNDROME)

Description

May begin any time from two days to two weeks prior to menstruation. Symptoms may include fluid retention, breast tenderness, headaches, nausea, anxiety, depression, irritability, sleep disturbances, food cravings, and other disturbances.

Aggravated by

Stress, lack of sleep, overwork, sedentary lifestyle, poor diet.

Recommended Essential Oils

Chamomile (Roman or German), citrus essences, clary sage, cypress, geranium, hops (but not if depressed), frankincense, juniper, lavender, marjoram, neroli, rose otto, sandalwood, vetiver, ylang ylang.

Methods of use

Baths, massage (preferably full body, otherwise head, neck, shoulders, or just back), vaporiser, dry inhalation (drops on a handkerchief), personal perfume.

Suggested Herbal Remedies

Diuretics: dandelion (decoction of the root), parsley. *Hormone balancer*: chaste tree (available in tablet form under its botanical name *Vitex agnus-castus*).

Nutritional supplements

As an alternative to *Vitex agnus-castus*, pre-menstrual formula of evening primrose oil plus a vitamin and mineral supplement (marketed as Efamol) is widely available from chemists and health shops.

Further suggestions

Seek to reduce stress and improve diet. A professional aromatherapy massage now and again will help to balance the nervous system, and thus reduce or alleviate symptoms.

SORE OR CRACKED NIPPLES

Description

Common during the first weeks of breastfeeding, before the nipples have become 'hardened' to the effects of continual sucking.

Aggravated by

Continuing to allow the baby to suckle on the sore nipple. But there is no need to give up breastfeeding, see Further Suggestions.

Recommended Essential Oils

Chamomile (German or Roman), rose otto.

Methods of use

Massage oil, aromatic ointment (see recipes on page 136).

Suggested Herbal Remedies

Calendula ointment (available from chemists and health shops).

Nutritional supplements

A good multi-vitamin and mineral supplement.

Further suggestions

To allow time for the sore skin to heal, try covering the nipple with a rubber teat from a baby's bottle during feeds. Baby will draw milk from the breast through the teat without causing you any discomfort! Purpose-designed nipple shields are also available from good chemists.

VAGINAL THRUSH (*Candida albicans*)

Description

Fungal infection of the mucous membranes of the vagina. Symptoms are a thick white discharge accompanied by intense itching.

Possible causes

Antibiotics: they destroy helpful colonies of bacteria and encourage resident thrush colonies to multiply. Also, the pill, high sugar/high yeast diet, sexual contact with an infected partner (men can carry candida but don't always show symptoms).

Aggravated by

Wearing synthetic fibres against the skin (e.g. nylon tights, lycra underwear) and tight jeans. They create a warm, moist and airless environment for candida to flourish. Also, harsh scented soaps and bath preparations.

Recommended Essential Oils

Lavender, garlic (see Nutritional Supplements), tea tree.

Methods of use

Bath, sitz bath.

Suggested Herbal Remedies

Oral doses: nettle, blackberry leaf.

Nutritional supplements

One or two garlic capsules daily (garlic has anti-fungal properties), and take lactobacillus acidophilis tablets (yoghurt bacteria), or eat 300 ml plain live yoghurt a day.

Further suggestions

Drastically reduce sugar, yeast and alcohol consumption and follow a well-balanced wholefood diet. If symptoms continue for more than a couple of months, seek the advice of a holistic nutritionist (see Useful Addresses, page 289).

AROMATIC PRESCRIPTIONS

The same combination of essences used in the following body massage blends can also be used in the bath and as mood-enhancing room scents (see Chapter 28). For best results, massage the oils into your skin immediately after a bath or shower.

MASSAGE BLENDS TO HELP PMS

Recipe 1

50 ml almond oil
10 drops bergamot
5 drops neroli
4 drops ylang ylang

Funnel the almond oil into a dark glass bottle, add the essences and shake well to disperse the aromatic droplets.

Recipe 2

50 ml almond oil
4 drops lavender
4 drops geranium
4 drops clary sage
8 drops sandalwood

Mix as for the previous recipe.

Recipe 3

50 ml almond oil
10 drops bergamot
6 drops juniper berry
4 drops vetiver

Mix as for the previous recipes.

MASSAGE BLENDS TO HELP MENOPAUSAL SYMPTOMS

Recipe 1 (hot flushes and night sweats)

50 ml almond oil
6 drops cypress
10 drops clary sage

Funnel the almond oil into a dark glass bottle, add the essences and shake well to disperse the aromatic droplets.

Recipe 2 (supportive/balancing)

50 ml almond oil
5 drops chamomile (Roman)
8 drops clary sage
5 drops rose otto

Mix as for the previous recipe.

GENERAL BALANCER

The following recipe is a good all-rounder for most menstrual problems, including spotting in-between periods, excessive menstruation and period pain.

50 ml almond oil
12 drops frankincense
5 drops rose otto

Funnel the almond oil into a dark glass bottle, add the essences and shake well to disperse the aromatic droplets.

AROMATIC OINTMENT

The following ointment will help sore and cracked nipples. The recipe suggests calendula oil as part of the base. This is a vegetable oil extraction of French marigold flowers and is available from herbal suppliers (see also the home-made version, page 32). In case of difficulty, you can use extra virgin olive oil instead. Beeswax can be obtained from herbal suppliers or direct from some bee keepers. If rose otto is prohibitively expensive for you, replace with three drops of the less costly Roman chamomile.

2 heaped teaspoonfuls grated beeswax
25 ml calendula oil
2 drops rose otto

Heat the beeswax and base oil in a heatproof dish over a pan of simmering water. Stir well until the beeswax has melted. Remove from the heat and cool a little before stirring in the rose oil. Pour into a spotlessly clean glass pot and cover tightly. Store in a cool dark place and use up within two months.

18
AROMATHERAPY FOR BABIES AND CHILDREN

Even though many aromatherapists advocate the use of essential oils for babies and children under the age of five, unsupervised home use is potentially risky (see Essential Oils Safety, Chapter 4). Generally, it is fine to vaporise your child's favourite essences around the home, and perhaps to put a few drops of decongestant oils on a handkerchief for him or her to sniff when they have a cold. But skin applications are another matter. Babies and young children have highly sensitive skin which is especially receptive to whatever is put on it, so it is inadvisable to apply aromatic oils regularly or to put essences in the bath for no better reason than for aesthetic purposes.

When treating older children, it is difficult to recommend standard quantities of essential oils according to age. Each child is an individual and does not necessarily develop at the so-called average rate. For example, while one ten year old may be the size of a small adult and tolerant of average quantities of essential oils, another may be very much smaller and consequently more sensitive to average quantities. Aromatherapists tend to play it by ear, generally advocating half the usual recommended amounts for children over five and under ten (refer to the Easy Measures chart on page 34).

Some aromatherapists recommend essential oils for newborn babies, say, one drop Roman chamomile or lavender in 50 ml almond oil for massage, or a single drop of the same essences diluted in one tablespoonful of full-fat milk (or even breast milk) and added to the bath. Others, like myself, prefer to use tiny amounts of soothing and comforting oils in the vaporiser instead. Choose an electric vaporiser rather than a nightlight candle version, as these are safer for children's bedrooms.

For babies under six months, I would suggest adding just one or two drops of neroli, Roman chamomile, rose otto or lavender to the water-filled reservoir of the vaporiser. After this age, add an extra drop of essential oil if you wish. A baby's sense of smell is especially acute; diffuse too much essential oil into the atmosphere – even a so-called relaxing essence like Roman chamomile – and your baby may become irritable and restless rather than happy and contented.

To protect against nappy rash, a generous covering of good old-fashioned zinc and caster oil cream at each nappy change is one of the best preparations available. However, if your baby actually develops nappy rash, try the proprietary calendula and hypericum ointment (usually labelled 'Hypercal'), which is available from most chemists and health shops. This gentle all-purpose cream is a marvellous treatment for most sore skin conditions.

With or without essential oils, massage is one of the finest treatments available for helping babies and children to feel happy and contented. In my own experience, it can also be of enormous benefit to hyperactive children, especially in conjunction with a diet free of artificial colourings and other chemical additives. As well as being a joy for both giver and recipient, massage has many physical benefits too. These include helping youngsters to grow stronger, encouraging deep sleep, better digestion and the relief of colic in infants (see Chapter 24).

TREATING CHILDHOOD ILLNESSES

Although there is growing concern in some quarters regarding jabs for diseases like mumps and measles (especially in children prone to allergies) it is beyond the scope of this book to put forward the arguments for and against vaccination. Suffice it to say, most childhood ailments are quite controllable and not at all serious if diet, hygiene and social conditions are adequate. It is a fact of life that the young are susceptible to all manner of germs and viruses. This is nature's way of strengthening the immune system. Complications are only likely to arise if the child was in poor health in general before contracting the infection. Although some children are born healthier than others, there is still a great deal parents can do to help their children cultivate a strong immune system. This is achieved by a good wholefood diet as outlined in Chapter 19, plenty of fresh air and exercise, adequate housing, and, above all, love. Sadly, many children in the world today (even in the so-called affluent West) are deprived of these basic requirements, so lasting health and happiness are bound to be in jeopardy.

Treatment for most illnesses is largely dietary with external applications of essential oils, including vaporisation to prevent the spread of infection during epidemics.

If a child's appetite has diminished, all well and good; a 24-hour semi-fast is the most appropriate treatment. During a fast, plenty of fresh water (preferably bottled spring water) should be taken as required until the appetite begins to return. A day or so on a diet of fresh fruit and fruit juice (preferably grape juice) diluted 50/50 with spring water should precede a gradual return to a wholefood diet.

Children over five years of age can benefit from skilful use of essential oils for a myriad of common ailments. Anything from coughs and colds to earache and chickenpox can be soothed with an aromatic remedy. Essences

can be used in baths, inhalations, compresses, massage oils, creams or ointments in concentrations about half that recommended for adults.

> **IMPORTANT** *I usually refer parents to a qualified homoeopath if a child is under the age of five years, or if the ailment is of a serious or chronic nature.*

The ailments outlined on the therapeutic chart are those generally regarded as 'children's illnesses' – though adults can also develop some of these if they escaped infection during childhood. Treatments for other common ailments such as colds, coughs and flu are to be found elsewhere in this section of the book. Instructions for the preparation of essential oils for the various recommended applications are to be found in Chapter 5.

THERAPEUTIC CHART: AROMATHERAPY FOR CHILDREN OVER 5 YEARS

Instructions for preparing essences for the various methods of use are to be found in Chapter 6.

CHICKENPOX

Description

A mild fever which begins with the appearance of blisters on the chest and back, later spreading to the rest of the body and causing severe itching. Chickenpox is more serious in adults.

Possible causes

The herpes zoster virus.

Aggravated by

Scratching can lead to bacterial infection of the skin and the subsequent formation of scars.

Recommended Essential Oils

Chamomile (German and Roman), eucalyptus, lavender.

Methods of use

To help reduce itching: Luke-warm bath with chamomile essence, aromatic lotion (see recipe, page 140).
To help prevent spread of infection: vaporiser.

Further suggestions

During the feverish stage of the illness (usually the first day) keep your child in bed. Otherwise, there is no need for bed rest.

GERMAN MEASLES (RUBELLA)

Description

A much milder version of measles. Manifests as a feverish cold, with mild aches and pains and tender lymph nodes in the neck. The rash appears on the first or second day, and lasts for about three days.

Possible causes

The rubella virus.

Recommended Essential Oils

See Measles.

Methods of use

See Measles.

Suggested Herbal Remedies

See Measles.

Nutritional supplements

See Measles.

Further suggestions

If you are pregnant and have not had rubella but have been exposed to the disease, seek medical advice immediately. Rubella can be dangerous to unborn babies. Gamma globulin injections may be indicated. Alternatively, consult a homoeopath who may pre-scribe a homoeopathic dose of rubella itself (called a nosode).

MEASLES

Description

Begins with loss of appetite and headache, followed by a feverish cold, sore throat and dry cough. The eyes become red and sensitive to light. The rash appears over the next few days, spreading downwards over the body.

Possible causes

The rubella virus.

Aggravated by

Bright light.

Recommended Essential Oils

Chamomile (German and Roman), eucalyptus, thyme (as a fumigant only).

Methods of use

Bath, vaporiser (to help prevent the spread of infection), aromatic lotion (see recipe, page 140).

Suggested Herbal Remedies

Garlic (see Nutritional Supplements), lemon balm, peppermint.

Nutritional supplements

For children over 12: one garlic capsule daily continu-ing for a week or two dur-ing the recovery period.

Further suggestions

Put your child to bed in a dimly-lit, but well-ventilated room. Seek medical advice as well.

MUMPS (EPIDEMIC PAROTITIS)

Description

Normally a mild childhood illness, but can be severe in adults, leading to sterility in men. Symptoms include painful swelling of the salivary glands on one or both sides of the face. In males, the testicles may also swell.

Aggravated by

Chewing is usually painful.

Recommended Essential Oils

Chamomile (German and Roman), lavender, lemon.

Methods of use

Warm compress of lavender or chamomile applied to the swollen cheeks.
For older children: Aromatic mouthwash with lemon essence (see recipe, below).

Suggested Herbal Remedies

Archangelica ointment (Weleda).

Further suggestions

Bed rest and a fluid diet of fruit or vegetable juices and spring water if chewing is painful.

AROMATIC PRESCRIPTIONS

AROMATIC LOTION TO HELP CHICKENPOX

To relieve itching between chamomile baths (refer to the Therapeutic Chart), make up the following lotion and sponge the skin as required. Incidentally, if the scalp is affected as well, add about six drops lavender to a large basin of warm water and pour a jugful at a time over your child's hair, taking great care to avoid the eyes.

100 ml distilled water
50 ml witch hazel
4 drops Roman chamomile (or 2 drops German chamomile)
4 drops lavender
4 drops eucalyptus.

Funnel the water and witch hazel into a dark glass bottle. Shake well each time before use and dilute 50/50 with warm water before applying.

AROMATIC LOTION TO HELP MEASLES

Sponge the body frequently with the following lotion.

100 ml distilled water
50 ml witch hazel
8 drops eucalyptus
8 drops lavender

Mix as for the previous recipe, remembering to dilute 50/50 with warm water before use.

MOUTHWASH TO HELP MUMPS

In older children who can be trusted not to swallow the mixture, the following mouthwash will help speed the demise of the infection. Use two or three times daily.

100 ml distilled water
10 drops lemon
3 drops Roman chamomile

Funnel into a dark glass bottle and shake well each time before use. Add two or three teaspoonfuls of the mixture to a teacup of warm water.

FUMIGANT

The following mixture can be vaporised in the home to help prevent the spread of infection during epidemics.

100 ml water
4 drops thyme (sweet)
4 drops eucalyptus
4 drops lavender

Funnel the water into a dark glass bottle, add the essential oils and shake well. Pour some of the mixture into the reservoir of an essential oil vaporiser. Remember to shake the bottle each time before use to disperse the oil droplets.

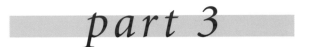

part 3

BODY, MIND AND SOUL

The cure of the part should not be attempted without treatment of the whole, and also no attempt should be made to cure the body without the soul, and therefore if the head and body are to be well you must begin by curing the mind: that is the first thing… For this is the error of our day in the treatment of the human body, that physicians separate the soul from the body.

PLATO, *Chronicles*

19

NURTURING YOUR WHOLE BEING

The term 'holistic' has appeared many times already, but so far we have barely scratched the surface of its meaning. The word itself has its roots in the Greek holos, which means whole or multi-dimensional (think of a hologram). Even though the word came into being in the late 1970s, the concept of holism can be traced back to the ancient civilizations of Egypt and Greece. Of course, the sages and physicians of the East have never lost sight of the reality of the whole and this is reflected in comprehensive systems of healing such as acupuncture and ayurvedic medicine, which have enjoyed an unbroken tradition for thousands of years.

Yet we in the Western world are only just beginning to awaken to the wisdom of the past. In our newfound realisation we are experiencing an upsurge of interest in traditional systems of healing whose incredibly complex philosophies were once dismissed as 'primitive' or 'superstitious'. In the light of recent research into psychoneuroimmunology or the interrelatedness of body and mind, it is increasingly evident that the knowledge of the ancients has been grossly underrated.

In all schools of holistic healing, the aim is to nurture the mind/body complex – and this includes the intangible, fluid areas of experience which we might call the spiritual aspect of our being. The spiritual aspect is hard to define, but is tied up with our sense of purpose and meaning. Without purpose we become depressed or apathetic; life then appears bleak and meaningless. Even when we do not follow a conscious spiritual path we may in fact be realising our purpose in some other way. It could be through music or some other art form no matter how humble, or simply through our work, family, relationships, or through a love of animals or nature – or more actively perhaps by working towards the realisation of a humanitarian ideal.

The vision of those who live and breathe the holistic ideal is that the expression of such qualities as compassion, intuition and nurturing will raise the consciousness of humanity as a whole. In so doing, we will once again begin to honour the earth, as did the healers and mystics of antiquity, realising that we and the earth move together in the one Dance of Life. However, putting sensitivity back into medicine does not mean we must leap into the wilderness of earth magic at the total expense of technological achievement and common sense. We need to integrate the best of orthodox medicine with the best of the gentler approaches, for the high-tech and strictly logical approach to treatment is dehumanised without the balance of intuition and feeling.

It should also be mentioned that even in cases where the pathological condition may have advanced beyond all hope of healing on the physical level, the person may still become healed in a spiritual sense. Indeed, this is the main aim of the hospice movement whose task is to enable terminally ill people to die peacefully in the knowledge that life is not without purpose and meaning. To die peacefully and without fear is the ultimate healing experience.

PUTTING IT INTO PRACTICE

The rest of this chapter is devoted to outlining some of the many ways in which we may begin to create favourable conditions within every level of our being, for in so doing we will enhance the action of the essential oils – and indeed, the efficacy of any other method of healing we may choose to employ.

FOOD

> 'Once upon a time there were three little sisters,' the Dormouse began…
> 'and they lived at the bottom of a well'
> 'What did they live on?' said Alice…
> 'They lived on treacle,' said the Dormouse…
> 'They couldn't have done that, you know,' Alice gently remarked, 'they'd have been ill.'
> 'So they were,' said the Dormouse, 'very ill.'
>
> From **Alice in Wonderland** by LEWIS CARROLL

Arguments abound as to what constitutes a 'well-balanced' diet. One minute we are told to avoid all animal fat because it is bad for the heart and to opt for polyunsaturated cooking oils and soft margarines such as sunflower or soya. The next moment we are told that, far from being healthy alternatives, many highly refined vegetable oils, low-fat spreads and other margarines actually contribute to a build-up of cholesterol in the body, and hence to the development of heart disease. So nutritionists are now urging that we go back to eating a little butter in preference to margarine, and to using moderate quantities of unrefined vegetable oils such as extra virgin olive oil and sunflower seed oil. Unlike processed fats and highly refined cooking oils, cold pressed or unrefined oils have been a dietary staple for thousands of years; therefore, they are much more compatible with the human digestive system. They also contain essential fatty acids and other nutrients in a naturally balanced form.

Similarly, we have been told to avoid all types of sugar, whether it be in the form of honey, unrefined muscovado or refined, white sugar. However, recent research suggests that a small amount of unrefined muscovado sugar is actually good for us. Moreover, far from being the number one enemy of teeth and gums, dark muscovado sugar (not the refined artificially coloured type which masquerades as the real thing) is said to *prevent tooth decay* – a view which was advocated by health food pioneers in the 1950s.

Then there is the question of whether it is healthier to be vegetarian, or even vegan. Or is the macrobiotic principle the ideal? And what about the Hay diet? Proponents of the Hay regime insist that a great deal of illness is caused by 'mixing foods that fight'. For example, we are told never to mix proteins with starches, say, bread with cheese, because protein requires acid digestive juices, while starch demands alkaline secretions. When proteins and starches are eaten at the same meal, so the theory goes, neither gets properly digested. Yet there are other health gurus who would refute such claims.

My own response to the mass of contradictions surrounding the question of diet is to suggest there is no one ideal diet suitable for everyone. We are each very different with varying physiological needs and personal philosophies. Whatever we may believe about diet, the only clear-cut rule, as far as I see it, is that our food should be as free as possible from harmful additives and the toxic residues of modern farming methods – no easy task nowadays.

It may be relatively easy to buy organically grown flour, but unsprayed organically grown fruit and vegetables are a rarity – unless you are able to grow them yourself. Even when they are available they can be expensive, prohibitively so for some people. The best thing we can do for the time being, until organically grown produce becomes the norm, is to eat foods as near as possible to their natural state – not out of tins and packets whose contents may be doused in white sugar, excessive salt, monosodium glutamate and additives.

A growing number of nutritionists are convinced that the food we eat also affects brain chemistry and thus the way we perceive the world. The first step in rebalancing body chemistry and freeing the spirit, we are told, is to alkalise the blood and keep blood sugar levels up. The former can be achieved by eating a wholefood diet largely comprising fresh fruits, salad greens, herbs and other vegetables. The timing of meals is also important; some people need to eat little and often to stabilise blood sugar levels and to keep their emotions on an even keel. These snacks should consist of complex carbohydrate foods such as wholemeal bread, dried fruits, nuts and seeds.

The following steps outline a wholefood diet as recommended by many aware nutritionists. It does not take into account food allergies – some people are allergic to wheat for example – or if you wish to avoid animal foods altogether (veganism) or whether, like myself, you prefer not to eat meat. It should, however, serve as a useful guide that can be adapted to suit individual needs. Aim to alter your diet *gradually* over a period of six months. Drastic overnight changes will certainly lead to digestive upsets.

Some excellent books on healing through diet are listed on page 288.

AT-A-GLANCE GUIDE TO HEALTHY EATING

Buy organically grown food if you can; but don't fret if you can't. Worrying too much about your diet will only lead to stress, which can be much more harmful than a few additives.

- Eat wholemeal bread and other complex carbohydrates such as dried beans, lentils, nuts, seeds (e.g. sunflower, sesame), wholemeal pasta, oats, brown rice and other wholegrain cereals. If dried beans, lentils, nuts and seeds cause excessive flatulence, try sprouting them in a purpose-designed salad sprouter (available from health shops) before cooking in the usual way. Sprouted bean can be eaten raw in salads. When legumes and seeds are sprouted, the chemicals responsible for causing intestinal gas are broken down in the process of germination and so the food becomes more digestible.
- Eat plenty of fresh fruit and vegetables – preferably unskinned, well scrubbed and raw in salads or lightly cooked.
- Cut down on all fats, particularly those from animal sources, especially lard, suet, double cream, butter and full-fat cheese. Use moderate amounts of cold-pressed vegetable oil such as virgin olive, sesame and sunflower seed, e.g. up to one tablespoonful each day.
- Sweeten your food sparingly with honey (preferably raw or unheated honey) or a little unrefined muscovado sugar, or more lavishly with dried fruits such as dates, figs, sultanas and raisins.
- Cut down on salt (even sea salt should be used sparingly) and use more herbs to flavour your food.
- Buy free-range eggs if possible.
- Eat red meat only occasionally, if at all. Instead, eat free-range poultry and fish, particularly oily fish, such as mackerel.

- Cut down on milk, whether full-fat or skimmed. The most digestible version is probably organically produced whole goat's milk, which those normally allergic to dairy products (eczema sufferers, for example) can often tolerate. However, live, full-fat plain yoghurt (preferably organic) is good for most people, whether it comes from the cow, goat or sheep.
- Try to avoid processed foods in cans and packets as far as possible because these are usually laden with chemicals. They will do no harm if used as an occasional stand-by but should not form the basis of your diet.
- A little white or red wine (preferably organic) is good for the digestive system and can help normalise blood cholesterol levels. One or two glasses a day is the recommended quantity.
- Drink plenty of water (bottled or filtered), herb teas, diluted fruit juices, and only one or two cups of ordinary tea or coffee a day if you cannot give it up altogether.
- It is fine to err once in a while, to indulge in the occasional chocolate bar, Danish pastry or fry up. And there is no need to feel guilty about it either. It is only when such indulgences become a daily habit, at the expense of more nourishing foods, that they constitute a health hazard.
- Throw away the scales and forget about counting calories, especially if you are stuck in a diet/binge cycle. Enlightened nutritionists now realise that people have very different metabolisms – while there are those who can eat vast quantities and remain slim, others certainly cannot. If you are very overweight for no apparent reason, you may be suffering from hidden food allergies, in which case, do seek the advice of a holistic nutritionist (see Useful Addresses, page 289).
- Eat slowly in convivial surroundings and, above all, enjoy your food!

MOVEMENT

Unlike a machine which eventually breaks down with use, the human body becomes stronger and more flexible if every muscle and joint is used frequently. It is interesting to note that osteoporosis (brittle bone disease) is on the increase in both men and women. Although the disease is related to poor health in general triggered by such factors as smoking, poor nutrition and low oestrogen levels in women after menopause, the disease can be prevented or lessened by taking regular weight-bearing exercise, such as brisk walking. Moreover, epidemiological studies suggest that as little as fifteen minutes exposure to sunlight (taken daily or as often as climate permits) enhances vitamin D levels, which in turn reduces fracture risk by a fifth. Vitamin D is needed for the absorption of calcium which is essential for healthy bones.

In relation to stress – whether it be the kind related to living in the fast track or that born of a monotonous existence – regular exercise increases the circulation which in turn increases oxygen levels in the blood and activates the endocrine system. This has a positive effect on our state of mind. Anyone who has recently taken up some form of exercise will tell you that it has brought them enhanced mental energy and concentration, the ability to sleep more deeply and a feeling of well-being.

My own approach is to favour natural outdoor activities such as hiking, hill walking, rowing and swimming – preferably in unpolluted rivers, lakes or seas. Of course, not everyone lives within easy access of such wild and beautiful places. For the city dweller, or for those who do not derive any special pleasure from communing with nature, other forms of movement such as dancing (any style to suit your own taste and stamina), cycling, keep-fit, football, tennis or some other energetic sport can be taken up instead. The only hard and fast rule is to go for something you enjoy doing, otherwise you are almost certain to give it up after the initial rush of enthusiasm has abated.

Before we go any further, if you are elderly, have a disability or are too ill to take vigorous exercise, do not despair: regular aromatherapy massage given by a friend or partner (see Part 4) can be almost as beneficial. Another excellent alternative is dry skin brushing (see Chapter 26). If such measures are supplemented by fresh air and moderate exposure to sunlight (up to an hour a day during the summer months) you will experience newfound vitality.

The safest times of the day to take your sunbathe is before midday and after four o'clock in the afternoon. At these times the rays are much longer and therefore less likely to burn. However, it may be necessary to use a high factor commercial sunscreen, especially if you have very fair skin. Unfortunately, natural sunscreen oils such as extra virgin olive oil and sesame offer relatively little protection and are only suitable for those whose skins do not burn easily.

One good all-rounder for body, mind and soul is the ancient discipline of yoga. Ideally, you should join a class headed by a qualified instructor who will monitor your progress and ensure that you do not pull any muscles. You will also be shown how to breathe correctly – a vital aspect of the art. There is no need to twist your body into weird and wonderful shapes or to stand on your head in order to benefit from yoga. Indeed, many people take up the art in their later years and have neither the ambition nor the ability to become contortionists. As you will discover, just learning the basics of good breathing, conscious relaxation and stretching is enough to enhance well-being. The following exercises will set you off on the right track.

COMPLETE BREATHING

The yoga 'complete breath' is one of the easiest ways to begin learning to use your lungs efficiently, and is extremely beneficial to those suffering from respiratory ailments such as asthma, hay fever and bronchitis.

Furthermore, by learning to breathe properly, we begin to strengthen the aura, or the body's immune system if you prefer to think of it in more down-to-earth terms. Try to do breathing exercises outside in the fresh air if possible, at least three times a week. The next best place is in a well-ventilated room, in which case, you could enhance the experience by vaporising any of the following essences which have an affinity with the respiratory system: cedarwood, cypress, frankincense, galbanum, myrrh, pine, sandalwood.

1 Lie on a rug on the floor or ground (in a garden, perhaps), or on a firm bed with your arms at your sides, palms face down.

2 Close your eyes and begin to inhale through your nose very slowly. Expand your abdomen slightly, then pull the air up into the ribcage, and then into your upper chest. Your abdomen will automatically be drawn in as the ribs move out and the chest expands. Hold for a few seconds, but try not to cork the air in your throat which will only create tension. Hold with an open throat and a relaxed chest and belly (much easier to do than it sounds).

3 Now begin to breathe out slowly through your nose in a smooth continuous flow until the abdomen is drawn in and the ribcage and chest are relaxed. Hold for a few seconds, again without straining. Repeat two or three times.

4 Now breathe in slowly as you did in Step 1 but gradually raise your arms overhead in time with the in-breath until the backs of your hands touch the floor.

5 Hold your breath for a few seconds while you have a good stretch from head to toe.

6 Slowly breathe out as you bring your arms back down to your sides. Repeat two or three times

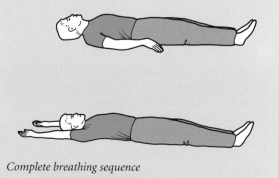

Complete breathing sequence

Full breathing can also be performed in a standing position. To enhance the stretch (Step 5) stand on tiptoes, with your heels coming back down again as you breathe out.

MOVING MEDITATION

The following yoga sequence is best described as a moving meditation. It differs from other yoga postures or *asanas* because each pose is held for no longer than two seconds, one following on from the other in a continuous movement. Yoga asanas are usually held for at least 30 seconds. Although it looks quite complicated, with practice you will soon be able to perform the sequence as a flowing movement with synchronised breathing. If you are reasonably supple, you should have little difficulty bending into each position.

However, if your muscles and joints are unused to this type of exercise, it is essential to take it slowly, only bending as far as your body will allow without causing pain. Indeed, the emphasis is not on perfect performance, but on the ability to focus inwards through breathing and movement. Whatever you achieve is right for you. After a short while you will find your muscles and joints loosening and allowing a free flow of movement. Repeat the entire sequence two or three times. As your stamina and flexibility increase, eventually you will enjoy performing ten or even twelve rounds, three or four times a week.

Perform the Sun Salutation in the morning before breakfast or, if more convenient, late afternoon before your evening meal. If practised regularly, it will lubricate the joints, improve circulation, massage the internal organs and increase strength and suppleness. At the same time, you will experience increased joy and vitality. To enhance the feeling, vaporise essences which suggest bright flowers, fruits and sunlight. Choose one or two of your favourites from the following possibilities: bergamot, coriander, geranium, grapefruit, lemongrass, mandarin, melissa, orange, palmarosa, petitgrain, rose otto.

SUN SALUTATION (SURYA NAMASKAR)

Take off your shoes and wear comfortable, loose clothing such as a T-shirt and leggings, a track suit or, if it is warm enough, just a pair of briefs. It is important not to restrict your breathing or hinder leg movement.

1 Stand erect with your feet together and your hands in a prayer position held at the solar plexus (midriff). Lift the chest and expand the ribs as you look straight ahead.

2 As you slowly breathe in, raise your arms overhead; bend back to arch your spine.

3 On the exhalation, bend forward as far as you can go without strain. If possible, place your hands flat on the floor beside your feet (or as far down as your body will comfortably allow). Let your knees bend and soften if this helps. Indeed, only very flexible people should attempt to do this movement with straight legs as it may cause pain and spasm in the lower back.

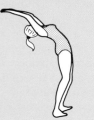

4 Inhale. Move your right leg in a backward step, knee touching the floor. The left knee should be between the hands with the foot flat on the floor. Look straight ahead. (When repeating the exercise remember to reverse position of legs.)

5 Holding on to the breath, and without shifting the right leg, raise the knee off the floor, then move the left leg in a backward step to meet the right foot. Toes are turned in and the body is elevated into a 'press-up' position, but with the arms fully stretched and palms flat on the floor. Look straight ahead.

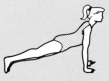

6 Exhale. Gently bend your knees to touch the floor and slowly slide the body down so that forehead and chest come into contact with the floor.

7 On the inhalation straighten your legs and bend backwards, looking up at the ceiling with arms straight, elbows close to the body and palms firmly on the floor.

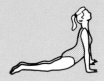

8 As you exhale arch your back into a cat's stretch, head down between your arms. Do not strain, keep your head limp.

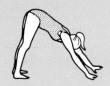

9 Inhale. Bring the right leg forward alongside the palms. The left foot and knee should touch the floor. (When repeating the exercise, reverse the position of the legs.)

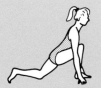

10 On the exhalation, bend forward until your hands are in line with your feet (or as far down as your body will allow). Tighten your abdomen and bring your head as close as possible to your knees, allowing the knees to bend a little to ease the movement.

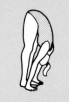

11 As you inhale, raise your arms overhead; bend back to arch your spine.

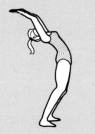

12 As you exhale, lower your arms to your sides.

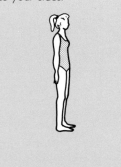

Once you have completed a few rounds of the Sun Salutation, with a 30 second rest between each cycle, lie down on a firm surface (preferably a carpeted floor covered with a blanket or yoga mat) and allow yourself to completely let go. Lie there for at least five minutes, allowing your breathing and pulse rate to return to normal. When you are ready, have a good stretch from fingertips to toes; roll over to one side and slowly get up.

DEEP RELAXATION

By inducing a slight shift in consciousness, deep relaxation enhances our ability to concentrate and to use imagery for self-healing and, indeed, for the healing of others (see Chapter 20). It is also the key which opens the door to the wisdom of the so-called higher self. When we access this part of our being, it may be experienced as sudden insight into a problem which may have seemed insoluble, or as a surge of creative energy, inspiration or enhanced intuition. Even though the relaxation response is relatively fleeting, the benefits are far reaching and accumulative. Each time you return from your sojourn, you will feel refreshed and revitalised, and thus better able to cope with the ups and downs of life.

Before you begin, find a quiet well-ventilated room with a pleasantly relaxing decor. Wear loose, comfortable clothing, and take off your shoes. If you live in a noisy area, it may also be helpful to play a tape of gentle music, but keep the volume down very low as your senses will be especially acute. Most important, ensure that you will not be disturbed for at least fifteen minutes.

Incidentally, if you have a friend or partner with a soft voice, perhaps they could be persuaded to guide you through the sequence – at least for a few sessions until you are familiar with the process. Or you could possibly record the instructions on to tape and listen to the sound of your own voice if you are happy with its tone. The instructions must be spoken very slowly, softly and clearly, pausing after each one to allow time for the breathing and stretching to be carried out.

The following essences, which are often included in traditional incense mixtures to enhance meditation, may be vaporised into the room to evoke a peaceful atmosphere and help deepen your breathing: cedarwood, frankincense, galbanum, juniper berry, myrrh, sandalwood.

DEEP RELAXATION SEQUENCE

1 Lie down on the floor or on a firm bed and have pillows for support if desired – one under your head and another under your knees which will support your lower back.

2 Close your eyes, take a few deep breaths through your nose, then breathe out through your mouth with a sigh … (If you are recording this or guiding a friend through the sequence, remain silent for about 30 seconds before moving on to the next instruction.)

3 Now become aware of your feet. Inhale through your nose, tighten your feet by first pointing your toes, and then flexing your feet towards your body. Hold on to this tension for a slow count of five…Now let them relax as you breathe out with a sigh.

4 Become aware of your knees. Inhale through your nose, tighten your knees, holding on to the tension for a slow count of five…Now let them go as you breathe out with a sigh.

5 Allow your attention to move to your thighs. Inhale through your nose, tighten your thighs, holding on to the tension for a slow count of five…Breathing out with a deep sigh of relief, let go of your thighs. Feel a wonderful sensation of release.

6 Now think of your buttocks. Inhale through your nose, tighten your buttocks, holding on to the tension for a count of five… Now let them go as you breathe out with a deep sigh of relief.

7 Now become aware of your abdomen. Inhale through your nose, tighten those muscles, holding on to the tension for a count of five… Then release, breathing out with a deep sigh.

8 Allow your attention to move to your chest. Inhale through your nose, tighten those chest muscles for a slow count to five… As you breathe out with a sigh, let go and relax.

9 Move your awareness to your shoulders. Breathe in through your nose, hunch your shoulders, pull them up towards your ears, holding on to the tension for a slow count of five… Now release your shoulders as you breathe out with a deep sigh.

10 Think of your hands. Breathe in through your nose, tighten your hands into fists, holding on to the tension for a count of five… Now release your hands as you breathe out with a deep sigh of relief.

11 Allow your attention to move to your arms. Tighten your arms, feeling the tension right down to your fingertips. Hold on to that tension for a count of five… As you breathe out through your mouth, let go and relax.

12 Think of your neck. Breathe in through your nose. Now arch your neck, holding on to the tension for a count of five… Release the tension as you breathe out through your mouth.

13 Allow your attention to focus on your face and scalp. Take a deep breath through your nose, now clench your jaw and screw up your face into a terrible grimace, holding on to the tension for a slow count of five… Now breathe out through your mouth with a deep sigh of relief. Experience a wave of deep relaxation moving over your whole body, from the top of your head right down into your toes. Experience a wonderful sensation of release… (If you are recording this or guiding a friend, remain silent for about a minute before moving on to the next instruction.)

14 Become aware of your body again and 'feel' around with your mind for any areas that may still be tense. Repeat the tightening and releasing of muscles until you feel deeply relaxed . Remain in this beautiful state for a while, perfectly at ease, perfectly at peace . (If you are recording this or guiding a friend, remain silent for five to ten minutes before moving on to the next instruction, which must be spoken very softly so as not to startle the listener.)

15 Now it is time to move out of your inner sanctuary, to return to everyday awareness. Raise your arms overhead and have a really good stretch from fingertips to toes. When you feel ready, roll over to one side before slowly getting up.

This exercise is most beneficial if practised once a day (twice a day if you have time) for the first two weeks, then three or four times a week thereafter, and at any other time when you feel stressed. For best results, do not carry out immediately after a heavy meal. Wait for at least two hours, or until you feel comfortable. On the other hand, if you do the exercise whilst very hungry, your rumbling stomach will distract your attention!

OTHER WAYS TO RIDE THE WAVES

Nature in her myriad forms is perhaps the most potent de-stressor of all, uplifting the spirits of the downhearted and offering tranquillity to the frenzied. So, whenever possible, get out into the countryside, or take a walk around the local park, breathe deeply and delight in the sights, sounds, textures and scents of the earth.

If you are suffering from the kind of stress born of a monotonous existence, make every effort to break the routine. This may sound obvious, but is easy to overlook when you are in a rut. Visit new places as often as possible; follow up sudden notions; take up a new hobby; read a different kind of book, newspaper or magazine from usual; join an adult education class; provide for compensatory physical activity.

- If you are suffering from low self-esteem, indulge in self-nurturing activities. Luxuriate in an aromatic bath; massage your body with aromatic oils; prepare a delicious meal and eat it in style – even if you are alone; buy yourself an attractive picture card, exotic fruit or scented candle; lose yourself in an uplifting film, novel, or play; listen to joyful music – or whatever else makes you feel good.

- Often we assume that all negative emotions are destructive, and so we try to put on a brave face. As a long-term option, however, this can lead to chronic negativity that festers beneath the surface and becomes the root cause of all manner of physical ailments. It is important therefore to express negativity in order to release it. So whenever powerful emotions such as anger begin to well up, especially if such feelings have become habitual, don't take it out on family and friends. There are ways of harmlessly discharging the aggression. If possible, find an isolated spot, such as the middle of a field, a hilltop, or perhaps beside a fast-flowing river or stream. Then take a deep breath and scream or shout with all your might, releasing the pent-up jealousy, anger, hatred, or whatever it might be. If isolation is impossible (as is often likely), the next best option is to scream or shout into a deep pillow or cushion to muffle the sound, then beat the hell out of it with your fists or a cricket bat.

- If your surroundings at home are dull, make every effort to improve the situation. Put fresh flowers or potted plants around the house. If possible, re-decorate at least one room in your home with positive and joyful colours such as shades of yellow and gold, peach, clear greens and pinks. Create a cheery atmosphere by vaporising your favourite essential oils. Similarly, try to wear uplifting colours instead of murky greys and a lot of black. According to colour therapists, dark hues can aggravate depression in susceptible individuals. It is a great pity that most school uniforms are based around black, navy and grey, colours which are hardly compatible with the exuberance of youth.

- Psychologists point out that those who are 'ultra-conforming' to a higher standard than society wants them to be, commonly suffer from chronic anxiety or depression. On the contrary, non-conformists tend to live longer and seldom get seriously depressed. The secret, we are told, is to be found in the healing power of laughter, especially that which takes the form of a mischievous sense of humour. So next time the going gets too serious, step back for a moment and have a good belly laugh at yourself and society – and glory in your individuality!

20

DEVELOPING YOUR HEALING POTENTIAL

So far we have concentrated mainly on self-healing, which is actually an important prerequisite for developing your innate ability to heal others. Here we shall delve a little deeper into the mind/body phenomenon. However, the exercises and techniques advocated may not appeal to everyone, for they demand a great deal of faith in one's ability to access the intuitive aspect of mind. Just in case you are thinking this chapter is going to be seriously weird, it should be mentioned that exploring your own innerscape may be somewhat out of the ordinary, but it can also be fun! We will begin with a brief survey of the human aura, then we shall explore one or two subtle methods of diagnosis and healing, and consider how these might be incorporated to enhance the experience of giving and receiving aromatherapy massage.

THE AURA

> *'Matter is the most spiritual in the perfume of the plant.'*
>
> RUDOLPH STEINER

Auras are real. All living beings have auras. Non-sentient manifestations of matter such as stones and water have auras too. The idea of the unity of all things in nature is embraced by quantum physics, which recognises a world of energy in the making, a subtle world where everything interacts and so influences everything else. At the molecular, atomic and subatomic levels even so-called 'dead' matter is buzzing with the same movement and energy which animates all life forms. The aura, or electro-magnetic field as it is known in science, is merely a reflection of this subliminal movement.

Interestingly, the word 'aura' is derived from the Greek

avra meaning breeze because it is said to be continuously in motion. Seers both ancient and modern describe the aura as a rainbow-coloured emanation radiating at least half a metre around the body, more or less ovoid in shape. The energy around the head is especially luminous, shimmering and altering in colour depending on our thoughts, emotions and physical state. Muddy colours in the aura indicate negative emotions or ill health; clear colours are generally a positive sign. Just as we can smell the ethereal fragrance or aura of a flower, some healers (especially acupuncturists) are able to smell the human aura; and this is quite apart from a person's usual body odour.

But is there any tangible evidence for the existence of the human aura? Up until recently if we wanted to find out about the state of our subtle body we had to take a psychic's word for it; a high-voltage technique known as Kirlian photography has been used since the 1930s to detect certain radiations from people, plants and material objects. But Kirlian photographs show only a small part of the aura, that which emanates just a few centimetres from the physical form. Much more advanced equipment has since been developed, along with a new diagnostic and therapeutic technique known as *electrocrystal therapy*. Quartz crystals are mechanically stimulated by high-energy, high-frequency radio signals (reputedly harmless) and are beamed into the body. The nature and frequency of the body's returning signals, which are displayed on a VDU screen in technicolour detail, indicates whether the tissues being scanned are healthy or otherwise.

Using this device, researchers were amazed to discover that certain energy centres or vortices of light exist within the body, and these coincide exactly with the chakra system, used in the East. The Sanskrit word *chakra* means wheel or circle. There are said to be at least seven major chakras, five of which radiate from points along the midline of the body, while the sixth and seventh are located between the eyebrows and just above the crown of the head. To the trained eye, the quality of light, colour and vibration of the chakras indicate whether there is dysfunction within the physical body.

Most interestingly, changes in the energetic body occur well before they manifest on the physical level, which means that subtle scanning techniques can be used as an early warning sign of impending illness. Steps can then be taken to nip the disease process in the bud, before it takes root in the body. Bio-electronic diagnostic and therapeutic techniques might even be the focus of medicine in the future.

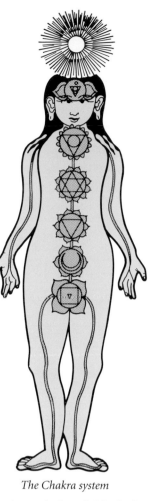

The Chakra system

The most popular aura-capturing technique is bio-feed-back imaging. The camera, which imposes the auric field on polaroid film, has been used in the USA since the early 1980s. It has been used to show the subtle effects of the Himalayan flower essences (similar to the Bach flower remedies, see page 50) on the aura. In fact, any holistic therapy, including aromatherapy massage, will influence the auric field for the better, usually within minutes of receiving treatment.

PERCEIVING AURAS THE NATURAL WAY

To see the aura without the aid of high-tech devices requires a certain amount of training, unless you are especially sensitive, but most people can *feel* the energy to a greater or lesser degree. The following method for detecting auric energy is sometimes demonstrated on introductory healing courses.

1 Find yourself a willing partner and sit or stand facing each other. Both of you need to hold out your hands in front and turn the right palm downwards and left palm upwards. Keeping your hands in this position, place them against the hands of your partner. Close your eyes, relax and become aware of your partner's hands; feel the warmth of their body and allow yourself to relax into the experience. After about 30 seconds of attunement, both of you need to raise your right hand above the other's upturned left hand, but it should remain loose and relaxed, not held stiffly because you will reduce any sensitivity. Stay there for a few minutes and you will begin to experience one of several sensations: it may be a slight breeze (as the ancient Greeks described the energy), or perhaps a tingling sensation, heat, especially in the palms, a sensation of cold, static or even a magnetic pull. Each of these sensations has a specific meaning to experienced healers, but for the purpose of this experiment it is enough to become aware of the energy.

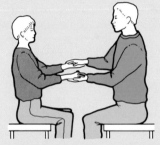

2 Now see how far you can move your hands away from each other and still experience the sensation. Move your hands back and forth or in circles, as if polishing a table, but keep your hands loose and relaxed. You may feel a curious pulling sensation, as though fluid were being drawn from your hands, or you might experience the movement as static.

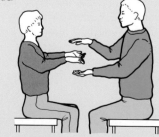

3 To break contact, move your hands close together again, slide them away and give them a good shake to remove any sensations you may have picked up.

AURIC CONTROL

If the above experiment proved successful, you will understand how easy it is for open and receptive individuals to pick up sensations from each other, both pleasant and unpleasant. This can also occur when giving ordinary physical massage, whether or not you are consciously aware of auric energy. Therefore, therapists of almost all schools of holistic healing employ certain 'grounding' and 'cleansing' visualisations to strengthen the aura and help prevent any lingering feelings of discomfort from distressed clients.

Whether or not you wish to become a professional health care practitioner, by learning to strengthen your own vibrations, you will help to uplift the spirits of those who may seek your help. Indeed, even though we may choose to overlook the fact, we humans are sensitive to the energy fields of others in our sphere. If this seems unlikely think how often you have felt inexplicably uneasy in the presence of another. Conversely, you have probably experienced joy in the presence of an unusually vibrant person.

GROUNDING

It is common to feel somewhat light-headed or 'distant' after giving or receiving healing in one form or another, whether it be the traditional aromatherapy massage or something much more subtle. To dissipate such sensations, most important if you are to carry out everyday activities immediately after a healing session, you must ground yourself. This simply means becoming aware of your physical body, especially your feet in contact with the ground. Close your eyes and imagine that your feet are like the roots of a tree, firmly in contact with the earth. Then feel that you are centred along a straight line running from the top of your head to your feet. This should have a calming and stabilising effect. But if it does not work, make yourself a warm drink and have a bite to eat; nothing will bring you back down to earth more speedily. (To help ground another person at the end of an aromatherapy massage, see page 192.)

VISUALISATION

To cleanse and strengthen your aura, close your eyes and imagine that you are centred within a sphere of white, blue or golden light which also permeates your body. If you cannot 'see' the sphere of light (not everyone has good visualisation skills) try to 'feel' that you are enclosed in a protective field (like the yolk within an egg) and that the energy around you is unbroken, especially over your head.

With practice, this visualisation (or feeling) of your auric space will become an automatic process. It can be carried out at any time when you feel the need, for example, when you are near anyone with a cold or flu, a strong aura is the metaphysical equivalent to a strong immune system; when you are experiencing any form of fear; when you feel distressed by noise; first thing in the morning and last thing at night; after a yoga or meditation session; or after giving intuitive aromatherapy massage.

OTHER WAYS TO CLEANSE YOUR AURA AND GROUND YOURSELF

If you find visualisation difficult, there are more tangible ways to cleanse your aura of unwanted sensations. However, in order for these to have the desired effect, they must be performed with conscious intent, not as empty ritual or in an absent-minded way. The simplest method is to wash your hands under a running tap, releasing any distress or tension that you may have picked up simply by thinking of it being washed away. Then become aware of your feet in contact with the ground; stamp your feet if this makes it easier. Alternatively, and if practicable, you could take a shower with the same intent.

Aromatherapists also wash their hands before giving massage, perhaps concentrating their attention into them and thinking of their hands as a conveyer of healing energies. You too may find this helpful.

The most natural way to balance and ground yourself is to commune with nature. If possible, go for a brisk walk after giving massage, preferably in the park or countryside, or do some gardening.

Yet another way to release negativity is to awaken to the spirit of the dance, especially that which is undirected and free. This is best performed alone, unless you feel you can be completely uninhibited dancing with others, in which case, dance with those who share the same purpose as yourself. Ignore any preconceived ideas you may have and put on some earthy music with a strong rhythmic pulse of at least 90 beats a minute – fast primitive drumming would be ideal – and forget how you look and move!

If none of the above appeals, or is impracticable, there is one other way. At the end of an aromatherapy massage, some aromatherapists ritualistically rub into their forearms a few drops of a 'psychically cleansing' essence such as juniper, rosemary or frankincense. Whether the efficacy of this practice lies within the subtle properties of the oil itself, or because of the aromatherapist's *belief* in the oil's healing powers, makes little difference. If it works, it works!

CREATING A HEALING CHANNEL

Without getting too deeply into the philosophy of intuitive healing, you may wish to take things a stage further. The aim of the following exercise is to connect your own consciousness with a universal source of healing energy, and to channel this force down through your body and out through your hands to the recipient. If done correctly, both parties will feel revitalised. A common mistake is to attempt to give your own vitality to the other person, which can result in you feeling drained afterwards.

Whether or not a universal healing energy actually exists does not matter. The important thing is to *believe* you are a conduit or a channel through which the healing energy can flow. The power of mind-over-matter is everything.

Of course, it is very important for both giver and recipient to feel at ease with each other, to experience a special empathy. Without empathy it is unlikely that much in the way of healing in the spiritual sense will take place. To empathise is not only to put ourselves in another's place, it is also to be able to connect both with our own and with the other person's inner strength. In so doing, we help to lift them from their negativity, without becoming engulfed by their suffering. It is vital to recognise the difference between empathy and sympathy. The feeling of empathy is closely linked with our intuitive self which is why it is extremely difficult to teach empathy as a skill, whereas sympathy hooks into our personal distress, thereby draining our emotional energy.

If the recipient of your healing feels wonderful afterwards, you cannot take all the credit for the success of the treatment. The healer is merely a catalyst in the process. No one can be healed (spiritually or physically) if at one level, perhaps unconscious, they do not wish to be healed, or if they cannot trust or let go of any fears that may be blocking the flow of healing energies. Indeed, every healer has come across the person who just does not get better, despite their doing everything 'right'.

The following visualisation for creating a healing channel and closing down afterwards is one which I use most often. If it feels appropriate to you, it can be practised a few minutes before giving aromatherapy massage, or prior to offering any other form of therapy.

1 Take several complete breaths (see page 145), either standing or lying down on a firm but comfortable surface.

2 Close your eyes and think of your aura as a sphere of white, blue or golden light surrounding and interpenetrating your body, or feel that you are protected within an energy field. Then imagine that you are centred along a straight line running from the top of your head to your feet. Feel perfectly balanced and calm.

3 Imagine or feel a source of energy above your head, a ball of white or golden light. You may find it easier to think of the energy source as either the sun or moon, whichever you feel most drawn to. At this point you can either address your 'higher self', think of this as a wise being, or say a prayer asking that you may draw down healing energy, or be given the ability to help the person in the way best suited to their needs.

4 Now take a few deep breaths. As you inhale, imagine you are drawing energy from the source of light, in through the top of your head, and out through your hands and feet as you exhale. You may begin to feel a tingling in your hands, or an expansive sensation around your head. Some people feel an 'opening' in the heart region. Even if you feel nothing at all this does not matter; it can take a great deal of practice to recognise subtle changes in consciousness. Simply allow yourself to feel balanced and relaxed. When you are ready, begin the massage (see Part 4).

5 At the end of the massage, send a closing thought to the other person; 'see' or feel that they are separate from yourself, safely enclosed within their own aura. Then, as in Step 2, think of yourself safely enclosed within your own auric space and centred along a straight line. Become aware of your feet in contact with the ground. Then, if you wish, imagine a spiral of white or golden light swirling clockwise from the earth and moving upwards from your feet to the top of your head. Feel that you are centred within the spiral of light.

THE SUBTLE APPROACH TO PRESCRIBING

Some aromatherapists employ subtle methods such as pendulum dowsing and muscle testing for determining which essential oils are safe and beneficial for individual clients. Although it can take time to perfect such skills, if you are drawn to this area of research you will find it both fascinating and rewarding. As well as being a tool for ascertaining the most appropriate essences for yourself (or another person), the same methods can be employed for identifying hidden food allergies.

PENDULUM DOWSING

The pendulum is simply one method of many for communing consciously with the intuitive aspect of your being. Even though there is a myriad of beautiful and intricately designed pendulums available from craft fairs and complementary therapy centres, it is easy enough to make your own. The simplest is to attach a wedding ring, pendant-shaped crystal earring, or a glass bead to an 8 inch piece of strong cotton thread. Alternatively, insert a needle into the centre of a cork (a wine bottle cork, for instance). The eye of the needle will provide a place for attaching the cotton thread.

Before you can use the pendulum, you will need to ascertain which direction of swing means 'yes', 'no' or neutral. Most pendulum users regard a clockwise motion as meaning 'yes', an anticlockwise movement as 'no' and a side-to-side movement, whether in a vertical or horizontal direction, as neutral.

To determine an aromatic prescription for yourself or for another, hold your pendulum over each of the essences to be tested. Cover the labels so as not to influence the outcome through auto-suggestion. Give yourself a 3 or 4 inch thread length or whatever length works best for you. While you are holding the pendulum with a relaxed hand and an open mind, ask silently or aloud whether the oil being tested is appropriate. If you are unused to working intuitively, you will be surprised to discover that after a minute or so the pendulum will begin to gyrate in one of the directions mentioned above, without any conscious effort on your part. It is estimated that nine out of ten people can cause a pendulum to move by the subtle power of the psyche. If, however, the pendulum remains still, the answer to your question is definitely 'no'. A neutral response could mean that the oil may be required at a later date.

If you get no response whatsoever, even though you may have tested a number of different oils, then dowsing is obviously not your forte.

Incidentally, if you have a large selection of essential oils you may prefer to dowse up to a dozen at one time. Those to be dowsed should be determined by your own experience and knowledge of the oils' therapeutic properties and/or via the aroma preference route. If the pendulum comes up with more than five essences, the maximum employed by most aromatherapists, simply trust your aromatic good taste and knowledge of compatible blending to make the final choice.

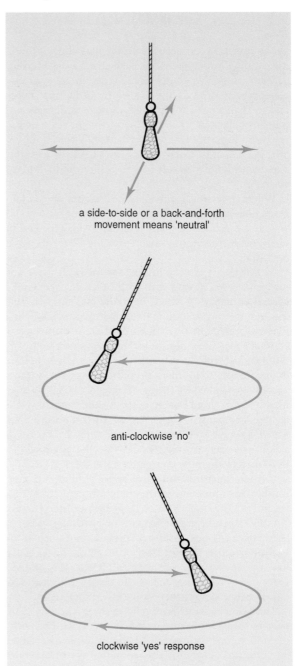

a side-to-side or a back-and-forth movement means 'neutral'

anti-clockwise 'no'

clockwise 'yes' response

MUSCLE TESTING

The muscle testing exercise given here is one of many employed by practitioners of kinesiology or Touch for Health. You will need to find a sympathetic partner with whom to work. You may wish to take turns at being tester and subject.

The subject needs to stand erect with their right arm raised to a horizontal position. With their right hand, the tester pushes gently down for two seconds, with the palm open, on the subject's extended arm, to feel the normal muscle strength. Then the subject holds a bottle of essential oil in their left hand. The tester then reassesses the subject's muscle power by gently pressing down on the raised arm. If the oil registers as positive, the subject's arm will stay up. However, if an essential oil is unsuitable the arm may shake or give way under the slightest pressure. In other words, the most beneficial essences will strengthen the muscle, or will have no effect, while those of no value at the time of the test will weaken the muscle.

Just because an essential oil appears to weaken a muscle, this does not mean it is necessarily toxic to the individual concerned. We might say that the all-knowing aspect of the subject's psyche decides whether or not an essential oil is appropriate for their needs at the time. The intuitive self then communicates its decision through the mind/body, answering 'yes', or 'no' in its own way. However, when using muscle testing, or dowsing, for detecting allergies to essential oils or food substances, a negative response may well indicate that a particular substance is potentially harmful.

Always remember that while subtle methods of prescribing can be remarkably accurate, in the right hands, they should not be relied upon at the total expense of the mundane approach to choosing oils. If you are an adept dowser or muscle tester, by all means use these skills to broaden the possibilities of aromatherapy. But it is enough to have a good knowledge of your chosen essential oils spiced with a little intuition.

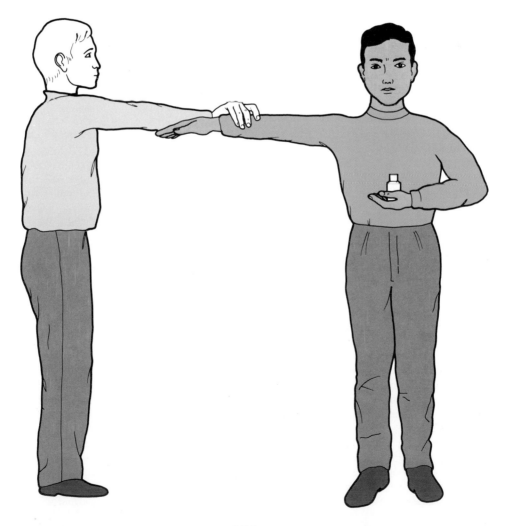

21
SCENTS OF MYSTERY AND IMAGINATION

Have you ever smelled a fragrance whose distantly familiar resonance elicited the frustrated response, 'It reminds me of something, but I can't think what', or tried to find the exact word or phrase to describe a certain scent whose essential nature was on the very tip of your tongue, yet remained unsayable? At such moments, scent has a kind of magical quality: a misty shape that emerges from the pool of forgetfulness just when you thought it had gone forever. In truth, once remembered, odours are rarely if ever forgotten, for they have the power to stir deep emotions. Indeed, catch a whiff of an aroma from childhood, for instance the shampoo your mother used, your father's tobacco, an old armchair, the garden shed, and you will be transported in an instant. But, just as one scent may summon to mind a joyful memory, another may cause the heart to move with grief.

When it comes to defining a particular aroma, be it apple pie, olive oil, honeysuckle or wet fur, could you describe the odour to someone who has never smelled it? At best, you might compare it with other scents, or with textures, colours, shapes, sounds or tastes, or even with a certain atmosphere or spirit of place. For instance, an aroma may smell sweetly mellow with a spicy kick, or fruity with a rounded edge, or like honey, vanilla fudge, wet leaves, or, more imaginatively, raucous like a scarlet-clad trumpet player, or mysterious and protective like an ancient forest. There is a place in the deep psyche where the senses intermingle and become a wonderland of perception. Those endowed with the condition known as *synaesthesia* will know what this can mean. For example, when subjected to loud sound, whether it be the noise of a train, a football crowd or the bombastic strains of the 1812 Overture, the synaesthete will experience a firework display of colours and shapes. Or there may be an idiosyncratic sensitivity to flashing neon lights whose garish display impinges upon the mindscape as a cacophony of sound.

Even though full-blown synaesthesia is rare, a great many people experience the phenomenon to some degree when exposed to fragrance. For instance, heavy scents like musk seed oil, patchouli and vetiver are commonly perceived as dark brown or olive green, resonating in harmony with the deep timbre of the cello. Lighter fragrances such as bergamot, lemon and geranium manifest to the synaesthete in various tones of bright orange, yellow and red, in tune with the high-pitched sound of the flute or piccolo.

SMELL AND THE MIND/BODY

Let us now consider exactly how odours are perceived and why they can have such a profound influence on the mind/body complex.

Any substance which has an odour gives off volatile scent molecules. Before these microscopic gaseous molecules can be detected, they must be drawn up with the in-breath to a yellowish patch in the roof of the nose. This is called the olfactory epithelium, which measures about five square centimetres and contains up to fifty million odour receptor cells, each bearing microscopic hair-like structures called cilia. These cells, technically speaking they are brain cells, are specialised sensory neurones embedded in a mucous membrane, each connecting directly with the brain by means of a single long nerve fibre.

Before the aroma molecules can be detected by the cilia, they must first be dissolved in the mucus. Responses to the aroma molecules are then sent in the form of electro-chemical impulses via the nerve fibres to the olfactory bulb, a part of the brain which actually extends into the nose.

The olfactory area of the brain is an aspect of the mysterious limbic system, which is sometimes called the 'old brain' or 'smell brain'. Evolutionists maintain that the two cerebral hemispheres of the brain, the 'right brain' and 'left brain', actually developed from the ancient olfactory lobes and that as the brain became more complex the instinctive smell brain remained at the forefront. Although the limbic area is largely uncharted territory, we do know that it is concerned with our instinctive drives: emotion, intuition, memory, creativity, hunger, thirst, sleep patterns, sex drive, and probably much more. Through the limbic system the interconnecting hypothalamus and pituitary bodies are stimulated, thus creating a cascade of responses in the whole mind/body complex (refer back to the Body Systems in Part 2).

So odour perception occurs mainly in the instinctive right hemisphere of the brain, virtually by-passing the cerebral cortex or left hemisphere which is concerned with language and other logical or conscious thought processes. Not surprisingly, then, we become somewhat lost for words in our attempt to make sense of that which is primitive and instinctive. However, within a moment of experiencing an emotional response to an odour, we attempt to regain our equilibrium by calling upon the left hemisphere for some kind of clarity, perhaps by trying to put a name to the scent. In fact, all too often we block our intuitive faculties by allowing the cerebral cortex to dominate. Ideally, we need to make full use of both aspects of mind.

To take a simple and well-known example of the primitive effect of aroma on the mind/body, catch a whiff of your favourite food, especially when you are feeling hungry, and your mouth will water, the digestive juices in the stomach will flow, and if it is a special festive dish, you will probably have many joyful memories to savour as well.

THE SHAPE OF SCENT

Despite a great deal of research into the study of olfaction, the precise mechanism which enables us to differentiate between odours is still largely a matter of conjecture. The best known explanation, and one which is popular amongst perfumers, is the *stereochemical* theory put forward in the late 1940s by the British chemist J.E. Amoore. Like primary colours, so the theory goes, all odours fall into a number of basic categories: floral, minty, camphoraceous, resinous, ethereal, musky, foul, acrid, burnt, mouldy, grassy and so on. It is suggested that there may be a connection between the geometrical shape of an odoriferous molecule and the odour it produces. The theory is that when an odoriferous molecule comes in contact with a corresponding receptor site on an olfactory neurone, it triggers a nerve impulse to the brain. For example, floral odours are said to have a disc-shaped molecule with a tail which fits a bowl-and-trough site. Camphoraceous odours have a spherical molecule that fits into an elliptical site, whereas minty odours have a wedge-shaped molecule that fits into a V-shaped site. Some odours appear to fit more than one site at the same time, producing a bouquet effect.

Even though other more complicated theories abound, the stereochemical theory certainly makes sense to the synaesthete who may perceive the scent of rose, for instance, as a pinky-peach oval, the earthy aroma of patchouli as square, and the pungent odour of sweaty socks as a cascade of sandy-coloured triangles. Strange? Not at all, for these are my own scent impressions!

SMELL RANGE

Although there are considerable differences between the smell sensitivities of individuals, generally speaking the healthy human olfactory sense can detect over 10,000 different odours. Perfumers and native hunters, however, may be able to detect several times as many odours, both in lower amounts and from a greater distance. This is because the sense of smell can be enhanced through training (see page 158).

There are individuals who have a remarkable olfactory sense. One famous person with a highly developed sense of smell was the American Helen Keller, who was deprived of most of her senses excepting touch and smell. She could identify friends and visitors by their personal odours. And simply by smelling people she said that she could decipher 'the work they are engaged in. The odours of the wood, iron, paint, and drugs cling to the garments of those who work in them…When the person passes quickly from one place to another, I get a scent impression of where he has been; the kitchen, the garden or the sickroom.'

Then there was Albert Weber who made a profession of using his nose. In the 1970s he had been with the US Food and Drug Administration (FDA) for over thirty years. His job was to protect the public from rank food and drink. The very early stages of decomposition are extremely difficult for the average human nose to detect. By sniffing, Weber could analyse twenty-four cans of tuna in two hours. To do the analysis chemically would take a couple of days.

What was especially unusual about Weber's sense of smell was that he appeared not to suffer from odour fatigue or adaptation, the perfumer's stumbling block. After short exposure to the same scent, the average person's olfactory cells cease to convey the odour to the conscious mind. Yet release a different scent into the atmosphere, and this will be detected immediately, only to fade within minutes. A detested odour, on the other hand, will seem to linger for an eternity – perhaps as a natural safety mechanism to alert us to the potential toxicity of certain unpleasant odours.

IDIOSYNCRATIC PERCEPTIONS

Odours are multifaceted; a single odoriferous material may be composed of many different overtones and undertones. For this reason you may perceive a particular scent quite differently from someone else, singling out just a nuance of the whole. Or you may lack conscious sensitivity to the entire odour. For instance, it is common to be odour-blind or *anosmic* to some musks or to sandalwood essence, which is possessed of a musky element. Some people, while not being totally insensitive to sandalwood oil, have a *partial anosmia* to the aroma. One person may pick up the soft woody overtone of the fragrance, whereas another may be repulsed by the 'urinous' note which lingers beneath the surface.

There is also a condition known as *cacosmia*. With this type of disorder, sufferers tend to avoid protein-rich foods which smell foul to them. Although it is generally thought that victims of the disorder experience a form of odour hallucination, it would seem much more likely that they hone in on the subthreshold sulphurous compounds present in proteins. Alcoholics frequently suffer from cacosmia.

Schizophrenia can sometimes be accompanied by a heightened sense of smell. Sufferers may also be especially aware of their own body odour, which they find offensive. In fact, there are a few reports of medical staff having commented upon the unusual, not necessarily unpleasant, odour emanating from certain mentally ill patients.

Sadly, there are those people who cannot smell anything at all. Although it is possible to be born without a sense of smell, *total anosmia* can be caused by a variety of reasons such as nutritional deficiencies, especially zinc deficiency, underactive thyroid, allergy, nasal polyps, ageing, head injury, a brain tumour or exposure to toxic chemicals. Whatever the cause, life without a sense of smell can be bleak. Apart from the dangers of being unable to detect the odours of something burning or spoiled food, even the most ambrosial foods are rendered tasteless, smell and taste being interrelated functions. According to one sufferer of my acquaintance, 'Without smell it seems that life itself has lost its spice and zest'. It is also reported that a quarter of sufferers of anosmia experience loss of libido, but not every sufferer. Loss of libido as a result of anosmia may be related to the associated depression which accompanies the condition, as depression is a well-known dampener of desire.

Just why the human nose should be able to smell one scent and not another, or perceive only an aspect of a particular scent, or indeed why we should like some fragrances and not others, is something of a mystery. As far as aroma preference is concerned, natural body scent, age, race and odour conditioning are thought to be contributing factors.

PSYCHIC SCENTS

While psychics talk of such things as clairvoyance (psychic seeing), clairaudience (psychic hearing) and clairsentience or psychometry (psychic feeling), rarely if ever do they seek to develop their psychic sense of smell. There may well be a word for psychic smelling, but I have yet to discover it. In our arrogance, we in the modern world have relegated the sense of smell to the 'primitive' animal level. Yet smell may turn out to be the most psychic sense of all.

Time and time again I have witnessed the psychic nature of smell. Quite recently I was reminded of the phenomenon having received a letter from an occasional correspondent, a person whom I had never met. The notepaper seemed to emanate a pine-like fragrance, yet no one else could smell it. After a tentative enquiry, it transpired that my distant friend loved the scent of pine essence. At the time of writing the letter she had run out of the essential oil and had been thinking of buying some more!

There is also a potent auto-suggestive element to smell. Strictly for research purposes, I have succeeded in hoodwinking others into believing that a disliked essence was present in a blend of aromatic oils. Having discovered the dupe, one person became most irate with disbelief; he was certain that the 'horrible' lavender had actually been present, and that the experiment was some kind of double bluff!

I remember reading somewhere that it is possible to convince a room full of people that a pervasive 'odour' is wafting from a suitably intriguing-looking bottle filled with nothing but water. If given the suggestion that the smell is unpleasant, those who are extremely sensitive may be so disgusted by what they conjure up that they will feel obliged to leave the room! The way to break the spell is to inform everyone of the dupe. You may find it interesting to set up some experiments of your own to prove the existence of odour hallucination; do let me know the results of your research. A word of warning: a known side-effect is the loss of all but the most forgiving of friends!

ENHANCING YOUR SENSE OF SMELL

It may be possible to learn to detect an odour to which you were previously 'blind' simply by repeated exposure. Odour researchers have shown that people with a total or partial anosmia to sandalwood essence, though having a perfectly normal sense of smell in other respects, have been able to generate new receptors for this particular scent. The secret is simply to sniff the aroma several times a day for up to two months.

My own suggestion for broadening odour perception is to enter into a relaxed and receptive state before sniffing. Breathe slowly and deeply and become aware of your aura, sensing that the energy around your head is expanding and merging with that of the flower or volatile essence. When you feel ready, hold the flower or essential oil sample, preferably on a smelling strip or piece of blotting paper near to your nose, and inhale slowly and deeply, concentrating on the idea that you wish to become aware of the scent. With this method, you may learn to detect a hitherto elusive odour within days rather than months.

PSYCHO-AROMATHERAPY

Psycho-aromatherapy aims to combine the physiological effects of essential oils on the central nervous system with the recipient's subjective responses to the aroma. However, it is a great pity that this area of healing has fallen prey to all manner of myths and fantasies masquerading as cast iron fact. Instead of stepping back and allowing the reality of the subjective to be of sole importance to the individual concerned, attempts have been made to categorise essential oils according to the *specific* emotions they are supposed to evoke or dispel. For instance, sandalwood will help us overcome egocentricity and procrastination; rose will sweeten the jealous heart; and chamomile will add a spark of interest to a bored mind.

When used as a tool for personal growth, plant essences may well have helped the initiator of such claims to deal with the same emotional issues. I do not doubt for a moment that others, having learned of the oils' fabled ability to influence specific feelings, have successfully employed the essences for healing the same states of mind. The truth is that any oil can bring about any desired emotional change if we truly believe it has the ability to do so. The role played by the power of suggestion should never be underestimated.

In some instances, even when a person is unaware of an essence's supposed emotional effect, if the oil has been prepared specially for them by an aromatherapist who believes the oil will influence the emotions in a specific and positive way, yet does not communicate this to the recipient, chances are that it will still have the desired effect. This may sound somewhat confusing in view of the previous dismissive remarks about the emotional influence of essential oils. Nevertheless, if there is a special empathy between client and therapist great things are

possible (refer back to Chapter 20). It seems that the all-knowing aspect of self is forever striving to enlighten the relatively naive conscious mind by whatever means it can muster, even if this means communicating through a mediator; that is to say, via the therapist and their chosen therapeutic tool. Indeed, this intuitive/telepathic connection between therapist and client is a well-known phenomenon in traditional psychotherapy.

Generally speaking, unpleasant scents trigger discomforting thoughts and mood states, whereas pleasant fragrances evoke happy memories or feelings and may also enhance creativity and inspiration. However, even the perception of 'pleasant' and 'unpleasant' is highly subjective. For example, while the German poet Schiller's muse resided in the odour of rotten apples – he kept them in the drawer of his desk and would take a whiff whenever he needed to find the right word – Coleridge's lurked in decay, 'A dunghill at a distance smells like musk, and a dead dog like elderflowers'. Moreover, a certain aroma may make us feel uneasy if we have learned to associate it with some unpleasant experience. An elderly friend of mine, for example, cannot abide the scent of rose. One whiff and she is back in the schoolroom disempowered by the glare of the harsh schoolmistress who always smelled of a rose-scented perfume.

SCIENTIFIC RESEARCH

When it comes to the physiological effects of essential oil on the central nervous system, a great deal of scientific research has been carried out in recent years using EEG instruments which record the electrical activity of the brain and skin. Without doubt, certain essences exert a relaxing effect on the mind/body, others have a stimulating effect, whereas a few are apparently capable of engendering relaxation or mental alertness depending on the state of the individual. At the same time, if an aroma is perceived as pleasant, odour stimuli in the limbic system cause a release of certain 'happiness chemicals' such as encephaline and endorphins, which help to reduce pain and create feelings of well-being. A disliked essence, on the other hand, will not gain the same access, hence the importance of selecting essences to suit individual preferences.

Sometimes the results of scientific research are contrary to expectation. As an illustration, according to studies carried out in the 1970s by Professor Torii of Toho University (Japan), neroli and rose, which are normally considered to be sedative oils, were shown to have a stimulating effect. The discrepancy may well be related to the concentration of oil used in the experiments. For instance, according to Gattefosse, angelica essence in low concentration stimulates the brain, whereas a high concentration becomes narcotic. Moreover, individuals are not always sensitive to the whole aroma but only to certain nuances. Both neroli and rose, for example, have an awakening top note which gives way to a narcotic undertone. Therefore, while one person may respond to the enlivening aspect of the aroma, another may experience its sedative effect. Receptiveness to the whole aroma may result in the recipient being stimulated and relaxed at the same time. In other words, they will feel spiritually uplifted, yet physically relaxed.

SUBTLE AROMATHERAPY

Just as the human ear is 'deaf' to high and low frequency sound, vibrations that animals can hear, it does not mean that we cannot be affected by them. Studies carried out at Warwick University by Drs Steve Van Toller and George Dodd have shown that we can also respond both physically and emotionally to highly diluted fragrances, so diluted that we cannot smell them. The results of EEG testing showed very clear skin and brainwave responses to subthreshold fragrance. In fact, responses may be even more profound because the conscious mind does not step in to block out or modify the psycho-physical effect.

This is an exciting area deserving of a thorough and exhaustive investigation, for it may lead to the discovery of a completely new branch of subtle healing with plant essences which we might call 'homeo-aromatherapy'. Although it would be a pity to miss out on the wonderful fragrances of essential oils, homeo-aromatherapy would compare with the Bach flower remedy system of healing (though only a few of the remedies are prepared from fragrant flowers) and traditional homeopathic medicine. These remedies are so highly diluted that only the energy pattern, vibration or 'memory' of the original medicinal material remains in the lactose tablet (homeopathy) or the liquid (flower remedies). Yet if the correct remedy is chosen, the healing effect on the mind/body can be remarkable.

ADVANCED SMELLING TECHNIQUE

Rather than be persuaded by the subjective responses of others, the smelling technique you are about to learn will enable you to find your own way along the path of psycho-aromatherapy. The technique also serves as a basis for developing and trusting your intuition, which is essential to healing work of any nature.

Since none of the senses is so easily fatigued as the sense of smell, you will have to limit yourself to smelling just a few essences per session, certainly no more than six. Each oil should also be diluted at around 6 per cent in a highly refined vegetable oil with little or no odour of its own, for instance, six to eight drops of essential oil in one teaspoonful (5 ml) of grapeseed oil. Undiluted essences, as well as those in high concentration as suggested here, are very powerful and may cause headaches or nausea if inhaled for too long, especially in a stuffy or overheated room. So always work in a well-ventilated area which is also moderately warm and free from cooking and other household smells.

Choose a time when you are feeling calm and receptive, perhaps after carrying out the deep breathing or relaxation sequence suggested in Chapter 19. Sit in a comfortable position. Dip a smelling paper or thin strip of blotting paper into the oil. It is also a good idea to write the name of the oil on the dry end of the paper, especially when assessing more than two essences. Waft the smelling strip around in order to encourage vaporisation, then inhale the fragrance slowly and deeply, allowing yourself to experience its effect fully.

Stay with the fragrance for a couple of minutes. What does the aroma make you think of? Is it a feeling, memory or image you would like to have more often? Write down your impressions in a notebook, even if this amounts to single words like 'jolly', 'bracing', 'apples', 'woody', 'medicinal', or even in terms of sounds, tastes, textures, colours and shapes.

Having emphasised the importance of working with aromas you enjoy, there is one exception to the rule. Should an aroma make you feel uncomfortable in any way, perhaps evoking an unhappy memory or a disturbing image, you can actually use the essence as a healing tool. Even though it may at first seem like masochism, try to write about your feelings in as much detail as possible. It is by viewing a negative feeling in the light of conscious awareness that it becomes less threatening, perhaps totally disempowered. For instance, have you ever written a venomous letter to someone, but decided in the end not to post it? You probably felt a great deal better for having vented your wrath, and relieved that there were no embarrassing repercussions. Here's wishing you joy!

PSYCHO-AROMATHERAPY CHART

The following essences and perfumery materials (absolutes) have been categorised according to the most likely effects they may exert on the central nervous system. A few of those essences categorised as 'aphrodisiac' may also have a subthreshold pheromonal influence (see page 232). Always remember to choose according to your aroma preference. If the aroma is disliked or conjures up unpleasant memories or feelings, the conscious mind can easily override the effect of the aroma on the mind/body.

Stimulating	Balancing	Relaxing	Antidepressant	Aphrodisiac	Anaphrodisiac
Angelica	(relaxing or	Cedarwood	Basil	Angelica	(quells sexual
Black pepper	stimulating	Chamomile	Bergamot	Cardamom	desire)
Cardamom	according to state	Clary sage	Carnation	Carnation	
Carnation	of individual)	Cypress	absolute	absolute	Camphor
absoluteé+		Galbanum	Chamomile	Cedarwood	Marjoram (?)
Cinnamon	Basil	Hops	Clary sage	Cinnamon	
Cloves	Bergamot	Juniper	Frankincense	Clary sage	* May be
Elemi	Frankincense	Mandarin	Geranium	Cloves	stimulating if used
Eucalyptus	Geranium	Marjoram	Grapefruit	Coriander	in concentrations
Fennel	Lavender	Melissa (true)*	Jasmine absolute	Galbanum	above 0.05 to
Ginger	Lemongrass	Mimosa absolute*	Lavender	Ginger	1 per cent (see
Grapefruit	Neroli	Myrrh	Lemon	Jasmine absolute	Easy Measures
Jasmine absoluteé+	Rose absolute	Petitgrain	Lime	Neroli	chart, page 34).
Lime	Rose otto	Sandalwood	Mandarin	Nutmeg	
Nutmeg	Rose phytol	Valerian	Neroli	Patchouli	**May be relaxing
Orange		Vanilla absolute	Orange	Rose absolute	if used in
Palmarosa		(also the	Palmarosa	Rose otto	concentrations
Patchoulié+		infused oil,	Patchouli	Rose phytol	at or below
Peppermint		see page 38)	Petitgrain	Rosemary	0.05 per cent.
Pine		Vetiver	Rose absolute	Sandalwood	
Rosemary		Violet leaf	Rose otto	Vetiver	
Spike lavender		absolute	Rose phytol	Ylang ylang	
		Yarrow	Sandalwood		
		Ylang ylang*	Ylang ylang		

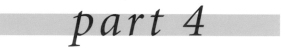

part 4

MASSAGE

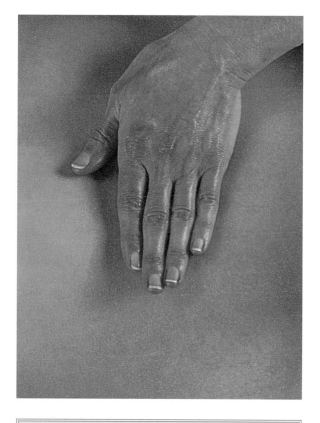

*The physician must be
experienced in many things but
assuredly rubbing… The way to
health is to have an aromatic bath
and scented massage every day.*

HIPPOCRATES

22
THE HEALING ART
OF MASSAGE

Throughout history therapeutic touch in some form or another, be it native shamanic or something much more technical, has been used to heal the sick and distressed. The healing power of massage was recognised and recorded by the physicians of ancient China, India, Egypt, Greece and Rome. And while most Eastern cultures have enjoyed a long tradition of massage therapy in this respect the West suffered a severe setback in the Middle Ages when the Church branded massage as a sinful 'pleasure of the flesh'.

At the beginning of the nineteenth century, massage made something of a come back when the Swedish gymnast Per Henrik Ling introduced his own style of massage which synthesised ancient Chinese techniques and passive gymnastic movements. Ling's methods were spread from his native Sweden by disciples and became immensely popular throughout Europe. Even to this day the term 'Swedish Massage' is used in tribute to Ling, and denotes a style of massage whose strokes are less vigorous than the deep tissue frictions and pummelling employed at the Turkish baths. Most other forms of massage which have developed since the nineteenth century (including aromatherapy massage) are at least partly influenced by the Swedish system.

Yet despite the current upsurge of interest in massage therapy, there are still those who cannot free themselves from the notion that massage is solely for tired sports enthusiasts or for clients of the dubious 'massage parlour'. Indeed, touch therapy is often undervalued, underused and sometimes grossly misunderstood.

In truth, massage is an advanced and conscious form of our instinctive and innate ability to offer healing through the laying-on-of-hands, whether it be the stroking of a furrowed brow or the rubbing of aching shoulders. In this respect, stroking and caressing may be just as important to our health as food and cleanliness. Indeed, psychologists tell us that tender loving touch, especially during infancy, is vital to our emotional and physical development.

When touching takes the form of skilled but sensitive massage, not only does it relax and revitalise an ailing or tired body, it is also a way of communicating warmth,

reassurance and a sense of self-worth. And when combined with the mood-enhancing properties of aromatic essences, we are nurtured on every level of our being, including the intangible spiritual level which may be embraced through our aesthetic appreciation of fragrance.

THE MIND/BODY EFFECTS OF MASSAGE

- Improves blood circulation and lymphatic drainage, and thus aids the elimination of tissue wastes such as lactic and carbonic acids which build up in the muscle fibres causing aches, pains and stiffness.
- Aids digestion and helps to prevent constipation.
- Can prevent and alleviate headaches.
- Encourages deep sleep and helps to prevent insomnia.
- Helps to reduce high blood pressure.
- Encourages deeper breathing and is therefore helpful for respiratory ailments. Deep breathing also brings about a sense of letting go, thus reducing stress levels.
- Triggers the release of mood-altering brain chemicals such as encephalin and endorphin which have the ability to reduce pain and engender a sense of well-being. Feelings of well-being also stimulate the immune system, and thus help in strengthening our resistance to disease.
- As tense muscles begin to relax, pent-up emotions are also sometimes freed. This may manifest as an overwhelming need to laugh or cry during the massage. Where there has been a great deal of stress and nervous tension the emotional release may be experienced as uncontrollable shaking, though this rarely continues for more than a few minutes. In every case, however, there is a subsequent feeling of renewed vitality.
- During massage or immediately afterwards, some people experience a light-headed sensation, as if they have had a few glasses of wine; a few fall into a deep sleep; many become tranquil; others who are prone to tiredness and lethargy suddenly feel more alert and energetic.

THE GIVER OF MASSAGE

Giving massage has its rewards too. As well as the enjoyment of knowing that we can help another person, we can lose ourselves in its rhythm and flow, and thus share in the recipient's experience of relaxation or elation. In other words, the giving of massage can be experienced as a form of active meditation.

To develop this concentration, you will need to attune to the needs of your partner. Although there are tangible signs of muscular tension which you can learn to recognise (see page 168) a good massage therapist also uses their intuitive faculties to sense which parts need soothing or revitalising. In order to build up this sensitivity, try not to talk too much during the massage. It is a great pity that some people chatter compulsively because they are afraid or embarrassed by silence or even of being touched. Yet it is usually during the quiet moments that subtle healing energies come to the fore. With practice and a genuine desire to help another, most of us can develop our healing potential. If you follow the sequence described in this chapter, you will soon acquire a good basic technique on which to develop your own intuitive style.

Before you begin the massage, however, it is important to be relaxed and in a positive frame of mind. Otherwise you may convey to your partner some of your own stress or negativity. Indeed, this is surprisingly easy to do in such intimate circumstances. You may find it helpful to do some deep breathing or yoga stretches such as those suggested in Chapter 19, or perhaps to carry out the aura strengthening visualisation described in Chapter 20 beforehand.

It is also important to wear loose, comfortable clothing. Remove jewellery and make sure your nails are cut short. Ask your partner to remove the necessary jewellery and clothes, but do respect their wishes if they feel happier wearing a pair of briefs, for instance.

THE RECIPIENT OF MASSAGE

To benefit fully from massage it is important to learn how to receive massage passively and with full awareness. If you constantly chatter and fidget, this is difficult to achieve. Instead, close your eyes, take a few deep breaths, then exhale with a sigh and relax into the experience. Concentrate your attention on your partner's touch and enjoy the sensation; allow your body to go heavy and limp. Allow your arms or your head, for instance, to be lifted and moved by your partner, rather than trying to help. Do speak up, of course, if something hurts, or if you feel cold or uncomfortable. Also, if your neck starts to feel stiff when you lie on your front, turn it to the opposite side.

CREATING A HEALING SPACE

Choose a peaceful room with a relaxing or uplifting atmosphere; certainly not a space screaming with busy zig zag patterns or garish colour clashes. Colour therapists tell us that jarring or harsh colour vibrations can affect us even when our eyes are closed. Equally, do not work in a room which emanates a morbid feeling, perhaps as a result of being decorated in murky hues. Most therapists would agree that neutral colours or pastel shades are far more conducive to relaxation and healing. The majority opt for soft greens, blues, pinks or mauves. However, there are a few therapists who would disagree with the pastel theme, preferring a single uplifting hue such as sunshine yellow or a warm peach. But whatever the colour scheme, do ensure that the room is spotlessly clean and uncluttered. It also needs to be very warm. It is surprisingly easy to become chilled when deeply relaxed, especially when the skin is coated in massage oil. Chilled muscles contract, causing a release of the stress hormone adrenalin, something you are trying to soothe away in the first place.

Give the massage in natural daylight if possible or under a soft lamp or candlelight. Harsh overhead lighting will remind you both of an operating theatre or a visit to the dentist! Even professional aromatherapists prefer to avoid too clinical a setting. Indeed, the healing power of aromatherapy stems from its ability to nurture all the senses, not just the sense of smell. A vase of fresh flowers, a potted plant or a bowl of fruit will enhance the healing space.

If you live in a noisy area, you may wish to block out background disturbance by playing relaxing music at low volume (the sense of hearing becomes especially acute when we are relaxed). Tapes or CDs of suitable music specially composed for relaxation or massage are available from good music shops, complementary therapy centres or New Age outlets. Although musical taste is highly subjective (just like our aroma preferences), specially composed music for relaxation has an unobtrusive air, a flowing quality whose rhythm deepens the relaxation response. If, however, your partner is one of the exceptional few who finds any form of music a distraction, do respect their wishes and turn it off.

THE MASSAGE SURFACE

Most professional aromatherapists use a purpose-built massage couch, which is ideal when doing a great deal of massage as it helps prevent back strain. However, it is more likely that you will have to work at floor level. Even though this can be hard work for the person giving the massage, it is actually better for the recipient because it will be easier for the giver of massage to apply beneficial pressure using their own body weight.

If you suffer from a weak back or poor muscle tone, but do not own a massage couch, it may be easier to give full-body massage on a solid wooden table – the old-fashioned farmhouse kitchen type is best. Ideally, it should be only a little wider than an average size single bed; otherwise it will be difficult to reach across in order to massage certain parts of the body. However, if you are very short or exceptionally tall, you may find that the table is at an awkward height. Professional couches are often custom built so that the top of the couch reaches to just below hip level.

Whether you are to give massage on the floor or on the kitchen table, a few blankets or perhaps a folded double-size duvet covered with towels will provide the necessary comfortable padding under your partner. You will also need one or two towels (a bath sheet is the best size) to place over your partner's body for warmth. It is necessary to expose only that part of the body you are massaging at the time. No matter what some of the glamorous massage manuals may indicate, professional massage therapists *never* leave a person completely uncovered, not only for reasons of warmth and modesty, but also because it can make the person feel vulnerable and isolated.

Massage can be given on a bed, but only if it has a firm mattress. If it is too soft, your partner will sink into it, and the mattress will absorb the beneficial pressure intended for their body. However, it is essential that you get on the bed and kneel beside your partner in order to carry out the massage, otherwise you will be forced to bend too much, which will cause discomfort to your back.

Similarly, when giving massage at floor level, never stand and bend from the waist. Apart from impeding the all-important flow of the massage, this will put an enormous strain on the lower back. Instead, kneel beside your partner. However, when giving back massage, some of the strokes can be performed whilst sitting astride your partner's thighs if you feel comfortable in this position (see the massage sequence beginning on page 169). The floor space where you intend to give the massage should, ideally, be carpeted to protect your knees. Alternatively, cover the area with a thick rug or a couple of blankets.

THE MASSAGE OIL

Prepare a suitable massage oil for your partner's physical and emotional needs. You will need about 1 to 1½ dessertspoonfuls of oil for a full-body massage, perhaps more if your partner has very dry skin, a great deal of body hair or is very big. If you intend to massage only one part of the body, the face, feet or hands, for example, you should need no more than one teaspoonful of oil. Put the oil into an attractive dish and place nearby, taking care not to knock it over as you work.

MASSAGE CAUTIONS

- Never massage a person who is suffering from fever or an infectious illness. Massage induces heat in the skin, muscles and joints which will exacerbate symptoms. More often than not, however, the person will feel disinclined to receive massage; an instinctive safety reaction.
- Never give firm massage directly over varicose veins.
- Never massage a person who suffers from thrombosis or phlebitis. Blood clots may become dislodged with the possibility of provoking a stroke.
- Never massage directly over skin rashes, skin ulcers, boils, swellings, bruises, sprains, torn muscles and ligaments, broken bones and burns. In any case, it is unlikely that the person would allow you to do so because any amount of pressure or friction will cause a great deal of discomfort.
- Even though massage is a marvellous pain reliever for arthritic and rheumatic complaints, never massage directly over swollen or inflamed areas (inflammation and swelling tends to flare up and die down at intervals) as this may cause further pain and tissue damage. However, regular massage over the vunerable areas at other times, when the pain and inflammation have subsided, will help to reduce the frequency of flare-ups.
- Always seek medical approval before massaging anyone suffering from a serious condition, such as advanced heart disease or cancer. In most cases, however, massage is an excellent therapy for soothing body and mind.
- Never massage a pregnant woman without first seeking the go-ahead from the woman's doctor or midwife.
- If something hurts, abandon the movement and move on to another area of the body.

MASSAGE TECHNIQUES

The basic sequence you are about to learn is a modified version of a professional aromatherapy massage. It is based on five massage movements: stroking (using the whole of the hand), kneading (rhythmic squeezing), pulling (a firm lifting stroke), friction (using the ball of the thumbs or heel of the hands), and feathering (light fingertip stroking). More vigorous strokes such as hacking and pummelling are rarely used in aromatherapy, though they do have a place in sports massage (see page 197).

Even if your first movements may seem uncertain, the more often you practise, the quicker you will gain confidence. Initially, you could try out the strokes on your own leg. Once you have developed a feel for massage, practise the strokes on your partner, preferably a person who is happy to try out the strokes on you too. By practising on each other, you will begin to develop a sense of how massage should feel, and what feels good to you should also feel good to your partner.

However, it can be daunting to attempt a full-body massage at the outset. Far better to practise on just one area of the body, preferably the back, where you have a large area to stroke.

TIPS FOR GIVING A GOOD MASSAGE

- Never give massage while feeling anxious, angry, depressed or irritable. Your partner will pick up your feelings and will begin to feel equally distressed.
- Ensure that your partner is not wearing spectacles, contact lenses or any jewellery that will impede the massage.
- Never pour the massage oil directly on your partner's skin; instead, pour a small amount into the palm of your hand, to warm the oil, then rub your hands together before applying. You need just enough to provide a comfortable slip. Too much oil will cause your hands to slide all over the body part, thus hindering any beneficial firmness of touch and sensitivity to areas of tension. Too little oil will create uncomfortable friction as a result of dragging the skin.
- Ensure that your hands are warm. Cold hands will shock your partner and may even cause their muscles to contract.
- When applying the oil in long smooth strokes, try to keep the whole of your hands in contact with your partner's body, moulding to its contours just as if you were sculpting clay.
- Generally speaking, strokes towards the heart should be firm, whereas strokes moving away should be much lighter.

- Try to keep in contact with your partner's body throughout the massage, even when you need to apply more oil. Keep one hand on their back, arm, foot or head, for instance. Ideally, the massage should feel like one continuous flowing movement. To break contact mid-flow will feel most disconcerting to your partner. However, it is fine to break contact once you have reached a natural break in the sequence, for instance when you have finished working on the back of the body and you wish your partner to turn over.
- Add interest by varying the pressure from very light to very strong. It should be lighter over bony areas, such as the shins and knees, but quite firm over large muscles such as those either side of the spine and the buttocks. But never apply pressure to the spine itself. Generally, slow movements are calming; fast movements are bracing; very slow and deliberate movements can be erotic (see Sensual Massage, page 206). However, the moderately slow movements employed by most aromatherapists tend to relax or stimulate according to the state of the recipient. In other words, aromatherapy massage has a balancing effect on the mind/body.
- Work with the whole of your body, not just your hands and arms. For instance, when you are kneading, move gently from side to side in time with your hands; when applying the long smooth strokes on the back or legs, lean into the movement, using your body weight rather than just your arm and shoulder muscles. The more relaxed and fluid your own movements, the more relaxed and at ease your partner will become.
- The key to working with the whole of your body is to become aware of your breathing. For instance, when gliding over the legs or the back, exhale slowly as you lean into the stroke; inhale as you release the pressure on the return stroke. Try not to hold your breath while doing the gliding strokes (a common mistake) as this creates tension in the whole of your body, especially in your hands. This tension will then be conveyed to your partner.
- Remember that sensitivity combined with the sheer joy of giving massage, no matter how basic, far outweighs a full routine of complicated strokes if they are carried out in a mechanical manner. The intent that goes with touch makes all the difference to its effect.

TIMING

A full-body massage can take up to one hour to complete. However, if you have only ten to fifteen minutes to spare, it is better to give a shorter quality massage to just one part of the body than to whizz through the whole sequence. The head, face, neck and shoulders, the hands and/or the feet, or a back massage, which includes the neck and shoulders, are good short-time areas. Interestingly, by giving good massage to just one part of the body, the relaxing or energising response will spread throughout the whole mind/body complex.

DEALING WITH MUSCLE TENSION

You may come across areas of the body that feel stiff, taut, grainy or even lumpy. Small nodules under the skin are caused by bunched-up muscle fibres and an accumulation of waste products. Sometimes these are so hard that beginners mistake them for bones! Soothe away any tension you may find by stroking the surrounding area. Once the area is sufficiently warmed and relaxed (after about five minutes of gentle rubbing and kneading), you can apply thumb pressure directly on the taut or lumpy area. Be sensitive to your partner's responses and ease or deepen the pressure accordingly. When applying the pressure, it helps if both you and your partner exhale with a long sigh whilst the pressure is being applied, and inhale as the pressure is released. Avoid causing intense pain. Instead, your partner should experience what can only be described as 'therapeutic pain', a dull sensation which will elicit a groan of relief. There is a world of difference between 'therapeutic pain' and that which causes one to shriek (and thus causes the muscle to contract even harder to protect itself). The only way to understand how freeing the sensation of 'therapeutic pain' can be is to experience it for yourself.

WHEN NOT TO APPLY PRESSURE

- If pain is severe and/or seems to be related to a vital organ, seek medical advice as soon as possible.
- Never use thumb pressure massage on a mole, wart, varicose vein, swelling, inflammation, or a scar that has not completely healed.
- Never apply pressure on the abdomen or on the breasts.
- Never apply pressure during pregnancy.
- Never apply pressure on fractured bones, torn ligaments, cuts or other trauma injuries.

THE MASSAGE SEQUENCE

MASSAGING THE BACK OF THE BODY

1 Position your partner on their front, head to one side, arms relaxed at the sides or loosely bent with the hands at shoulder level. Some people feel more comfortable with a rolled up towel or cushion under the chest and ankles.

2 Cover your partner from neck to toe with one or two towels. If you are working on the floor or on a bed, kneel with your knees slightly apart. If you are using a massage couch or table, stand with your feet slightly apart so that you are able to bend at the knees, thus enabling you to lean into the strokes.

Attunement

1 Before oiling your hands, move to the right of your partner and place your left hand gently on the back of their head. Place your right hand on the base of the spine.

2 Breathe slowly and deeply, asking your partner to follow your lead so that you are breathing together in unison.

3 Allow yourselves to relax into the experience. Continue for about thirty seconds. This will calm you both and will enable your partner to become accustomed to your touch.

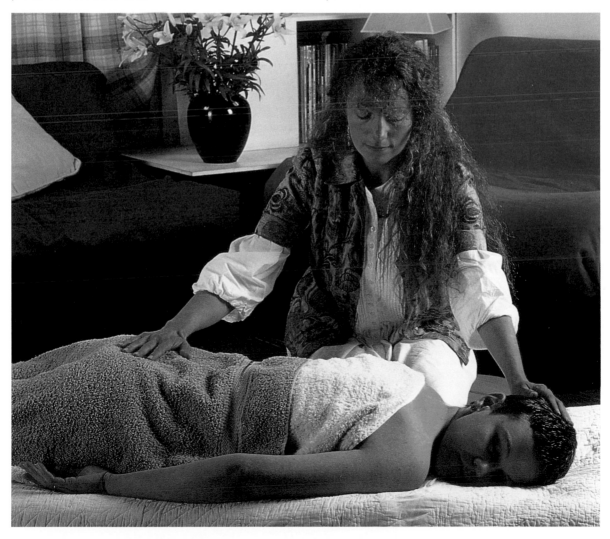

Feathering

Feathering, as its name suggests, is an extremely light stroke which is barely perceptible to the recipient. Nevertheless, it can have a profoundly soothing effect, especially to those suffering from nervous tension or pent-up anger.

1 Without peeling back the towel, begin feather-light stroking from the top of your partner's head and downwards over the whole body.

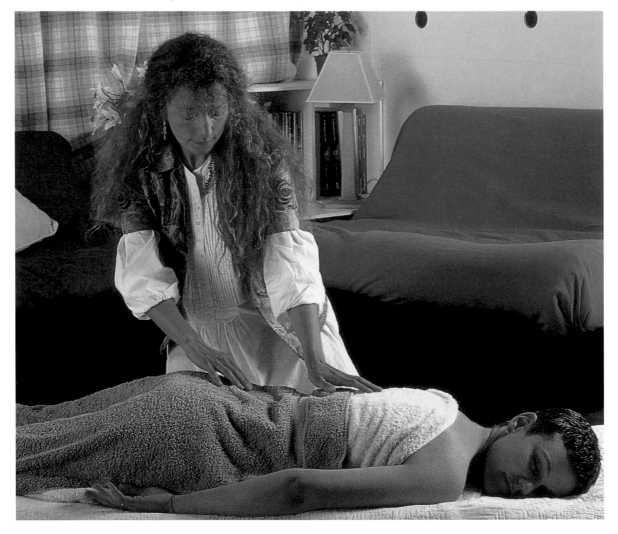

2 With hands very relaxed, fingers loosely separated, feather-weight brush with your fingertips in one long sweeping movement down the body and off at the toes.

3 Take your hands back to the head and sweep downwards again. Do this at least a dozen times.

hint

If you are working in a kneeling position, and if your partner is much taller than you are, it may be easier to feather the top half of the body first, say, from the head to the hips, then to position yourself further down the body in order to feather from the hips to the feet.

Gliding (effleurage)

This is the simplest and most instinctive of all the massage strokes. It is used on all parts of the body at the beginning and at the end of a massage, and to ease the flow from one movement to another. Stroking is also used when applying oil.

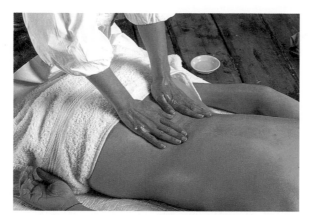

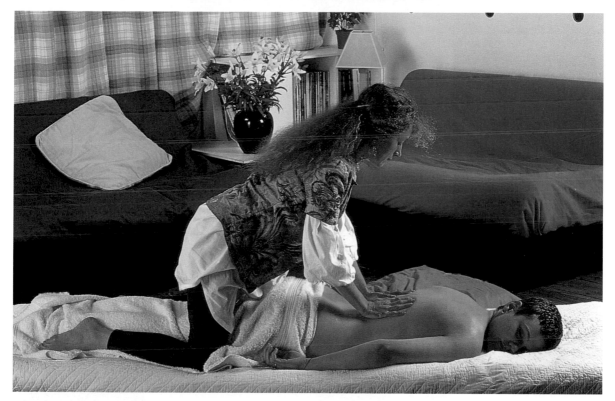

1 Peel back the towel, exposing the whole of the back. Place your hands at the base of the back, on either side of the spine, with your fingers fairly close together, but relaxed and pointing towards the head. Never apply pressure to the spine itself, but to the strong muscles on either side of the spine.

2 Now glide your hands up the back, leaning into the stroke until you reach the neck.

3 Fan out your hands firmly across the shoulders, then glide them down. When you reach the waist, pull up gently and return smoothly to the starting position.

4 Repeat several times.

---

hint

If you are giving massage at floor level or on a bed, you can sit straddling your partner's thighs for this stroke if you wish. Otherwise, kneel to one side of your partner as you did for the feathering strokes.

---

5 Starting with your hands on the lower back as before, glide firmly upwards. When you reach the shoulders, move your hands in circles over the shoulder blades. Then continue to make connected circles down the back, until you reach the original position. Repeat several times.

Kneading (petrissage)

Kneading is carried out on the fleshy muscular parts of the body. It consists of alternately squeezing and releasing handfuls of flesh in a broad circular motion with the heels of your hands and fingers, rather like kneading dough. The same kneading action can also be carried out with just the forefingers and thumbs on small areas, for instance between the shoulder blades. The purpose of kneading is to relax the muscles by draining away waste products and aiding venous and lymphatic circulation.

1 Position yourself to one side of your partner. Starting from the hips or the buttocks, begin to knead. Using the whole of your hands, alternately grasp and squeeze the flesh (but do not pinch).

2 Work up the sides of the body and across the upper arms and shoulders, paying special attention to areas of tightness (muscle tension).

3 Work back down the body to the buttocks, an area which often holds a great deal of tension and is deserving of extra attention.

4 Move to the other side of the body and repeat.

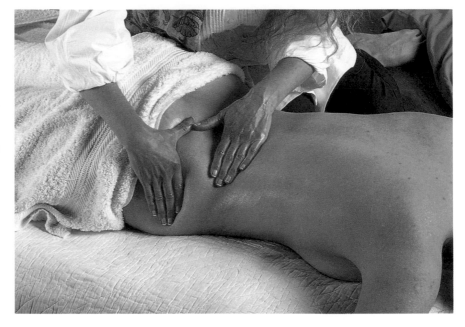

Pulling

This is a firm lifting stroke used on the sides of the torso and the limbs.

1 Remain in position to one side of your partner's back. With your fingers pointing downwards, gently pull each hand alternately straight up, each time overlapping the place where the last hand was. Start at the buttocks and work your way slowly up to the armpit and back down again.

2 Move to the other side of the body and repeat.

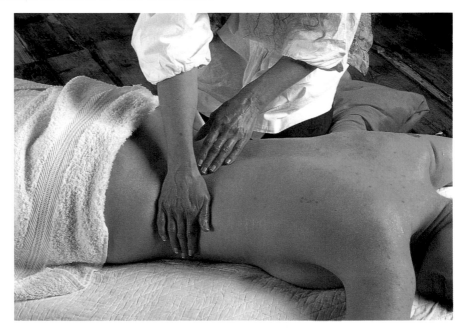

Friction

The following movements make use of the thumbs to reach deeper into the tissue where hidden tensions lie. Only use friction after you have relaxed your partner's muscles with the previous strokes.

1 Position your hands, the thumbs pointing towards each other, as illustrated, on either side of the spine. Keeping your whole hand in contact with your partner's body, lean into the stroke as you glide up the back to the neck. When you reach the top, fan out your hands across the shoulders, ease the pressure and slide them back down to the original position. Repeat two or three times.

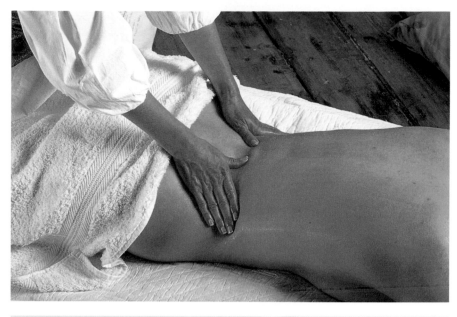

2 Position yourself to one side of your partner. Starting from the small of the back, with both thumbs together on the left side of the spine, make small circular movements with your thumbs into the muscles all the way up the spine until you reach the neck. With your thumbs on the upper back continue the circular movements. Do not press on the spine itself. Work on the muscles just above the shoulder blades and those lying between them. Move your hands back down to the base of the spine. Repeat the same frictions on the right side of the body. Soothe the whole back by returning to the gliding stroke and repeat two or three times before moving to the next stroke.

3 Apply some fairly strong friction to the lower back by placing your hands on either side of the spine and circling with the heels of your hands. Then, using your thumbs as before, work on any tension you may find there. Continue with several gliding strokes up the entire back before moving on to the neck and shoulders.

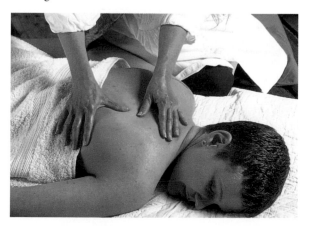

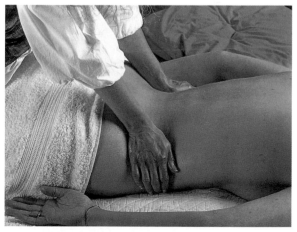

KNEADING THE NECK AND SHOULDERS

1 Position yourself to one side of your partner, and ask them to rest their forehead in their own hands as illustrated. Using both hands, knead the neck muscles, working up and down the neck to include the muscles at the base of the skull.

2 Ask your partner to release their hands and place their head to one side as before. Place your right hand on your partner's right shoulder, your left hand on their left shoulder, and begin to knead both shoulders at the same time. Then place both hands on your partner's right shoulder and knead. Repeat the movement on the left shoulder.

hint

If you are working on the floor or on a bed, you can sit astride your partner's thighs for this stroke if you wish. Otherwise, position yourself to one side of their body so that you can reach the shoulders.

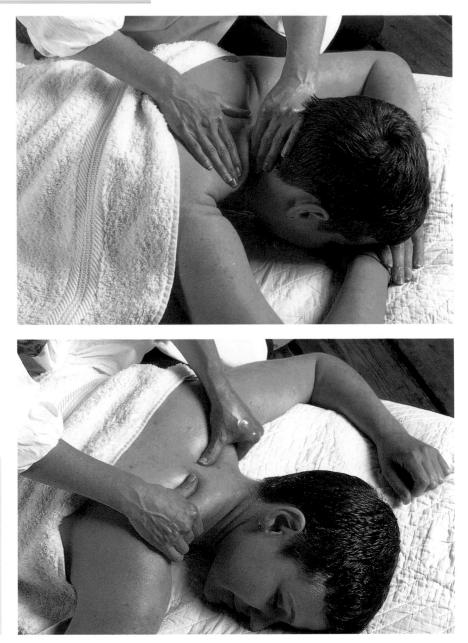

3 Finish the back sequence by returning to the long gliding strokes, but this time let the stroking become gradually slower and lighter until you move into the feathering stroke. Repeat several times. When you feel ready, cover your partner's back with a towel before moving on to the next stroke.

If you wish to end the entire massage here, return to the attunement position with which you began, placing your left hand on the crown of your partner's head. Place your right hand on the base of your partner's spine as before. Hold for about thirty seconds, breathing slowly and deeply together with your partner. When you feel ready, gently move your hands away.

MASSAGING THE BACKS OF
THE LEGS

Before applying the oil, place your hands flat on the soles
of your partner's feet, the heels of your hands at the base
of the toes, your fingers pointing towards the heels. Hold
for several seconds (not illustrated).

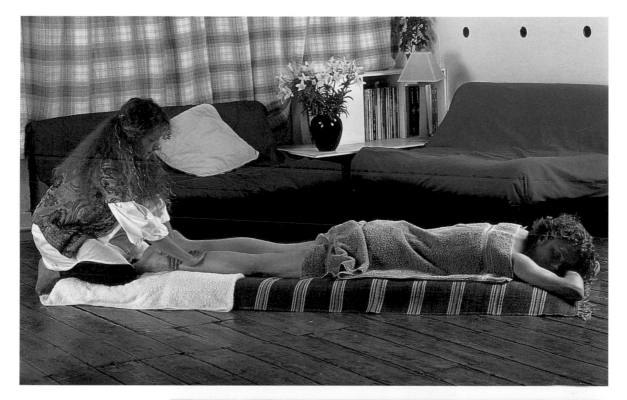

1 Oil your hands.
Starting with the left
leg, cross your hands over
and, moving both hands
together, stroke firmly up
the leg from the ankle,
going lightly over the back
of the knee, to the start of
the buttocks.

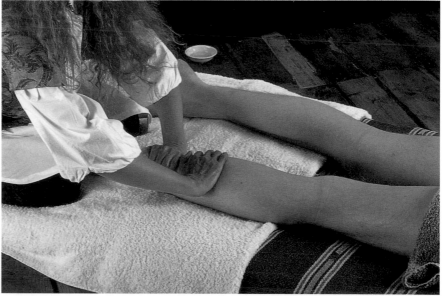

2 When you reach the top of the leg, fan out your hands and, with a lighter stroke, glide down either side of the leg. Repeat several times, applying more oil as necessary. Still working on the left leg, use your thumbs to apply friction to the calf muscles. Press firmly, moving your thumbs in tiny circular strokes all over the area up to the start of the knee. The back of the knee is a very tender spot, so never apply pressure there.

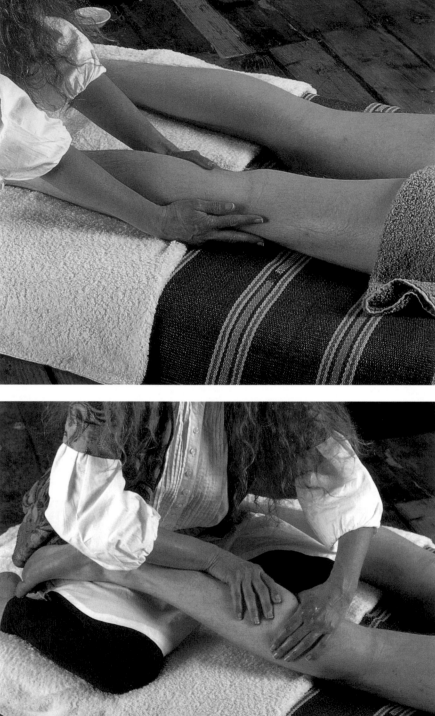

3 Begin to knead the calf muscles, using rhythmical movements. Then begin to knead the thigh, gently on the inner part, more strongly on the outer part where the muscles are larger.

4 Soothe the legs by returning to the gliding movement with which you began. Repeat two or three times. Cover the leg with a towel and repeat the entire sequence on the right leg.

Once you have massaged both legs, place your hands flat on the soles of the feet, as you did at the beginning of the leg sequence and hold for several seconds before quietly asking your partner to turn over.

MASSAGING THE FRONT OF THE BODY

Position your partner on their back with a cushion or rolled up towel under the knees to prevent any strain in the lumbar region. Your partner may also appreciate the support of a rolled up towel under the ankles (optional).

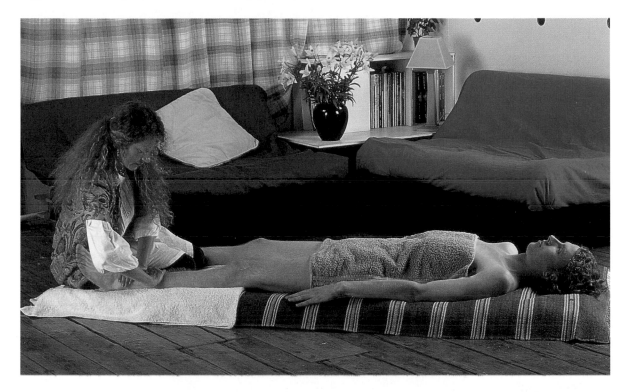

The Legs

1 Oil your hands. Beginning on the left leg, cup your hands over the ankle and stroke up the front of the leg. Do not apply direct pressure to the shin bone as this can be painful.

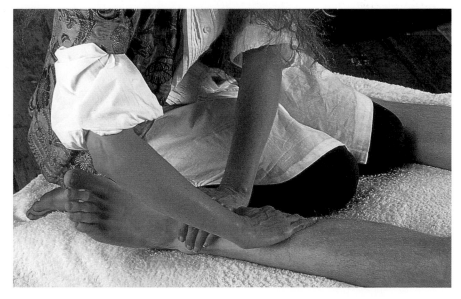

2 When you reach the top of the thigh, fan your hands out and glide them lightly down the sides of the leg. Repeat several times.

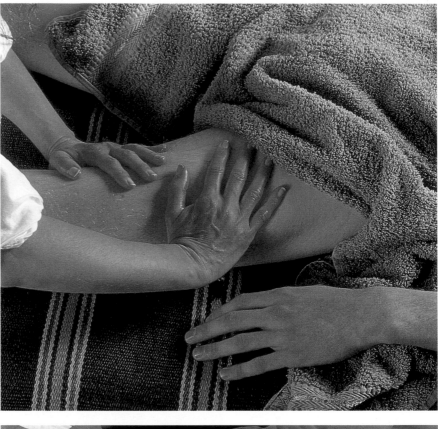

3 Then place both hands flat and side by side on the thigh. Begin to squeeze the muscles along the whole of the upper leg rhythmically, from just above the knee to the hip. When you reach the top of the leg, continue the stroke by squeezing down the thigh to the knee. Repeat several times, moving up and down the thigh.

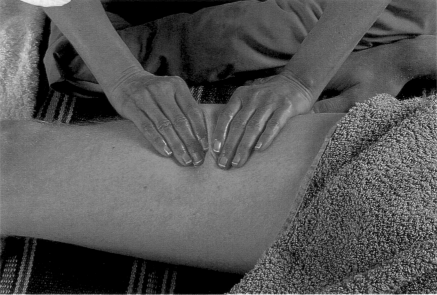

4 Begin to knead the thigh muscles, gently on the inner part, more strongly on the outer part. Then soothe the whole leg by returning to the gliding stroke with which you began. Repeat two or three times before massaging the right leg.

THE KNEE

1 Start with your thumbs crossed just under the knee cap. Stroke up the sides of the knee to the top, one thumb on each side, allowing your thumbs to pass at the top.

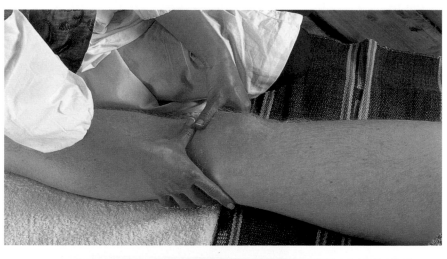

2 Now stroke each thumb down the opposite side, both thumbs completing a full circle, passing the other at the top and bottom. Repeat several times. Continue with circular thumb pressures around the knee.

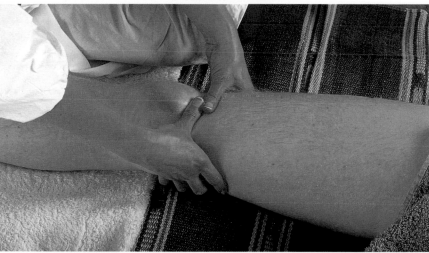

3 Gently stroke the sides and the back of the knee with the fingers of both hands at once. Finish by holding the palm of your hand over the knee for several seconds.

4 Return to the gliding stroke with which you began, stroking from ankle to thigh, repeating several times. Cover the leg with a towel before repeating the sequence on the other leg.

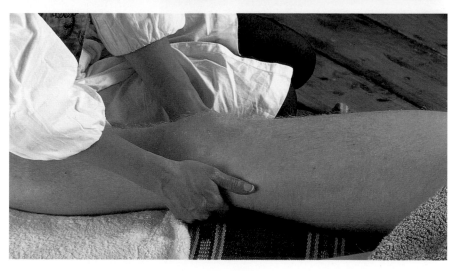

THE FOOT

1 Unless your partner's skin is very dry, the foot requires very little oil. Beginning with the left foot, stroke firmly with both hands from the toes towards the body. When you reach the ankles, return your hands to the toes with a light stroke. Repeat several times.

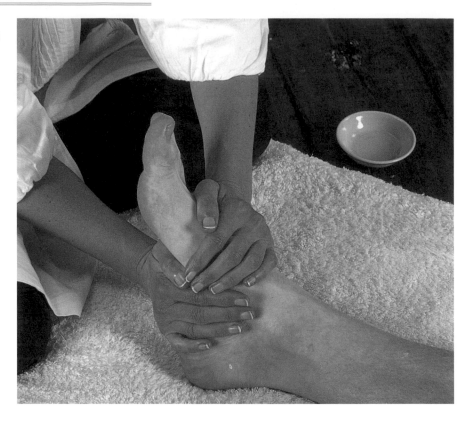

2 Support the foot by placing your fingers underneath it with your thumbs on top at the base of the toes. Moving towards the ankle, make broad thumb circles all over the top of the foot.

3 Work on the soles of the foot with the thumbs of both hands. Make small circles covering the entire sole.

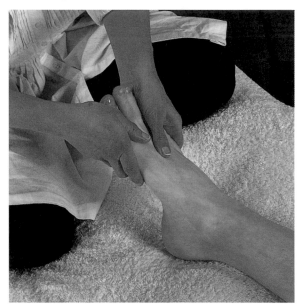

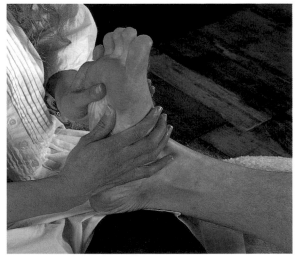

Stroke the whole of the foot as you did at the beginning then, using your middle fingers with one hand on each side of the foot, begin to circle the ankle. This is a very sensitive area, so use only light pressure.

4 Now work on the toes. Starting with the big toe, gently squeeze and roll each toe between your thumb and index finger; rotate in both directions, then gently pull them towards you until your thumb and index fingers slide off the top of the toe.

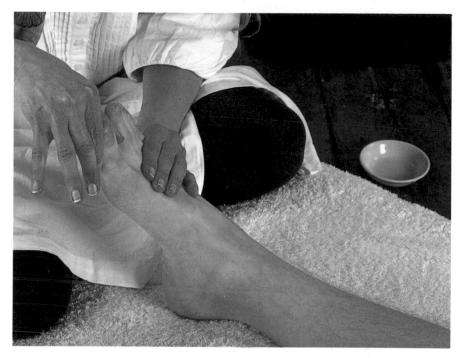

5 To encourage flexibility, clasp all the toes with one hand and bend them gently backwards and forwards.

6 Then return to the stroking with which you began. Repeat two or three times. However, the last stroke should be performed extremely slowly, allowing your hands to slide right off the toes. Cover the foot with a towel, then repeat the sequence on the right foot.

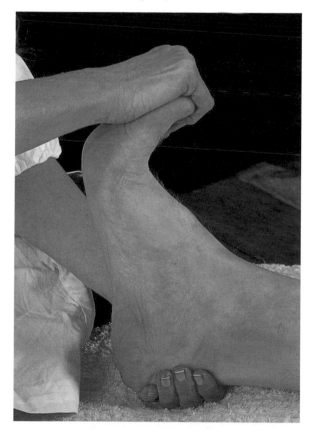

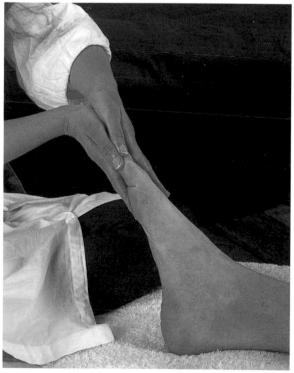

THE ARMS

1 Oil your hands. Cup both your hands around your partner's wrist and lower arm. Pressing firmly, glide both hands together up the arm.

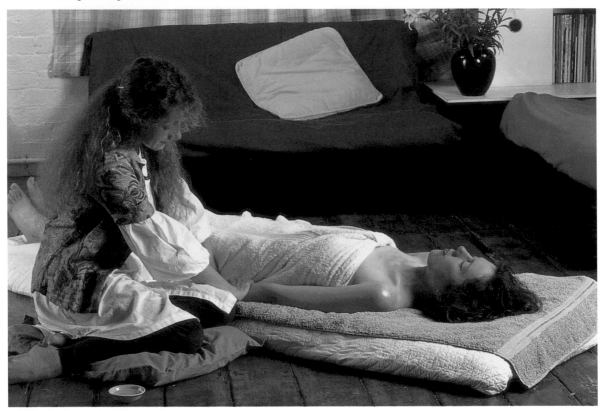

2 When you reach the top of the arm, separate your hands and glide them back down the full length of the arm and over the hands. Repeat several times.

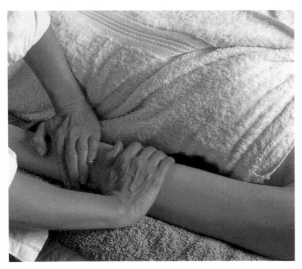

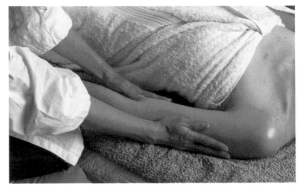

3 Using both hands, knead the forearm and then the upper arm. Soothe the whole arm by returning to the gliding stroke with which you began. Repeat the entire sequence on the other arm.

THE HANDS

The hand, like the foot, usually requires little oil. Unless the skin is exceptionally dry, the oil left on your hands after massaging the arm will be sufficient.

1 Begin by holding your partner's hand in your hands to leave your thumbs free to work on the back of the hand. Make tiny circular thumb pressures all over the area, including the wrist.

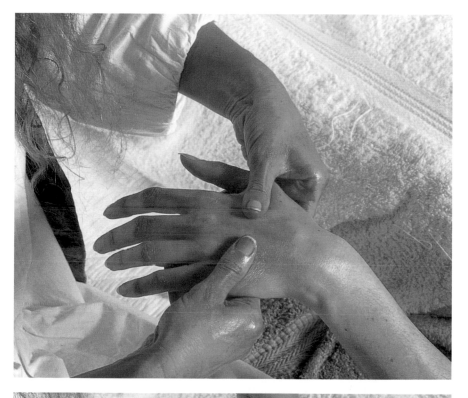

2 With both thumbs lying horizontally over the knuckles, press down and at the same time flex the fingers towards you, giving the hand a good stretch.

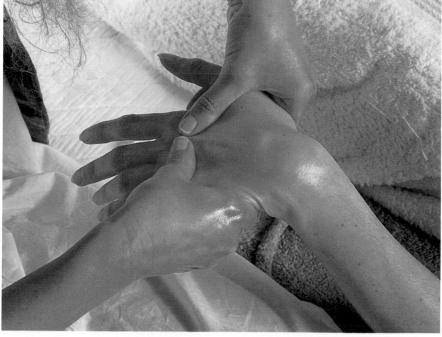

3 Turn the palm uppermost, then, paying extra attention to the muscular area at the base of the thumb, firmly circle the thumbs all over the palm.

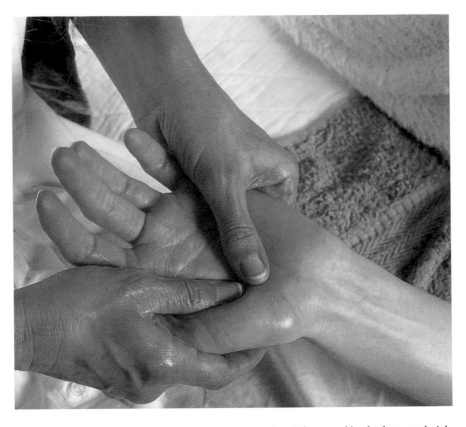

4 Hold your partner's hand with their palm down in one of your hands and use your other to work on each finger. Paying particular attention to each joint, do circular thumb pressures along the top of each finger, from the tip to the knuckle. Squeeze the outer edge of each finger, then gently pull them, giving them a little twist as you slide your hand down and off at the fingertips.

5 Stroke the whole hand, front and back, then sandwich your partner's hand between your own. Hold for a few seconds, then slide your hands very slowly off at the fingertips. Repeat a few times.

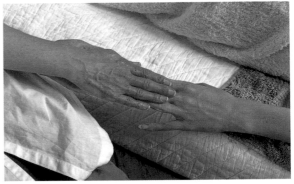

6 Repeat the sequence on your partner's other hand.

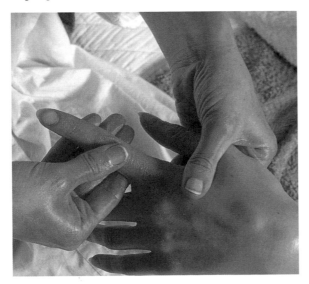

THE ABDOMEN

Some people are apprehensive about having this sensitive area massaged. If your partner agrees, use only light pressure.

1 Oil your hands, then move to one side of your partner. Let your hands rest very gently over the navel for a few moments. Begin to massage the whole belly lightly, moving both hands (fingers and palms) clockwise around it, following the coil of the colon. You will find that one hand can complete a full circle, but the other will have to break contact each time the hands cross. Repeat several times before coming to rest over the navel.

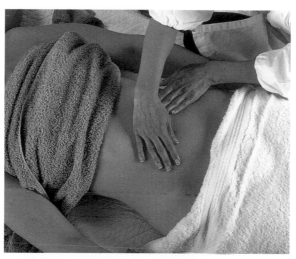

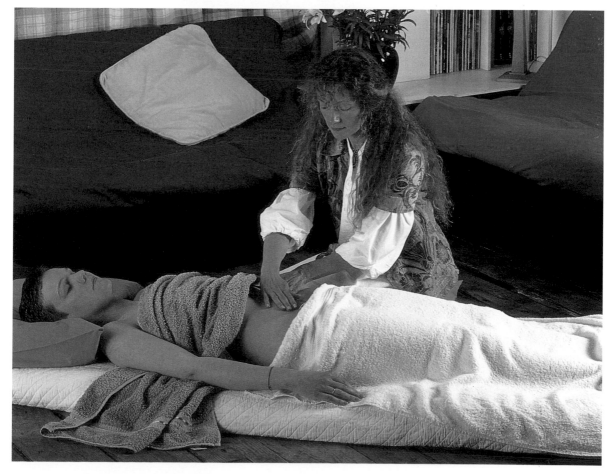

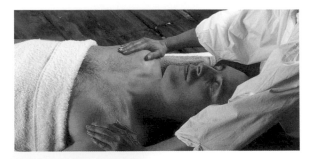

CHEST AND NECK MASSAGE

1 Position yourself at your partner's head. If you are kneeling, your knees should be parallel with your partner's ears. Apply the oil to your hands. Place them on the upper chest with your fingers facing each other. Hold for several seconds. When you are ready, slowly glide your hands away from each other towards the shoulders.

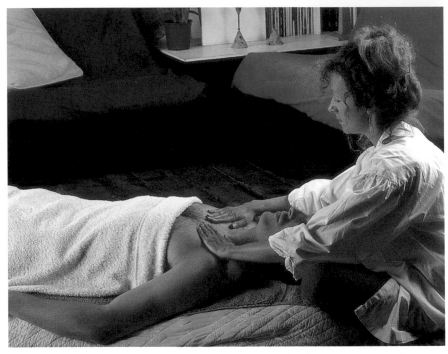

2 Continue the stroke by gliding your hands across the shoulders and up the back of the neck. Repeat several times.

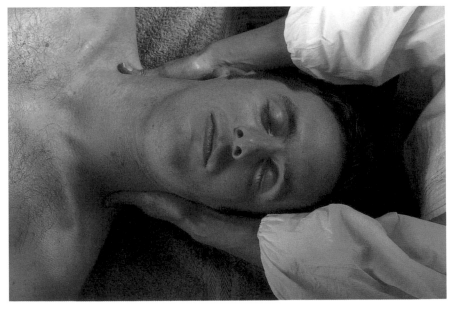

3 Gently turn your partner's head to the right. Place your right hand on their forehead, or, if you prefer, support the head by letting it rest in your right hand. Place your left hand on your partner's left shoulder and glide your hand firmly all the way up the neck. When you reach the base of the skull, use all your fingers and gently circle the area several times to release any muscle tension. Return to the gliding movement and repeat several times before slowly turning your partner's head to the left. Repeat the sequence on the right side.

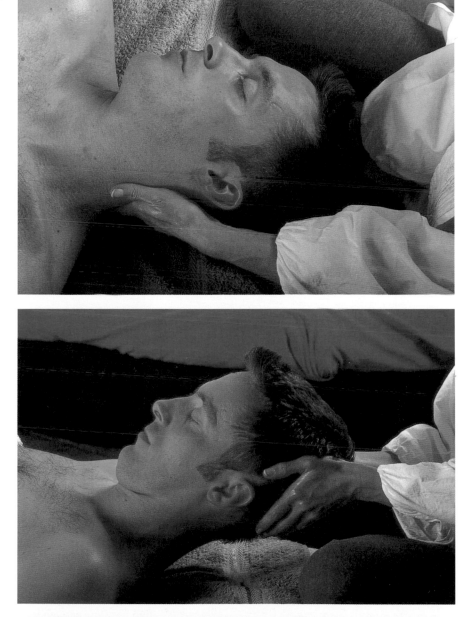

4 Gently move your partner's head to the middle so that they are lying in a straight position once more. Now give the neck a good stretch. Clasp your hands together at the back of the neck and lift the head very slowly and gently a few inches from the massage surface; then pull from the base of the skull towards you. Still supporting your partner's head, allow it to come back down gently. Repeat several times.

CAUTION *Do not use sudden or jerky movements, which may cause muscle spasm resulting in a stiff neck. Work slowly and gently, encouraging feedback from your partner. If performed correctly, this passive movement releases a great deal of tension in the neck and shoulders.*

FACE AND SCALP MASSAGE

A good face and scalp massage can ease away tension headaches like magic! At the same time, by improving the circulation, it imparts a healthy glow to the complexion. Only the lightest fingertip pressure is required for the face, for it is important not to drag the skin. However, it feels good to receive firm strokes over the scalp.

1 Before oiling your hands, place them on either side of your partner's head, the heels of the hands covering the forehead and the fingers extending downwards, anchoring the sides of the head. Hold them there for a few moments.

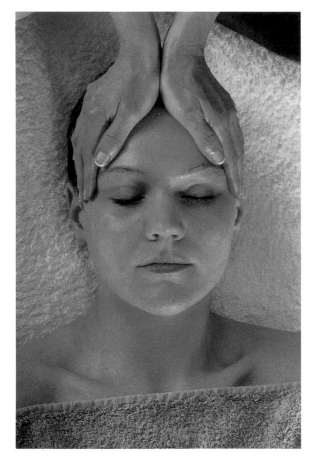

2 Then move your hands to the forehead and smoothly stroke the brow, hand-over-hand, up and over the hair to the crown of the head.

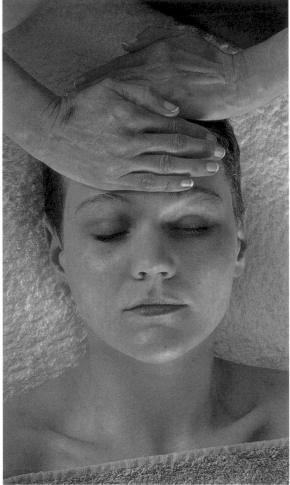

3 Move your hands gently away and oil them (using a blend suitable for your partner's skin type, see page 218). Gently starting from the throat and sweeping up to the chin, use the whole surface of your hands and slide your hands over your partner's face. Circle the cheeks, moving around the eyes (but not close enough for oil to seep in) and over the forehead. This is to oil the skin before you begin the main part of the massage.

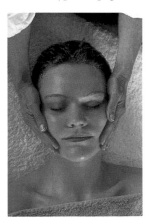

4 Place your thumbs in the centre of the forehead between the eyebrows. Slide both thumbs apart and, when you reach the temples, finish with a little circular flourish before gliding off at the hairline. Return to the starting position, but this time a little higher up. Continue to stroke the forehead, a strip at a time all the way up to the hairline.

6 Place the middle fingers on each side of the nose near the bridge, crossing your thumbs to steady your hands. Using tiny circles, work down the sides of the nose, on the cheeks at either side of the nostrils, over the upper lip and across the chin.

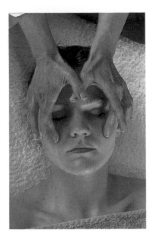

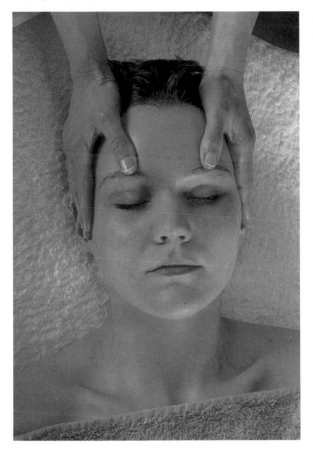

7 Place your thumbs on the chin and pull them slowly and firmly outwards and upwards along the jaw bone to the ear. Then hold the point of the chin between your thumbs and forefingers and squeeze along the whole chin, using a 'milking' action.

5 Place the balls of your thumbs at the inner corners of the eyes just below the eye socket. Smooth lightly outwards and upwards towards the temples. Repeat a little lower down, a strip at a time, until you reach the edge of the cheekbone. Repeat the same movement again just below the bone, pressing lightly upwards.

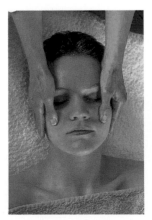

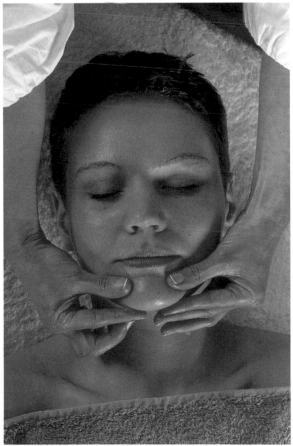

8 Gently pinch the edges of each ear at the same time, from the top down to the ear lobes. Repeat once or twice, and finish by pulling the lobes gently downwards several times. Then, with the tips of the forefingers, trace around the spiral of the ears.

9 Allow your partner to bathe in darkness for a few moments. Place the heels of your hands gently against both eyes with the fingers extending downwards. Hold them there for no less than ten seconds. Gently stroke the entire face and neck as you did at the beginning, before moving on.

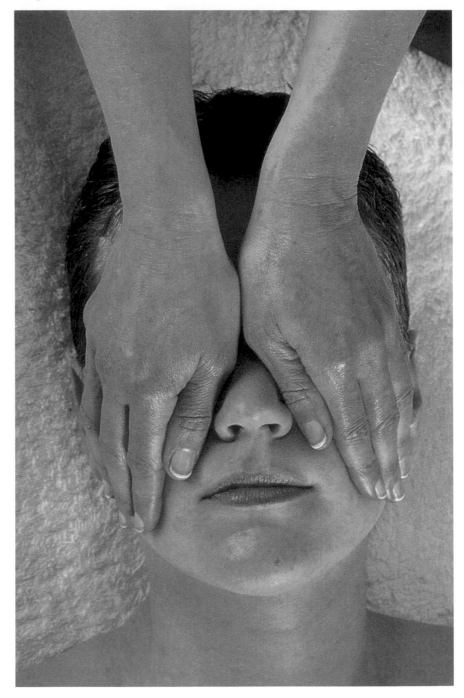

THE SCALP

1 Unless you wish to apply a pre-wash hair conditioning oil, there is no need to oil the scalp. Using your fingers, press quite firmly and move the scalp over the bone. Do not simply slide your fingers through the hair over the scalp. Work up and down the head, covering the whole area. You will also need to place your partner's head gently to the right, and then to the left in order to massage the entire skull.

2 If your partner has sufficient hair, run your fingers through it several times, allowing your fingertips to brush the scalp.

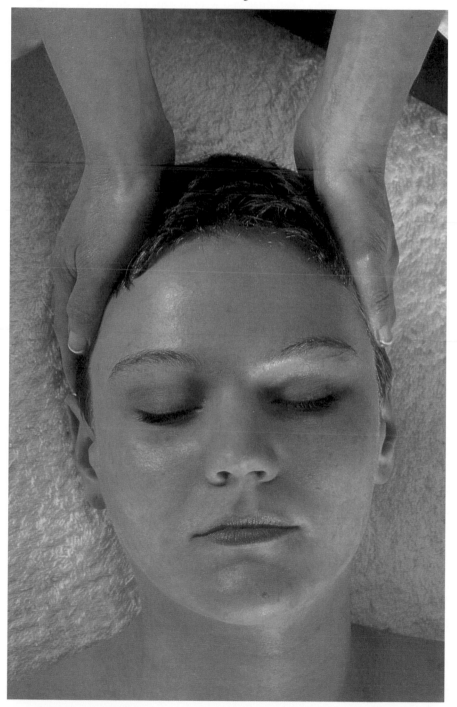

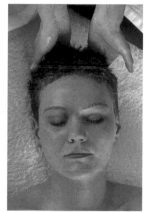

3 Finish the scalp massage by holding your palms lightly against your partner's forehead with your fingers extending down the temples (as you did at the beginning). Hold your hands in this position for several seconds, then gently move away.

ENDING THE MASSAGE

Whether or not you have massaged the entire body, conclude with full-body feathering as described on page 170. This is best carried out when your partner is warmly covered from neck to toe.

You may also wish to 'massage' your partner's aura. To do this, allow the feathering strokes to become lighter and lighter until your hands are moving through the space several inches above your partner's body. Both of you may perceive certain sensations such as tingling or warmth as your hands sweep through the electromagnetic field. Focus your attention on the idea of brushing away stress and tension and any physical pain, allowing the negativity to pass out through the soles of your partner's feet. Every time your hands move off at the toes, give them a little flick as though you were shaking off droplets of water. This will help to counter any static (or nervous tension) you may have picked up from your partner's energy field.

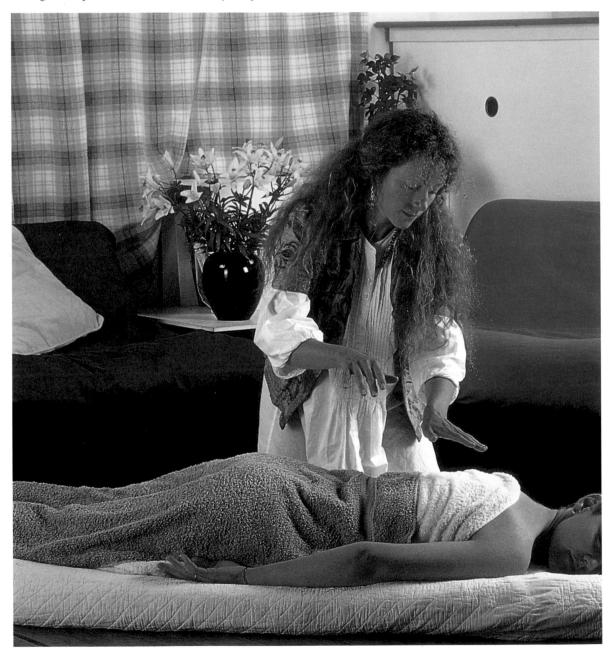

Whether or not you have massaged the aura, it is important to ground yourself and your partner at the end of a massage. Grounding is explained in Chapter 20 where you will also find out how to ground yourself. Suffice it to say here, some people feel a little light-headed or 'distant' after receiving a good massage. To counter this, you will need to encourage your partner to focus on different parts of his body, especially the feet.

Place your right hand over your partner's abdomen, and your left hand on the crown of their head. Unless your partner is asleep (this can happen!) encourage them to take two or three deep breaths and to exhale with a sigh (it will help if you breathe in unison with your partner). Hold your hands in this position for several more seconds, breathing normally. Then place the palms of your hands over the backs of your partner's hands, holding for several seconds. Move to your partner's knees, placing the palms of your hands over the knee caps, and holding for several seconds. And finally, place your hands flat on the soles of your partner's feet. Hold for several seconds while both you and your partner take two or three deep breaths as before.

When you are ready, quietly move away, allowing your partner to rest for a while and to 'come round' in their own time. Incidentally, it is always good to share a warm drink (and perhaps a light snack) at the end of a massage. This will ensure that both of you are well and truly back down to terra firma.

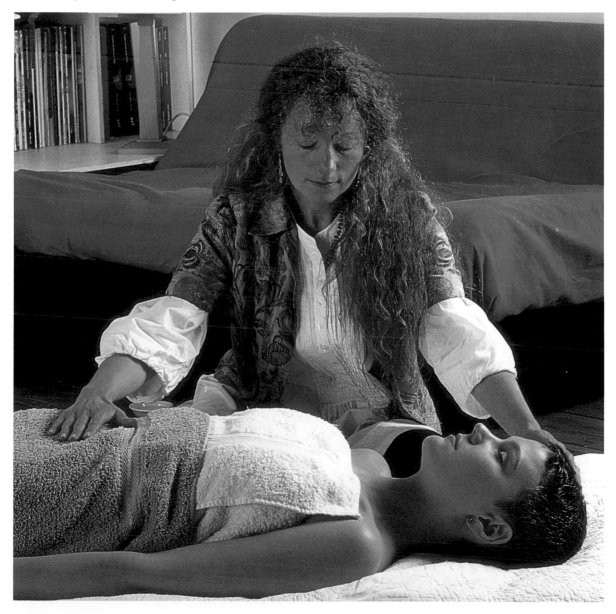

SELF-MASSAGE

It has to be said that self-massage is not quite the same as receiving a good aromatherapy massage from a friend or an aromatherapist. For instance, you cannot completely drift off, and neither can you reach all parts of your body without strain. None the less, if there is no one around to give you a massage, or if you cannot afford a professional treatment, self-massage with aromatic oils is a wonderful self-nurturing activity. It is particularly beneficial for PMS, mild depression, tiredness or simply for those days when you wake up feeling bad about yourself. Apart from the healing properties of the essences used, the massage strokes can be geared to suit your needs. Fast, stimulating strokes can be applied when you need a wake-up treatment, whereas slow, soporific movements will help you wind down at the end of a hectic day.

A good time to give yourself an aromatherapy massage is immediately after a warm shower or bath because the oils will penetrate the skin more readily if it is slightly warm and damp.

THE LEGS, FEET AND BUTTOCKS

Begin the massage on your legs. It is easier to do this whilst sitting on a large towel spread out on the floor. With your leg slightly bent at the knee for comfort, begin by stroking your whole leg from ankle to thigh. Even when you need a bracing treatment, always begin with gentle movements, gradually letting them become firmer and faster.

Once you have improved the circulation by firm stroking, you may begin gently and rhythmically to knead your calves, thighs and hips. Using the whole of your hands, alternately grasp and squeeze the flesh with one hand releasing its hold as the other starts to gather a new handful. Rock smoothly from hand to hand as if you were kneading dough. Then massage your feet, referring to the foot massage sequence on pages 180–181, and adapting the movements as necessary.

Stroke and knead your buttocks whilst lying on your side. Try also to stroke oil over the whole of the lower and mid-back. You will find this area easier to reach if you broadly circle the area using the back of your hand. Roll on the other side and repeat.

THE ABDOMEN, ARMS AND HANDS

Roll on your back with your knees bent and massage your abdomen, using the whole of your hand and gently circle the area in a clockwise direction.

Sit up to massage your arms. Stroke your whole arm from wrist to shoulder, then knead the forearm and the upper arm, gently squeezing and releasing the flesh. Massage the area around your elbow with your fingertips, using extra oil if necessary.

Now massage your hands. Stroke the back of each hand pushing firmly up towards the wrist. Then squeeze and stretch each finger (see the hand massage sequence on page 183). Turn your palm uppermost and do firm thumb circles all over the palm and around the wrist. Finish the hand massage by stroking both the palm and the back of your hand from fingers to wrist.

THE NECK AND SHOULDERS

Using the whole of your left hand, broad circle the back of your neck and around the right shoulder blade. Then, starting at the base of your skull, stroke down the side of your neck, over your shoulder and down your arm to the elbow. Repeat several times. Then change hands, using the right hand to work on the opposite side of the neck and shoulder.

THE FACE AND SCALP

Now work on your face and scalp. Lie down (or sit up) and stroke the whole of your face from forehead to chin, working from the centre outwards. Pinch along your eyebrows from the centre of the temples with your thumbs and index fingers. Hold the point of your chin between thumbs and index fingers and squeeze along the whole chin using a rhythmical 'milking' stroke. Return to the stroking with which you began, then cover your eyes with the palms of your hands and allow yourself to bathe in darkness for several seconds. When you are ready, slide your hands slowly apart and off at the sides, gently stretching your face.

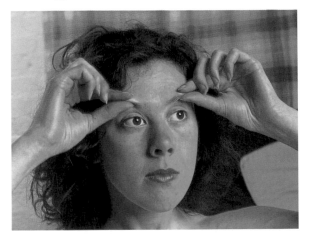

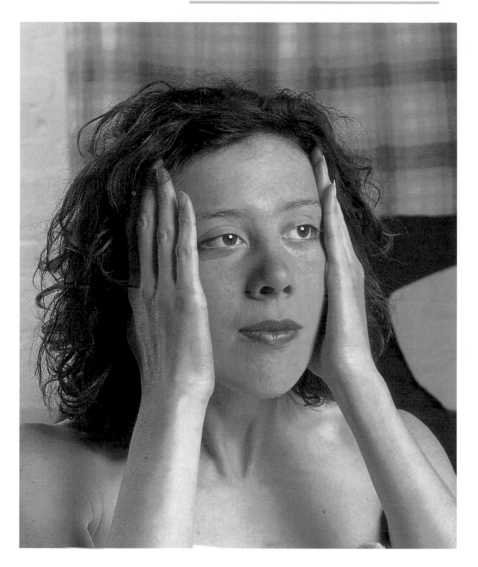

BASK IN A SUNBEAM

If you are fortunate enough to have a sunny room in your home, a wonderful way to enhance self-massage and to uplift your spirits is to bask in a sunbeam immediately afterwards. Time of day and weather permitting, place a thick fluffy towel on the floor, in a shaft of sunlight, then lie down and bask for at least fifteen minutes. The sensation of the warm sun on your body and the scent of the aromatic oils emanating from your skin is an incredibly sensuous and uplifting experience. It is especially beneficial during the winter months when you may be experiencing some degree of light deprivation (see also SAD, page 108). Moreover, provided the window is kept shut, the glass will prevent the possibility of sunburn and will intensify the warmth of the winter sunshine.

MASSAGING OLDER PEOPLE

While aromatherapy massage cannot replace a sensible diet and lifestyle, it can be used as an adjunct to these things, and thus can ease many of the health problems associated with ageing, the most common being stiffness and coldness in the joints and extremities, coupled with poor circulation. Regular massage and aromatic baths will enhance skin and muscle tone, increase flexibility in the joints and improve circulation.

Later in life, it may no longer be comfortable to receive massage on the floor, so if you do not have a massage couch, offer to massage the recipient in a chair. For a back massage, ask the person to sit astride the chair, facing its back. The recipient may then lean forwards against a cushion placed over the back of the chair. When you come to work on the lower back, kneel on the floor or sit in another chair of equal height. Foot or hand massage can be given whilst you are seated next to or in front of the recipient, with their hand or foot placed in your lap. It is also important to ensure that the room is warmer than usual, and that the parts of body you are not massaging are warmly wrapped with a towel.

Prepare a massage oil suitable for the person's needs (see the therapeutic charts in Part 2).

WORKING ON THE SHOULDERS AND NECK

1 Tense, fibrous tissue in the shoulders can be felt quite easily and will need plenty of deep kneading to release the tension. Cup your hands over each shoulder, stroke and knead from the base of the neck to the outer edge. Massage all over the upper arms as well. Once you have warmed the area, you could also add deep rotating thumb strokes and larger strokes with the heels of your hands.

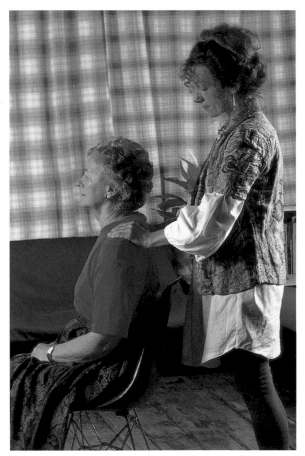

2 To massage the neck, support your partner's forehead with one hand and use the other to massage the back of the neck. Use small rotary movements with your thumbs and roll the flesh between thumb and fingers.

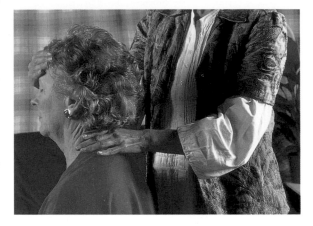

3 To give foot massage (see pages 180–81), your partner needs to be seated in a comfortable upright chair. It may be necessary to place a cushion at the base of the spine, to support their back. Sit in a chair of a similar height, positioned slightly to one side of your partner. Cover a pillow with a towel (to protect it from oil stains) and place it across your lap. Gently lift your partner's lower leg and place it on the pillow, ensuring that the knee is slightly bent. This position is much more comfortable for the recipient than when the leg is held straight out.

4 To give hand massage (see pages 183–184), position two chairs of equal height opposite each other. Cover a pillow with a towel and place it across your lap. If your partner's chair has wooden arms, ensure that the pillow also covers the arm of the chair to cushion your partner's elbow and forearm. Make sure your partner's feet are flat on the floor. It may also be necessary to place a supportive cushion in the small of the back. Then gently lift your partner's bent arm, placing it across the pillow as illustrated.

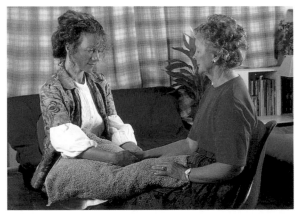

23
SPORTS MASSAGE

You need not be an athlete to benefit from the conditioning and performance-boosting effects of sports massage. Anyone who is physically active, whether they jog, cycle, hike, dance or perhaps have a physically demanding job, will appreciate its healing effects.

Studies have shown that the main benefits of massage for the physically active are as follows:

- If given immediately before exercise, massage warms and loosens the muscles and joints, thus helping to prevent cramp and injury.
- If given soon after strenuous exercise, massage stimulates the flow of blood and lymph which act in tandem to remove waste products that accumulate between the fibres of hard-working muscles. In so doing, pain and stiffness are markedly reduced.
- Massage can boost conditioned muscles to an even higher level of performance, significantly increasing the amount of work they can do while decreasing recovery time.
- The uplifting effect of massage upon the emotions is also a contributing factor in its ability to enhance performance.

There are four basic categories of sports massage, and each is important in enhancing physical fitness and decreasing recovery time: conditioning massage; warm-up massage; post-activity massage; massage to aid healing of injuries.

Instructions for preparing essential oils for massage and other applications are to be found in Chapter 5.

THE CONDITIONING MASSAGE

This is simply a relaxing, full-body aromatherapy massage (as described in Chapter 22) carried out 24 hours before participating in strenuous activity. Its main purpose is to relax the central nervous system and to aid restful sleep. If possible, have the massage towards the end of the day after a warm aromatic bath. Choose between one

and three essences from any of the following categories: *balancing* – bergamot, geranium, lavender, rose otto; *light and soporific* – clary sage, chamomile (Roman), neroli, petitgrain; *heavy and soporific* – cedarwood, sandalwood, vetiver.

THE WARM-UP MASSAGE

This is to be carried out after a warm shower, just before strenuous activity. If there is no time to carry out a full-body treatment, just concentrate on the muscles the person will be using, such as the back, buttocks, legs and arms. Use fairly light gliding strokes, gradually becoming faster and more stimulating. Then do plenty of kneading, followed by some rapid percussion strokes (see below). The most appropriate essences to use for the warm-up massage should be balancing or enlivening rather than very warming and analgesic (too much heat in the muscle may result in a degree of sluggishness rather than optimum performance).

Choose between one and three of the following essences: eucalyptus, geranium, grapefruit, juniper berry, lavender, lemon, lemongrass, peppermint, pine, rosemary.

PERCUSSION (TAPOTEMENT)

Percussion encompasses a range of brisk rhythmic strokes performed repeatedly with alternate hands. The main value of percussion is to stimulate soft tissue areas such as thighs and buttocks, thus toning the skin and improving circulation. As well as helping to condition extremely worked muscles, when used in conjunction with good nutrition, percussion can also be helpful for breaking down cellulite. Although there are several other percussion movements, we shall concentrate on the easiest to master: pummelling and hacking. Incidentally, before trying out the strokes on a partner, practise them on your own leg, ensuring that your hands are relaxed and your wrists loose. This can be achieved by giving your hands a good shake before you start.

Pummelling

1 Loosely clench your fists, bouncing the fleshy sides of your fists alternately and rapidly against the skin.

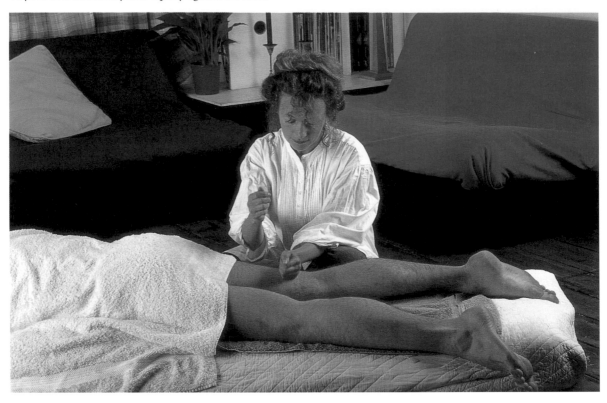

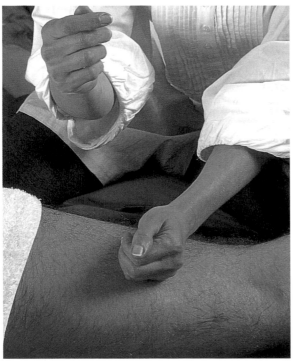

Hacking

2 With your palms facing each other, and your fingers loosely together, bounce the sides of your hands alternately and rapidly up and down against the skin.

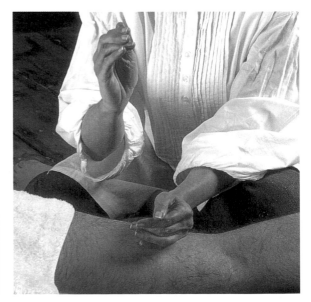

Cupping

3 Cup your hands, arching them at the knuckles, with your fingers straight. With every strike, your cupped hands will trap air against the skin, resulting in an amusing sucking sound. Keep repeating the same rapid movements. Although it is hardly conducive to meditative massage, cupping usually makes people laugh — a great way to release physical and emotional tension.

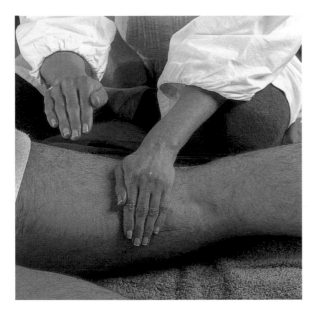

POST-ACTIVITY MASSAGE

The purpose of the post-activity massage is to prevent extremely worked muscles from going into spasm. After a warm shower, give a full-body massage if possible, otherwise concentrate on the muscles that have been worked the most. Always massage from the extremities towards the heart. Do plenty of smooth gliding strokes, followed by gentle squeezing and kneading. Avoid causing pain to overworked muscles.

Choose one of the following warming essences: black pepper; coriander; ginger; marjoram; nutmeg; vetiver.

MASSAGE TO AID HEALING OF INJURIES

The first approach to dealing with common injuries such as strains (overstretching of the muscles), sprains (wrenching and twisting of a joint) and bruises is to apply a cold compress to ease the pain and reduce any swelling.

Even though you must never massage directly on an injury, it is beneficial to massage very gently above and below it, working towards the heart . Gentle massage helps to disperse excessive fluid and generally aids the healing process.

Choose one of the following cooling essences: chamomile (German or Roman), cypress, geranium, peppermint.

MUSCLE CRAMPS

An overworked muscle in the foot or leg may suddenly go into spasm causing excruciating pain. The first step in relieving the pain is to stretch the cramped muscle. In many cases, simply walking on the affected limb is enough to release the spasm. If this does not work, however, you will need to flex and massage the affected area.

FOOT CRAMP

To relieve cramp in the foot, grasp the toes and gently bend them back towards the body whilst holding the heel with the other hand. Then stroke the sole of the foot with the heel of your hand or your thumb.

CALF CRAMP

Calf cramps can be eased by flexing the entire foot so that the toes are pointing towards the body and there is a pulling sensation in the affected muscles. Then knead the calf muscles firmly, working up the leg to the knee and back down again.

HAMSTRING CRAMP

To relieve hamstring cramp, the sufferer should lie on their back and raise the affected leg with the knee straight and the toes of the foot bent towards the shin bone. Then stroke the back of the thigh firmly towards the buttocks.

Usually there is no need to apply an aromatic oil to ease cramp. However, if the pain returns, despite carrying out the above treatments, apply a massage oil containing any of the following essences: cajeput; chamomile (German or Roman); lavender; marjoram; rosemary.

24
MATERNITY, BABIES AND CHILDREN

MATERNITY

Gentle massage can be enjoyed throughout pregnancy. As well as soothing away tension and fatigue, it can alleviate minor ailments such as fluid retention, backache, aching legs and insomnia, all of which are common during pregnancy. However, do seek the approval of a doctor or midwife first.

Essences suitable for use during pregnancy can be vaporised as room perfume to enhance the experience of massage for both giver and recipient. For the reasons given on page 24, it is advisable to avoid skin applications of essential oils during pregnancy unless under the guidance of a qualified aromatherapist. However, virtually any good quality vegetable oil can be used for massage, though some mothers-to-be have noticed that they develop fewer, if any, stretch marks by massaging with extra virgin olive oil. Although this is a heavy textured oil, if used sparingly it will be absorbed into the skin within half an hour of application.

If you are massaging a pregnant woman, most of the strokes described in Chapter 22 can be safely employed. However, it is important to avoid deep pressures and percussion strokes such as pummelling and hacking. In the later stages of pregnancy, when the recipient is unable to lie on her front, you can massage her back whilst she lies on her side with her upper leg propped on a cushion. Or she could sit astride a chair leaning forward on to a pillow. Pay special attention to her legs, especially the thighs, which can become quite tensed during late pregnancy as a result of carrying the extra weight. You can gently and smoothly massage her abdomen by stroking the whole area in broad clockwise circles, with your strokes gradually becoming lighter and lighter until you are barely touching the skin. This has a soporific effect on both mother and baby.

PREPARING FOR CHILDBIRTH

If you are pregnant, it is important to strengthen the pelvic floor muscles to help prevent tearing of the perineum during childbirth. To test the strength of these muscles, try to stop yourself from urinating mid-flow. If you can accomplish this several times consecutively you are in good shape. If not, practise the same squeezing and releasing action several times a day (not necessarily when you need to urinate), holding on to the contraction for as long as you can, without holding your breath or tightening your thighs and abdomen. With regular practice, you will be able to hold each contraction for a slow count to ten. It is by consciously relaxing your pelvic floor muscles at the moment of birth that you help prevent tearing the perineum. Moreover, strong pelvic floor muscles are a good insurance against painful menstruation, painful intercourse, difficulty in achieving orgasm, prolapses and incontinence later in life.

THE LAST SIX WEEKS

During the last six weeks of pregnancy, it is also helpful to prepare the perineum for childbirth by massaging the whole of the vaginal area with extra virgin olive oil after a warm bath or shower. Some midwives recommend stretching the perineum with your fingers. However, it is important to seek professional advice before attempting to do this.

Prepare your breasts during pregnancy by massaging with unrefined almond, sunflower or olive oil after your bath. Use your thumb or finger pads and massage with gentle circular strokes towards the nipple. Avoid using soap on your nipples as this tends to dry up the natural oils.

MASSAGE DURING CHILDBIRTH

Even though many women appreciate being massaged by their partner during labour, others prefer not to be touched. The way a woman will feel during labour is almost impossible to predict, especially if it is her first baby. Nevertheless, if you are about to become a father, or if you have been invited to support a friend during childbirth, it is as well to practise the basic sequence given in Chapter 22 beforehand. Chances are that your partner will be only too pleased to receive your loving touch at this special time.

Being the final stage of pregnancy, essential oils can be added to the vegetable base oil if you wish. Lavender, chamomile (German or Roman), marjoram or clary sage can be massaged into the sacral area to reduce pain. Using the flat of your hand, make slow rhythmic circles all over the lower back. Although some women find that light stroking given during a contraction takes the edge off the pain, others prefer to be soothed and comforted with firmer strokes in between contractions. Some women find massage helpful at any stage of labour.

The same aromatic oil can be massaged into the abdomen using very light, circular strokes moving in a clockwise direction. However, most women appreciate this stroke in between contractions. Others find that very light fingertip stroking downwards over the lower abdomen and upper thighs helps to buffer the pain during a contraction.

Some women experience shaking legs at the end of the first stage of labour, and also immediately after giving birth. This can be helped by stroking the thighs from the upper part to the knee and back again. Press firmly down the leg, and lightly as you move upwards. Always keep your movements flowing and rhythmic.

It is important that your partner makes her likes and dislikes known to you, so do encourage her to ask for what she wants, for this is the surest way to discover how best to help.

MASSAGE AFTER THE BIRTH

Gentle massage to the shoulders, neck, face and scalp can help alleviate the depression that commonly follows childbirth. Vaporise your partner's favourite essential oils into the room and apply a low concentration of essences suitable for her skin type (refer to the Skin Care chart on page 218). It is through caring and nurturing that she will begin to regain her equilibrium.

MASSAGE FOR NURSING MOTHERS

To help stimulate a good flow of milk, it is important to breastfeed your baby as soon as possible after birth. It is the instinctive sucking reflex of the baby that causes the milk to flow, as well as helping the uterus return to its normal size. Breast massage, in conjunction with adequate rest, nourishing food and copious amounts of bottled water, will help to promote the supply for as long as you wish to continue breastfeeding. Massage will also greatly reduce the likelihood of problems such as mastitis (inflammation and infection of the milk ducts) and the development of a breast abscess.

Massage your breasts once or twice a day throughout the nursing period. Cupping the breast with one hand, and massaging with the other, apply a light base oil such as almond or sunflower seed. Then begin stroking very gently with your thumb or fingertips from the periphery down to the edge of the areola. Before feeding your baby, however, it is important to remove any oil that may have seeped on to the nipples.

BABY MASSAGE

In parts of the East and in many tropical countries, baby massage is regarded as one of the essential skills of motherhood, and is passed down from mother to daughter. Oiling, stroking and stretching the body is believed to help babies grow stronger by encouraging deep sleep, better feeding and the relief of colic. Research carried out by natural childbirth gurus would support this claim, hence the increasing popularity of baby massage. Indeed, many hospital maternity units now encourage parents to massage their babies.

You can begin stroking your baby lightly with plain almond or virgin olive oil (but not the 'extra' grade as this may be a little heavy for a new baby) after the first week after birth. Try to massage your baby every day, perhaps just before bathtime, and at least half an hour after a feed. As your baby grows a little older, he or she will take an active part in the massage, wriggling, kicking and gurgling in response to your touch. So make it a game between the two of you!

When massaging, Indian mothers sit on the floor with their legs outstretched to form a cradle in which they lay their babies. If you find this position uncomfortable, support your back with cushions propped against the wall. Alternatively, massage your baby whilst kneeling on a carpeted floor with your baby on a towel. Remember to cover your lap (or the floor) and the surrounding area with extra towels, just in case! Ensure that your hands and the room are very warm.

As a baby's body is so small, you will tend to use stroking movements most often. The following simple massage sequence does not have to be done 'by the book', just do whatever your baby enjoys.

THE SEQUENCE

1 Begin on the front of the body. Apply a little massage oil with long strokes all over your baby's body, shoulders to feet, but avoid the face to prevent the possibility of oil seeping into the eyes. You could, however, gently stroke the crown of the head. Repeat the stroking several times.

2 Next massage your baby's belly with your fingertips, stroking clockwise around the navel.

3 Hold your baby's hand in one of your hands, gently stretching the limb. Stroke the entire arm from shoulder to wrist, then squeeze all the way down the arm. Repeat several times.

4 Uncurl your baby's fist and gently stroke the back of the hand, and then the palm. Gently squeeze and rotate each finger. Repeat the sequence on the other arm and hand.

5 Move on to the legs. Hold your baby's foot in one hand, gently stretching the limb. Stroke the leg from thigh to ankle, then squeeze the leg all the way down. Repeat several times. Stroke the foot, front and sole, with the pad of your thumb, then squeeze and rotate each toe. Then massage the other leg and foot.

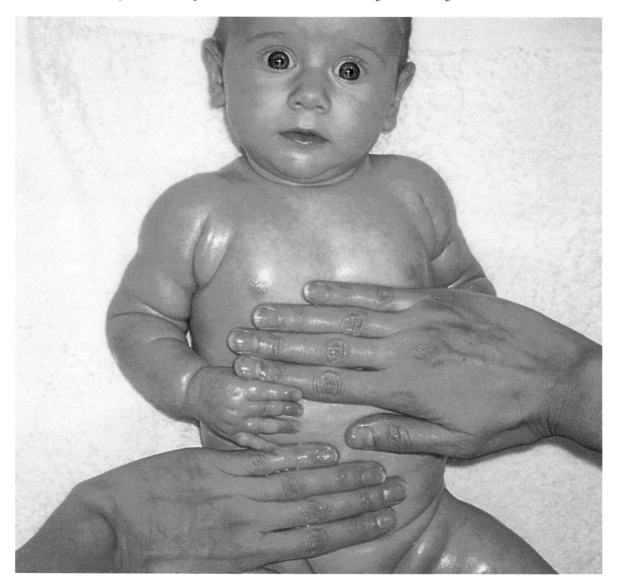

6 Turn your baby over and oil the back of the body. Stroke up the back of the legs, over the buttocks and up the back. Slide your hands across the shoulders and down the arms, then glide them down the sides of your baby's body to the feet. Repeat several times.

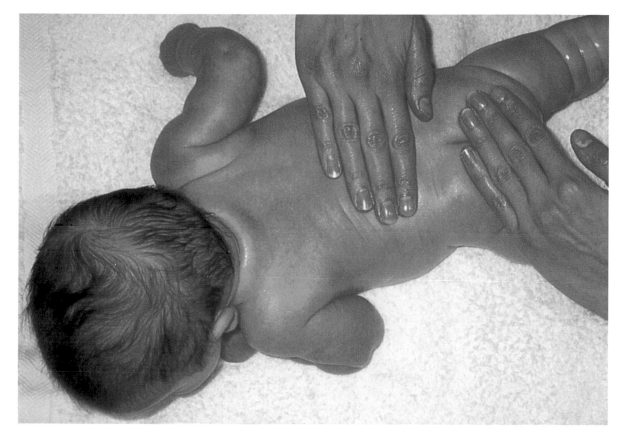

7 Stroke over and around each buttock, then very gently press the buttocks together. Babies also love having their bottom patted, so with four fingers of one hand, gently pat all over the buttocks.

8 Finish the massage by sliding your hands very gently and smoothly down your baby's back, one hand following the other. As one hand reaches the legs, lift it off, return it to the top of the back and repeat. Gradually stroke more and more slowly and lightly. This smooth continuous stroke has a calming, soporific effect. After the massage, wrap your baby in a warm towel. He or she will probably be content to lie in your arms for a while, and will perhaps even fall asleep. There are few experiences so delightful!

MASSAGING CHILDREN

Although children love being massaged, they may not lie still for more than ten minutes, twenty minutes at the most. They may wriggle and giggle at first, but after a while even a hyperactive child settles down. The best time to massage your child is shortly before bedtime, after a bath. This will ensure a good night's sleep for everyone! Set out to do a shortened version of the full-body massage sequence described in Chapter 22, gently stroking and kneading according to your child's preference. Alternatively, concentrate on a back and/or foot massage.

For children over five years of age, you can use a low concentration of essential oils in the vegetable base oil if you wish. Otherwise, simply vaporise their favourite essences.

As you will discover, massaging babies and children is fun for both giver and recipient, so relax and enjoy it!

25
AROMATHERAPY MASSAGE FOR LOVERS

Aromatherapy lends itself most readily to erotic plea-sure. It combines massage with scent, thus awaken-ing the most primitive of senses: smell and touch. Add music, delicious food and a seductive setting and you are nurtured in every sense. Share these pleasures with your lover, and you may even transcend the boundary of the senses to experience ecstasy!

In reality, however, passion may have been off the menu for some considerable time. Unfortunately, just about any long-term relationship can fall prey to sensual deprivation. This is hardly surprising if a couple must channel their energies into caring for young children or holding down a demanding job outside the home. Indeed, if this reflects your own lifestyle, then you may well be thinking that you have neither the time nor pri-vacy to caress each other with aromatic oils.

Yet, even though it may mean a juggling act, it is pos-sible to capture some time to be alone with your partner if you really want to. If you are a parent, try to enlist the help of family and friends, perhaps building a supportive babysitting network. Parents of older children may even manage an afternoon of pleasure while the children are at school. It may mean taking a day off work, but what bet-ter way to use up your holiday entitlement? Or better still, you may even snatch the odd weekend away, taking your precious oils with you, of course.

The reward will be worth far more than the effort expended in stealing those precious moments. As well as engendering relaxation, heightening intimacy and enhancing mood, these qualities are bound to affect oth-ers in your sphere positively, especially children. As chil-dren are so receptive to the changes in mood of their par-ents, they will respond by becoming more joyful and relaxed themselves.

COUPLES HEALING

For a couple going through a bad patch in their relation-ship, loving touch (not necessarily erotic massage) can impart that vital element of mutual trust and relaxation that may have fallen by the wayside, or perhaps never quite developed in the first place. Indeed, too many peo-ple equate cuddling, touching and massage as a prelude to sexual intercourse rather than as a means to fulfilling a need for sensual contact independent of an ultimate goal.

When orgasm is no longer expected, those who suffer from 'performance pressure' will experience new found freedom. For example, if one partner is perceived as being too demanding sexually, the other may withdraw from sex altogether, thus causing a rift in the relation-ship. However, by learning to enjoy giving and receiving non-sexual touching (through the exchange of therapeu-tic aromatherapy massage), a great deal of tension is released. The 'demanding' partner will relax enough to enjoy passively the sensations for their own sake. The 'unresponsive' partner, finding themselves in a non-threatening situation, will become awakened to pleasure, and most likely to their own sexual needs.

So it is essential to avoid erotic massage in the early stages of the healing process. Instead, concentrate on tra-ditional aromatherapy massage until such time as your relationship is ready to move on. It is far more important to share and explore increasingly subtle levels of em-pathy, which can be experienced through loving touch. Where there is empathy, there is also spiritual compati-bility, as reflected in the feeling that there is no real dis-tance between partners. Yet there is also the realisation that both partners are individuals in their own right. Neither partner has power over the other. Without this seemingly paradoxical state of intimacy and freedom, sex can never be totally fulfilling.

It is also true that before we can truly love another, we must first love ourselves. We might 'need' someone, cling to them, pity them, idealise them, but only when our own cup is full to the brim can it overflow to others. Positive self-esteem is the foundation for enjoying life and creating healthy relationships. However, loving your-self in this way does not mean being narcissistic and dis-regarding of others. Rather, it means regarding yourself as a person worthy of the love and respect that you would feel for a good friend.

For a couple who already have a wonderful relationship, massage (erotic or therapeutic), will enhance and intensify the loving bond in a way that words cannot possibly describe. Each will take delight in the other's joy: the secret of a deep and lasting relationship.

CREATING A MAGICAL SPACE

Just as you learned to create a healing space for giving traditional aromatherapy massage, the room in which you intend to share erotic massage needs to be warm and cosy with its own special atmosphere. You could simply clear the room of any clutter, unplug the phone, dim the lights and let your imagination do the rest. Or you may prefer the enchanting atmosphere created by the warm, flickering glow of candlelight. If, however, you are spending the afternoon together, natural daylight diffused through muslin curtains can be as romantic as moonlight.

FRAGRANCE

If you have a nightlight vaporiser, this too will add to the ambience of enchantment. Vaporise essences whose auras are suggestive of magic and sensuality, aromas such as enigmatic resins with fruits, earthy fragrances with spice, or woody scents with exotic florals (see the recipe suggestions on page 206). Alternatively, you could perfume the room with richly fragrant flowers. Certain blooms emanate a decidedly erotic fragrance. The scents of jasmine, orange blossom, lilac, white lilies or orchids are reputedly the most erogenic fragrances on earth, for they are possessed of certain odour nuances that whisper of our own sexual secretions (see also page 232). However, some people can detect the subthreshold 'animal' note in the scents of such flowers, which is why the blooms may elicit disgust rather than delight. So you must choose most carefully the flowers for your magical space.

MUSIC

If you wish to play music in your erotic sanctuary, think of the songs or melodies that are especially evocative of peak moments in your relationship; almost all lovers have their special music. However, while this can be played before, during and after love making, it may not be suitable while giving sensual massage. In order to build up an erotic charge, sensual massage needs to be performed with slow, smooth and flowing movements. Likewise the most appropriate music for massage is flow-

ing and rhythmic, not loud, erratic or jerky. You are almost certain to find yourself massaging to the same rhythm as the music. Indeed, it is almost impossible not to. Imagine then what it would be like to be massaged to the strains of 'Jumping Jack Flash', or to the '1812 Overture', cannon fire and all. Great fun for a few maybe, but nerve-racking or exhausting for lesser mortals!

THE MASSAGE 'BED'

The most seductive surface on which to massage each other is a firm bed or a futon. Or you could use cushions on the floor, covered with a cotton sheet or a couple of fluffy bath towels. You may also need a second sheet or bath towel to cover areas of the body you are not working on, thus preventing your partner from becoming chilled. This may not be necessary, however, if the room is extremely warm, or if your lover is hot-blooded!

THE MASSAGE OIL

The basic instructions for preparing massage oils and room scents are to be found in Chapter 5. Although personal preference is vital when choosing oils for erotic massage, the following recipes contain a few sensual blends which you may find inspiring. The same combinations of essences can be used in the vaporiser if you wish, in which case, you will need to adjust the quantity of essential oil accordingly, adding about 6 drops altogether to the water-filled reservoir of the vaporiser (exact quantities and ratios of essences are not at all crucial for room scents). For further advice on creating blends with Aphrodite in mind, see Chapter 27.

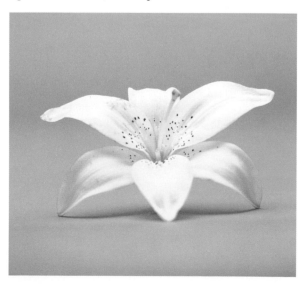

SENSUAL MASSAGE BLENDS

Choose one of the blends suggested below, or mix one of your own creations. You may prefer to use infused oil of vanilla (see page 235) as a base for your essential oil blends as it has a particularly sensual aroma. Quantities of essential oil are given in drops for 30 ml of base oil.

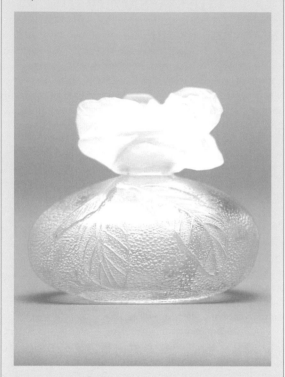

Tonight

6 drops coriander
2 drops lime
2 drops rose otto
2 drops frankincense

Freya

3 drops petitgrain
3 drops bergamot
3 drops lavender
2 drops vetiver

Firebird

3 drops lemon
3 drops orange
1 drop ginger
3 drops frankincense

Interlude

3 drops mandarin
4 drops sandalwood
3 drops ylang ylang

Rhapsody

2 drops clary sage
3 drops bergamot
2 drops neroli
4 drops cedarwood

Moments

2 drops rose otto
5 drops sandalwood

EROTIC MASSAGE TECHNIQUES

Unlike ordinary aromatherapy massage, the main purpose of which is to bring about deep relaxation, sensual or erotic massage aims to tease and awaken desire. The erotic 'extras' you are about to learn can be incorporated into the basic massage sequence described in Chapter 22 if you wish. However, it is enough to give a slow, rhythmic massage based on stroking, kneading and feathering, which also includes attention to the erogenous zones: the lower belly, the insides of the thighs, the backs of the knees, the buttocks, the lower back, the breasts, the ears, the lips, the back of the neck, the palms, the insides of elbows, the armpits, the soles of the feet and in between the toes and fingers.

The three basic massage movements in themselves are not necessarily erotic, but add very light scratching, licking, hot breath on the skin, and other diversions – fired with a passionate desire for your beloved – then before you know it, you are courting Eros! Generally, what feels good to you should also feel good to your lover. However, the ancient erotic texts proclaim that women are more responsive to lingering, gentle stimulation, while men prefer firmer handling. But you must discover for yourself what you and your lover find erotic.

Erotic massage can be a leisurely affair or a brief encounter; whatever turns you on, as they say! Nevertheless, without actually giving massage by the clock (a dampener of desire if there ever was one) do try to give each other at least fifteen minutes of exquisite teasing before moving on to other things.

EROTIC MASSAGE

Erotic diversions can be incorporated into the main sequence described in Chapter 22 if desired, or you may prefer to invent your own sequence, spiced with any of the following delights.

BACK, BUTTOCKS, ARMS AND HANDS

1 As an erotic variation on the back massage routine (see page 169), position yourself at your lover's head. Place your hands horizontally on either side of the spine on the uppermost part of the back, fingers pointing towards the spine. Using a sliding stroke, move your hands down the length of the back, and over the buttocks.

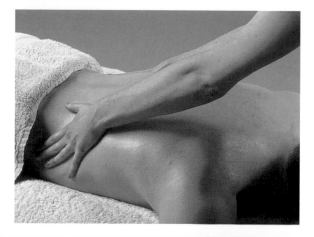

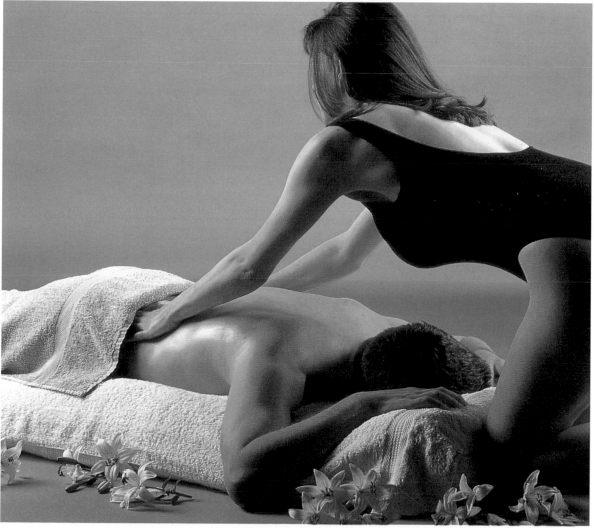

2 Then glide your hands over your partner's hips and slowly pull them up the sides of the body and into the armpits. Fan your hands out over your lover's shoulders, then lightly glide them down the outer edge of the arms. When you reach the hands, slide your fingers in between your lover's fingers, then lightly glide your fingertips up the inside of the arms. When you reach the shoulders, pivot your hands back to the original position. Repeat several times.

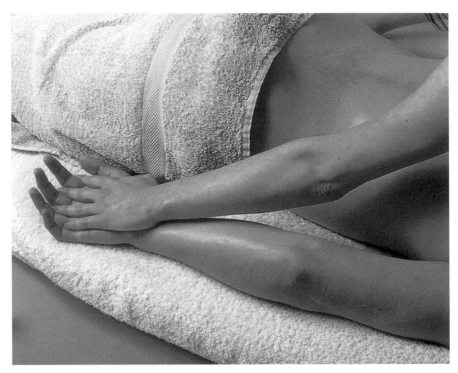

FEATHERING WITH LONG HAIR

1 Feathering or light caressing can be done with long hair. So if you or your lover qualify, slowly caress the other's body by sweeping your hair over it. Brush from the top of the neck and down the body to the tops of the toes before starting again. Do not forget to sweep down each arm as well. Repeat as many times as you wish. The only part of the body that does not appreciate being caressed with hair is the face. Indeed, it is most irritating to get hair in your eyes or mouth.

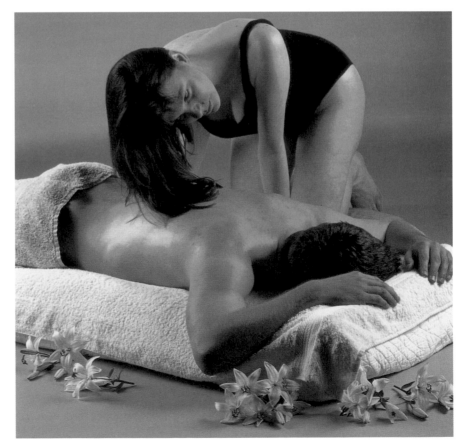

EAR CARESS

If your lover enjoys ear caressing, linger here for some time. Lightly circle one ear at a time with your finger. Nibble and kiss the earlobe, tracing the shell-like crevice with your tongue.

THE BELLY SLIDE

1 After caressing your lover's ears, slide your hands very lightly over the throat and on to the chest, with your fingers pointing towards the feet.

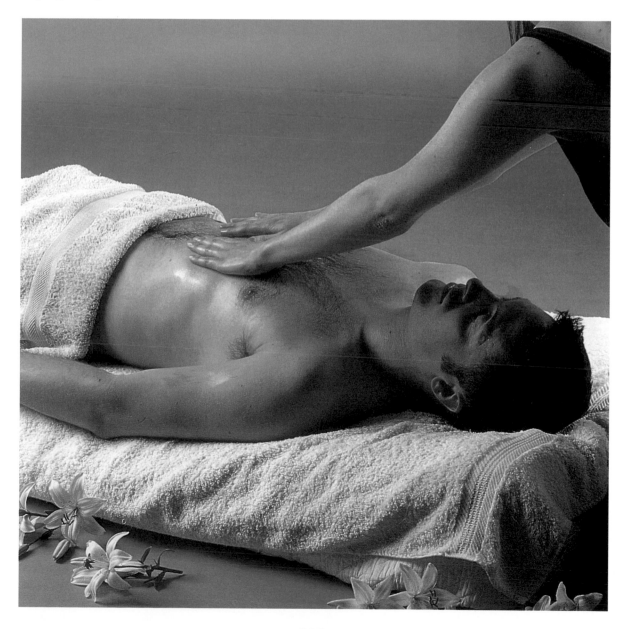

2 Slide your hands very slowly over the breasts or chest, down towards the abdomen, keeping the pressure light, but increasing slightly as your hands pass over the navel. When you reach the pubic bone, fan your hands out and bring them very slowly up the sides of the body to the armpits. Slide your hands over the shoulders, and bring them back to the original position. Repeat as many times as you wish.

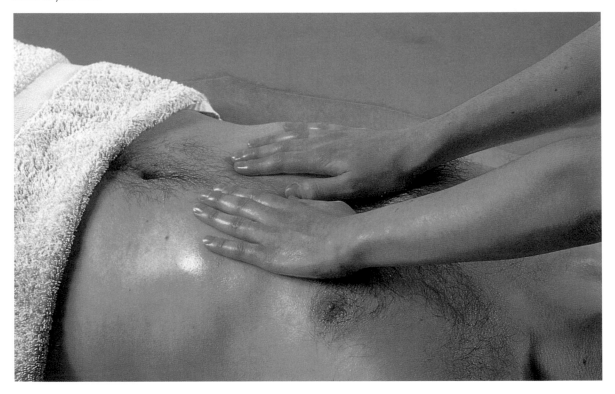

STROKING AROUND THE BREASTS

As a variation, begin as before with your hands placed on the upper chest, fingers pointing towards the feet. Then slowly and gently slide your hands down between the breasts, then around and underneath them and up towards the armpits. Slide your hands over the shoulders back to the original position. Repeat as many times as you wish.

TOE TEASER

Many people find foot massage (and also hand massage) very sensual. An impish way to drive your lover wild is to finish the foot sequence (see page 180) by running the tip of your little finger slowly in and out between the toe… exquisite torture if your lover has ticklish feet!

ENDING THE MASSAGE

Do some featherlight stroking with your fingertips barely touching the skin, paying special attention to the inner thighs and backs of the knees. Breathe on your lover's neck, circle the navel with your tongue, stroke behind the ears, touch the eyelids and lips. Caress your lover's arms and hands with soft lips and hot breath on the skin. Then do fingertip feathering downwards over the whole body, grazing the nipples, lips and genitals until your lover is tingling with erotic sensitivity… caress with your imagination!

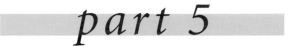

part 5

AESTHETIC AROMATHERAPY

Things are pretty, graceful, rich, elegant, handsome, but, until they speak to the imagination, not yet beautiful.

EMERSON ON 'BEAUTY', FROM
THE CONDUCT OF LIFE, *1860*

26
AROMATIC BEAUTY CARE

At one time the search for 'beauty' was confined to superficial treatments comprising weird and wonderful concoctions, spiced with exotic extracts and finished off with a plastering of make-up. The most important attribute of beauty — good health — was largely ignored. It is by practising the healthy lifestyle regime suggested in Chapter 19, and without becoming obsessive about your appearance, that a clear complexion, shiny hair, strong teeth and a supple body can be yours. Viewed from this perspective, the aromatic beauty treatments revealed in this chapter will work more efficiently, adding far more than just the polish.

Until recently men have shied away from the whole idea of 'beauty care', but things have changed, and now a great many men are happy to experiment with all manner of enticing concoctions. Most of the recipes and treatments given here are suitable for both men and women, but even if you are one of the lucky few, blessed with a fine trouble-free skin, good teeth, sparkling eyes and shiny hair, the use of the finest natural body care preparations will help to preserve these attributes for as long as possible.

You will be pleased to hear that the beauty preparations are quick and easy to make, often from ingredients that you will have in the larder or the fridge. What is more, creating your own skin care preparations is not only enjoyable, but the fruits of your labour may also be better for your skin than some commercial products, and at a fraction of the cost.

> **IMPORTANT** If you suffer from a skin complaint such as eczema, psoriasis or acne, you may need to seek further advice from an aromatherapist, herbalist or nutritionist who will devise for you a personalised healing programme. We are all different; what may work for one individual will not necessarily work as well for another.

THE FOUNDATIONS

THE FREE RADICAL CONNECTION

In recent years the health and beauty gurus have been extolling the virtues of skin care products containing 'free radical fighters'. Free radicals are acknowledged to be the number one enemy of skin. They are highly reactive particles which form toxic peroxides in the presence of oxygen. If left unchecked, they can damage collagen and elastin fibres (proteins which keep the skin resilient and muscles firm) and destroy cells throughout the whole organism. What is more, they have even been implicated as the primary cause of the ageing process itself. Yet free radicals are formed naturally during a wide variety of biological processes, from respiration to the carrying out of enzyme activities. It is only when they get out of control that they become problematic. Whatever can be done to neutralise the potentially damaging effect of wayward free radicals will also help to preserve skin and muscle tone and prevent premature ageing.

What causes free radicals to go on the rampage? The main triggers are:

- Over-consumption of highly processed fats and oils such as sunflower margarine and refined vegetable oils whose natural complement of nutrients has been drastically altered by the refining process. If your diet is also deficient in natural anti-oxidants such as vitamin E, which acts to buffer free radical activity, you run the risk of premature ageing and the development of degenerative disease.
- Skin applications of oils and creams (whether prepared from refined or unrefined oils) already damaged by free radicals. Unfortunately, this can occur well before the product begins to smell rancid. Commercial formulas contain preservatives which certainly help to slow down oxidation and prolong the shelf-life of the product, but they can also cause allergic reactions in

susceptible people. Home-made cosmetic creams and oils are free from potentially risky preservatives. However, it is essential that they are prepared from high quality oils which have not passed their best before date. They must also be stored in a cool dark place (preferably the fridge) and used up within a couple of months.

- Excessive exposure to ultraviolet light (including sunbeds). Radiation emitted from such sources can penetrate the skin and destroy its network of supporting elastin and collagen fibres. However, moderate doses of sunlight (up to one hour a day) is good for you. It stimulates circulation in the skin, triggers the formation of vitamin D and makes you feel well.
- Prolonged emotional stress.
- Air pollution from sources such as exhaust fumes, chimney smoke, industrial chemicals and cigarette smoke.
- Toxic metals such as lead and mercury which are increasingly being traced in drinking water and in our food.
- Pesticide residues in the environment and in food and water.
- Chemical food additives and foods lacking in freshness.

Free radical activity can be neutralised in the following ways:

- By ensuring your diet is supplying you with enough vitamin E. The nutrient acts as a free radical scavenger, mopping up these destructive particles and neutralising their effect. Many unrefined cooking oils, such as extra virgin olive and sunflower seed, contain appreciable quantities of the vitamin in a naturally balanced form. Other good sources of vitamin E are green leafy vegetables, egg yolk, wholegrain cereals, fresh peas and beans.
- Certain oils, for example evening primrose which is used for medicinal rather than culinary purposes, are supplemented with natural source vitamin E before being encapsulated. This acts to retard free radical activity in the human body, and not just within the oil capsule itself. If you wish to take an oil supplement, evening primrose is one of the finest. The usual maintenance dose for healthy skin and hair is 2 x 250 mg capsules a day.
- While it is essential that your diet is rich in all nutrients, vitamin C is especially important. Just as the anti-oxidant vitamin E appears to work particularly on the fat-based membranes of the body, vitamin C works on its fluids. It enhances vitamin E's protective abilities and helps shield the body from damage due to environmental pollutants. Ensure that you obtain enough vitamin C by eating plenty of raw fruits and vegetables.

- Other known anti-oxidants include beta carotene (the precursor of vitamin A) and selenium. Beta carotene is found in all orange-coloured fruits and vegetables and in green leafy produce such as spinach and cabbage. Good sources of selenium are fish, seafood, meat, wholegrains and dairy produce.
- By applying high quality unrefined vegetable oils and essences to the skin.
- By using a sunblock or high factor sunscreen whenever you go out in the sun. However, if your skin is not especially sun-sensitive, it is my own belief that it is preferable to apply a natural sunscreening oil such as extra virgin olive oil or sesame oil (see the Repertory of Base Oils on page 35). The chemicals used in commercial sunscreen formulas may turn out to be problematic in themselves. Nevertheless, whether you use a proprietory sunscreen or a natural oil, it is essential to stay out of very hot sunshine. You can, however, take a short sunbathe (one hour maximum) in the morning before midday or after four o'clock in the afternoon when the sun's rays are longer and weaker and therefore less likely to burn.

THE MIND/BODY EFFECTS OF DRY SKIN BRUSHING

The benefits of this old and well-proven nature cure technique are amazing. Not only does dry skin brushing help the condition of the skin itself by whisking away the build-up of dead skin cells on the surface, it stimulates lymphatic drainage and the elimination of as much as one-third of body wastes. Complaints such as arthritis, cellulite (characterised by dimpled 'orange-peel' skin which is cold to the touch), high blood pressure and even depression have been linked to poor lymphatic drainage. Although dry skin brushing cannot totally replace adequate exercise, it is in fact the same in body stimulation terms as a good massage or twenty minutes jogging!

You will need a purpose-designed vegetable bristle brush with a long, but detachable handle so that you can reach your back. These are available from many good health shops or from some chemists. The brush must always be kept dry but washed in warm soapy water every two weeks. If you cannot obtain a body brush, a hemp glove is a good alternative. The body needs to be brushed once a day for a few minutes *before* your morning bath or shower (twice if you have cellulite). It is a good idea to take a week's break every month as skin brushing, like many natural detoxification techniques, is more effective if the body does not become too accustomed to it.

THE DRY SKIN BRUSHING TECHNIQUE

To brush your skin, make sweeping movements over each part of the body. Be gentle; brush too vigorously, especially if you are unused to body brushing, and you will scratch your skin. Begin with your feet, including the soles, then move up your legs, front and back, with long sweeping strokes. Brush over the buttocks and up to the mid-back. That is, always work towards the heart and bring toxins towards the colon. Then brush your hands, front and back, up the arms, across the shoulders, down the chest (avoiding the nipples if you are a woman) and then down the back of the neck to the upper back. Finally, brush the abdomen (avoiding the genitals), using a clockwise circular motion following the shape of the colon.

The skin on the face and neck is too sensitive for the body brush treatment, but you could use a soft bristle shaving brush for these areas if you wish. Using just the tips of the bristles, sweep across the forehead, gently around the eyes, down the nose, cheeks and chin towards the neck. Then brush the neck, back and front, towards the chest.

Skin brushing need take no longer than five minutes each time and can be done while you run the bath. After the bath or shower, apply your favourite aromatherapy massage oil to nourish your skin, or simply use a fine-textured vegetable oil such as almond or safflower, without the addition of essential oils.

CAUTION
- *Skin brushing is safe for almost everyone. The exceptions are those suffering from skin disorders such as eczema or psoriasis and those with areas where there is infected or broken skin. You can brush where the skin is healthy, but avoid any areas where you have bad varicose veins.*
- *If, during the first week of skin brushing, you break out in pimples here and there, do not be put off. This indicates that your body is throwing off toxins and eliminating these through the skin. After a week or two of dry skin brushing, your skin will look healthier than ever before.*

THE FACE

DAILY ROUTINE FOR ALL SKIN TYPES

Wash your face twice a day with a mild pH balanced soap or cleansing bar which helps to balance the skin's acid mantle. The mantle is a mixture of sebum (oil) and fluid supporting a microfloral of bacteria (the skin's defence against infection). It has a pH value of 5.5 which means it is slightly acid. Ordinary soaps and cheap facial preparations are alkaline and in some people can lead to dry, flaky skin.

After washing, particularly if your skin is oily, you will benefit from a mild astringent such as rosewater or one of the skin-tonics suggested on page 222. Although not essential, skin tonics make the skin feel fresh and invigorated.

While the skin is still damp, apply a moisturiser made from beeswax and plant oils or a light-textured vegetable oil such as almond, apricot kernel or jojoba. Alternatively, use a good commercial product, preferably a cream or lotion that does not contain mineral oil. Mineral oil clogs the skin and contributes to the development of blackheads and pimples.

WEEKLY TREATMENTS FOR ALL SKIN TYPES

Exfoliation

Although dry skin brushing with a shaving brush is good for stimulating lymphatic drainage which helps to reduce puffiness, some skin types need a slightly more intensive treatment to remove dead skin cells from the surface of the skin. A build-up of dead skin cells causes uneven skin tones and a dull appearance. Younger skins tend to shed skin cells without help, but as we age, the reproduction processes under the skin slow down. New skin cells are formed more slowly and worn out cells, which are pushed to the surface, tend to stay around in patches.

To make a simple exfoliating rub for sloughing off dead skin cells, moisten a handful of medium ground oatmeal (cornmeal if your skin is dry) and use as a *gentle* rub. Massage into all parts of your face and throat, paying particular attention to the area around the nostrils. Rinse off with warm to cool water. If you are a man and you shave, you need only exfoliate the hairless parts of your face, such as the forehead. Shaving is a highly efficient method of exfoliation. Incidentally, you may find it easier to use an exfoliating washing sachet. Put the ground oatmeal in the middle of a cotton handkerchief or piece of muslin, tie up the corners, then moisten with lukewarm water before use.

> **CAUTION** *Although exfoliating products are generally known as 'scrubs', this is certainly not what you should be doing to the fragile skin of your face. Even the mildest irritation or inflammation of the skin triggers free radical activity. So gently rub, don't scrub!*

Facial Sauna

Most skins benefit from the deep-cleansing effect of an aromatic steam bath, especially congested or oily skin that is prone to blackheads and blemishes. Fill a heat-proof mixing bowl with near boiling water, then add two or three drops of an essential oil suitable for your skin type (refer to the Skin Care chart on page 218). Hold your head over the steam and cover your head and the bowl with a towel to trap the aromatic vapours. Stay there for about five minutes. Finish this treatment by splashing your face with cool water to remove wastes accumulated on the skin's surface. You can follow this treatment with a face pack if you wish (see the recipes on page 222), or wait half an hour for your skin to settle down and apply your usual moisturiser.

> **CAUTION**
> - *Facial saunas should be avoided if your skin is prone to thread veins. Intense heat causes the blood vessels under the surface of the skin to dilate, thus exacerbating the problem.*
> - *Avoid facial saunas if you suffer from asthma; concentrated steam may trigger an attack.*
> - *American studies on skin health have indicated that the over-use of facial saunas (more than twice a week over several months) can cause 'jungle acne', a disorder brought about by the presence of too much moisture in the skin. Those who already have acne should be careful too. Excessive use of steam treatments (including walk-in saunas) can exacerbate the condition. However, the judicious use of steam treatments is extremely beneficial for acneous skin.*

Face Packs

The purpose of face packs is to deep cleanse and brighten the complexion. They can be applied after ordinary cleansing, or after an aromatic bath or facial sauna while the skin is still warm and moist and, therefore, more receptive to whatever you put on it (see the face pack recipes on page 222).

PERIODIC TREATMENTS

You may be surprised to learn that it is not advisable to apply an aromatherapy skin care oil to your face every day. The best results are achieved by doing it the French way: by applying the oils as a periodic 'cure', either once a week or daily for two weeks with a three to four week interval before resuming again. This prevents the skin from becoming too accustomed to the essences and failing to respond positively to them.

Choose an aromatic formula suitable for your skin type (refer to the Skin Care Charts on pages 218—221). There are four ways of applying the oils for skin treatments:

1 Apply a fine film of oil just after a bath or shower when your skin is still warm and moist. Do not wipe off any excess for twenty minutes; it can take this long for the oils to be absorbed.
2 Apply at least half an hour after a facial sauna or deep-cleansing face pack. The skin needs time to settle down after these treatments in order to absorb the essences (and the fat-soluble nutrients from the base oil) more efficiently.
3 Apply immediately after a five-minute warm compress. Half fill a heat-proof mixing bowl with hand-hot water, then immerse three face flannels in the bowl. Wring out and cover the face (except the nostrils, mouth and eyes) with two of the flannels. As one cools, replace it. Then massage the aromatic oils into your skin while it is still warm and damp.
4 Apply shortly before going for a walk in the open air (preferably the park or unpolluted country air). The combination of fresh air and essential oil is a superb skin rejuvenator.

If you choose the once a week regime, apply the oils three times a day if possible, otherwise once a day will suffice.

FIRST AID FOR CONGESTED SKIN PROBLEMS

BLACKHEADS, WHITEHEADS AND PIMPLES

Blackheads (cosmedones) are caused by a build-up of sebum (the skin's lubricating oily fluid) which forms a hard plug over the entrance to a pore or hair follicle which then blackens due to exposure to oxygen in the air.

Blackheads do not disappear of their own accord, but they can be removed by steaming the skin or by applying a warm compress. This acts to open the pores and loosen the oily material. The blackheads can then be eased out with scrupulously clean fingers wrapped in a tissue. Afterwards, dab the area with witch-hazel.

Whiteheads (milia) look like tiny white lumps on the skin. They are similar to blackheads except that, where the blackhead is exposed to the air, the whitehead remains closed due to an accumulation of dead skin cells covering the opening of the duct, making it impossible for the oil plug to move out of the pore. Unfortunately, the removal of whiteheads is beyond home treatment. If you attempt to squeeze them, this can cause inflammation and the formation of raised spots which will take a long time to clear up. If you have whiteheads and wish to get rid of them, it is advisable to consult a beautician who will open the milia with a very fine stylet, which leaves no scar.

A pimple or spot is formed when oil-blocked follicles become irritated and inflamed. White blood cells, which move into the area to fight the inflammation, create pus. This type of spot usually heals within a couple of days. If, however, the inflammation takes place deeper in the skin, the pimple is more severe and can turn into an acne cyst, in which case, the blemish will take much longer to heal, perhaps lurking beneath the surface for several weeks.

Ideally, the best action is to leave well alone, to allow the pimple to take its natural course. Fiddling with your skin and squeezing spots can make the problem worse, spreading the infection and possibly even causing scarring. Realistically, it is difficult to resist the temptation to speed-up the healing process, in which case you should steam your skin (or apply a warm compress), then apply a yoghurt or clay face pack to the affected area, or to your whole face if preferred. Afterwards, dab the spot with undiluted tincture of calendula (available from herbal suppliers) and continue to apply several times a day until the spot dries out. Most aromatherapists advocate dabbing spots with a drop of neat lavender or tea tree oil. Although this can work well for some people, in my own experience, the drying effect of an alcohol-based preparation is far more effective.

As a preventative of skin eruptions, experts on skin health advise those who suffer from severe acne or problems with recurrent blackheads, whiteheads and pimples to give up (or drastically reduce) animal fats in their diet and to replace these with cold-pressed or unrefined vegetable oils. Too much animal fat in the diet is believed to clog the pores and hair follicles with fatty deposits that encourage bacteria-based spots.

THE KITCHEN COSMETICIAN

AROMATIC OILS AND SKIN HEALTH

It is rarely acknowledged that essences used in baths and general massage will help the complexion whether or not they are applied directly to the face. This is because they reach the bloodstream via the lungs and skin and work systemically, influencing the body as a whole. Very congested skin (especially if it is acneous) cannot absorb essential oils efficiently anyway, but when used in the bath and in general body massage they will be more easily absorbed through the softer skin of the abdomen, the inner sides of the thighs and the upper arms.

When an appropriate essential oil for your skin type is combined with a high quality base oil, the positive effects are significant. The tiny molecules of both the essential oil and the nutrients in the base oil (especially vitamin E) can penetrate the deepest layers of the skin. It is from here that they act to stimulate the growth of healthy skin cells, increase the amount of moisture retained, promote the elimination of cellular wastes and generally support the function of blood capillaries.

A SELECTION OF BEAUTY OILS

The speciality base oils profiled below are those which are increasingly used in aromatherapy beauty treatments. Other vegetable oils suitable for body massage as well as beauty care are featured in the Repertory of Base Oils in Chapter 5.

Apricot Kernel Oil
Prunus armeniaca
A light, finely textured oil extracted from the seed kernel of the fruit. It is possible to obtain unrefined versions which contain small amounts of the free radical fighting anti-oxidant, vitamin E.
Availability
The oil is obtainable from some health shops and by mail order from essential oil suppliers.

Avocado Oil
Persea americana
The finest quality oil is cold pressed from the flesh. It has a sludgy appearance (indicating that it has not been damaged by heat and excessive refining) and a delightful emerald green hue. Refined avocado oil is pale yellow with very little odour and few nutrients. Cold-pressed

avocado oil is rich in essential fatty acids and contains appreciable quantities of beta carotene and vitamin E. Despite its viscosity, the oil has excellent powers of penetration and skin regeneration. It is therefore a superb treatment oil for dry, dehydrated or ageing skins. It can also be taken internally in capsule form to prevent skin dryness and dehydration, such as that caused by excessive sunbathing.

Availability

Unrefined avocado oil is available in capsule form from most chemists and health shops. It is possible to obtain bottles of avocado oil from essential oil suppliers, but do specify that you want the unrefined green oil. Unfortunately, I have come across refined versions of avocado oil labelled 'cold-pressed'. By getting to know the difference between refined and unrefined oils, and broadcasting this knowledge to suppliers, unscrupulous merchants will think twice before attempting to hoodwink the public.

Borage Oil
Borago officinalis

The oil is warm-pressed or solvent extracted from the tiny seeds of the plant, which is also known as starflower, due to the pointed star shape of its exquisite blue flowers. The oil is rich in essential fatty acids which are vital for skin health. Being an expensive oil, a small amount is usually added to aromatherapy blends to boost the skin-rejuvenating properties of other oils. However, the most effective skin-enhancing action of borage oil comes from taking it as a nutritional supplement.

Availability

Borage oil (sometimes labelled 'Starflower') is available in capsule form from chemists and health shops. For topical applications, pierce a capsule with a pin and squeeze out the contents.

Castor Oil
Ricinus communis

Apart from its use as a laxative, castor oil is a popular ingredient in protective hair and skin care products. It comes from the castor plant, an attractive shrub native to West Africa. The oil is cold-pressed from the glossy brown seeds and has wonderful lubricating and waterproofing properties, which is why it is included in many commercial hair conditioners and nappy rash creams. Its main use in aromatherapy is in hair conditioning formulas. However, it does have a very sticky texture and a strong odour which can be off-putting to some people.

Availability

Widely available from chemists.

Jojoba
Simmondsia chinensis

Jojoba (pronounced ho-ho-ba) comes from an evergreen desert plant native to South America. The oil (actually a liquid wax) is virtually colourless and odourless. It is extracted from the beans of the plant and is semi-solid at room temperature. It is a marvellous substance because it needs little or no refining, and is extremely stable. I have never known the oil turn rancid. The chemical structure of jojoba resembles the skin's own oily secretion, sebum. As well as being an excellent moisturiser for all skin-types, when massaged into the skin it combines with sebum and acts as an emulsifier, gently unclogging the pores and freeing embedded grime. So it can even be used on oily or acneous skin. Jojoba also contains myristic acid, which has anti-inflammatory properties.

Availability

Available from most health shops or by mail order from essential oil suppliers.

Macadamia Nut Oil
Macadamia integrifolia and M. ternifolia

Macadamia nut oil is relatively new to aromatherapy. The finest quality oil comes from Australia. Although most of the oil produced has undergone extensive refining, it is possible to obtain a superior warm-pressed version. The oil is special because it is the only known plant oil to contain palmitoleic acid, an essential fatty acid found in sebum, so it has a natural affinity with the skin. Unrefined macadamia oil has a fine texture and a golden hue, with very little aroma. It is highly emollient making it especially beneficial to dry and ageing skin.

Availability

Not generally available, so you will need to obtain the oil from an essential oil supplier.

Passionflower Oil
Passiflora incarnata

The oil is warm-pressed from the seeds found in the orange fruits of the passionflower, a fast-growing climber native to South America. The oil contains appreciable quantities of linoleic acid which acts to prevent moisture loss. Taken orally, it helps to promote and maintain skin elasticity.

Availability

Available in capsules from chemists and health shops. Although primarily used as a nutritional supplement, you could also add the contents of one or two capsules to an aromatherapy skin care oil to boost the beneficial effects (pierce the capsule with a pin and squeeze out the contents).

Peachnut Oil
Prunus persica

The highest quality peachnut oil is cold-pressed from the kernels of the fruit. It has a pale golden colour and a delicately sweet aroma. Peachnut oil has a fine texture and is easily absorbed into the skin. Taken as a supplement, it helps to strengthen the hair and promote shine. The oil also contains useful quantities of vitamin E.

Availability
Can be obtained from health shops, though usually as a nutritional supplement in capsule form. Bottled peachnut oil can be obtained from essential oil suppliers.

SKIN CARE CHARTS

You can prepare your own skin care blends from the choice of base oils and essences shown here (instructions for mixing your own body and facial oils are to be found on page 34). Do remember not to exceed the recommended $\frac{1}{2}$ to 1 per cent dilutions for facial treatments.

SKIN TYPE
Normal

DESCRIPTION
Soft, smooth and finely textured. Few problems like spots and flakiness.

RECOMMENDED ESSENCES
Chamomile (German and Roman), geranium, lavender, neroli, rose otto.

RECOMMENDED BASE OILS
Almond, apricot kernel, extra virgin olive (diluted 50/50 or more with a lighter base oil), jojoba, passionflower (contents of one capsule to every 10 ml of another base oil), peachnut, safflower, sesame, sunflower seed.

SUGGESTED FORMULAS

1 drop chamomile (Roman)
1 drop geranium
3 drops lavender
15 ml almond oil
10 ml sunflower seed oil

3 drops lavender
2 drops neroli
25 ml jojoba oil

2 drops chamomile (Roman)
1 drop rose otto
2 capsules passionflower oil
20 ml apricot kernel oil

SKIN TYPE
Dry

DESCRIPTION

Close-textured and fine, but can feel tight after washing with soap. May also flake and is predisposed to developing facial lines.

RECOMMENDED ESSENCES

Chamomile (German and Roman), lavender, neroli, rose otto, sandalwood.

RECOMMENDED BASE OILS

Almond, avocado, borage (contents of one capsule to every 10 ml of another base oil), evening primrose (one capsule to every 10 ml of another base oil), extra virgin olive (diluted 50/50 with a lighter base oil), jojoba, macadamia nut, passionflower (contents of one capsule to every 10 ml of another base oil), peachnut, safflower, sunflower seed, wheatgerm (5 ml to every 30 ml of another base oil).

SUGGESTED FORMULAS

1 drop rose otto
3 drops sandalwood
10 ml extra virgin olive oil
15 ml macadamia nut oil

2 drops neroli
2 drops lavender
1 drop rose otto
2 capsules borage oil
20 ml safflower oil

1 drop chamomile (German)
4 drops lavender
10 ml avocado oil
25 ml peachnut oil

SKIN TYPE
Oily

DESCRIPTION

Has a characteristic shiny look with large pores; usually prone to developing blackheads and pimples (see also page 215).

RECOMMENDED ESSENCES

Bergamot FCF, cedarwood, cypress, frankincense, geranium, juniper berry, lavender, patchouli, rosemary, vetiver.

RECOMMENDED BASE OILS

Jojoba, passionflower (contents of one capsule of passionflower to every 10 ml of jojoba).
Important Apply after a bath, shower or warm facial compress for maximum penetration. Wipe off any excess after 30 to 40 minutes.

SUGGESTED FORMULAS

2 drops frankincense
3 drops cedarwood
25 ml jojoba oil

2 drops cypress
1 drop geranium
2 drops bergamot FCF
25 ml jojoba oil
2 capsules passionflower oil

1 drop patchouli
1 drop frankincense
2 drops lavender
25 ml jojoba oil

SKIN TYPE
Combination

DESCRIPTION
The chin, nose and forehead form an oily T-zone of the face, whereas the skin around the eyes, cheeks and neck is dry.

RECOMMENDED ESSENCES
Chamomile (German or Roman), frankincense, geranium, lavender, rose otto.

RECOMMENDED BASE OILS
Extra virgin olive (diluted 50/50 or more with a lighter base oil), hazelnut, jojoba, passionflower (contents of one capsule to every 10 ml of another base oil), peachnut, sesame.

SUGGESTED FORMULAS

2 drops chamomile (Roman)
2 drops geranium
5 ml extra virgin olive oil
20 ml seasame oil

2 drops frankincense
3 drops lavender
15 ml hazelnut oil
10 ml jojoba oil

1 drop frankincense
2 drops lavender
1 drop geranium
25 ml jojoba oil

SKIN TYPE
Sensitive

DESCRIPTION
Can be of any type, and may become sensitive from exposure to harsh soaps and cosmetic materials. Always carry out a patch test before using any skin care product (see page 23). Use essences in very low concentration e.g. $\frac{1}{2}$ per cent or less.

RECOMMENDED ESSENCES
Chamomile (German or Roman), lavender, neroli, rose otto.

RECOMMENDED BASE OILS
Almond, apricot kernel, evening primrose (contents of one capsule to every 10 ml of another base oil), jojoba.

SUGGESTED FORMULAS

1 drop chamomile (German)
30 ml almond oil

1 drop rose otto
2 capsules evening primrose
25 ml jojoba oil

2 drops lavender
25 ml apricot kernel oil

SKIN TYPE
Thread veins

DESCRIPTION

Broken veins usually occur around the nostrils and across the cheeks. Can affect all skin types, but especially sensitive skin.

RECOMMENDED ESSENCES

Cypress, frankincense, geranium, neroli, rose otto.

RECOMMENDED BASE OILS

Apricot kernel, calendula (an infused oil, see page 39), evening primrose oil (contents of one capsule to every 10 ml of another base oil), extra virgin olive (diluted 50/50 or more with a lighter base oil), jojoba, passionflower (contents of one capsule to every 10 ml of another base oil), peachnut.

SUGGESTED FORMULAS

1 drop chamomile (Roman)
1 drop neroli
1 drop geranium
5 ml extra virgin olive oil
20 ml apricot kernel oil

2 drops cypress
1 drop frankincense
25 ml peachnut oil

1 drop geranium
3 drops frankincense
25 ml apricot kernel oil

SKIN TYPE
Ageing

DESCRIPTION

In need of nourishing and toning.

RECOMMENDED ESSENCES

Frankincense, galbanum (in less than $\frac{1}{2}$ per cent concentration), geranium, myrrh, neroli, rose otto, sandalwood.

RECOMMENDED BASE OILS

Almond, apricot kernel, avocado, borage (contents of one capsule to every 10 ml of another base oil), extra virgin olive (diluted 50/50 or more with a lighter base oil), jojoba, macadamia nut, passionflower (contents of one capsule to every 10 ml of another base oil), peachnut, safflower, sunflower seed, wheatgerm (5 ml to every 30 ml of another base oil).

SUGGESTED FORMULAS

4 drops sandalwood
2 drops frankincense
2 capsules passionflower
5 ml wheatgerm oil
30 ml sunflower seed oil

1 drop rose otto
1 drop myrrh
10 ml avocado oil
15 ml sunflower seed oil

2 drops neroli
1 drop myrrh
1 drop geranium
10 ml macadamia nut oil
15 ml apricot kernel oil

FACE PACKS

Face packs or masks are designed to balance skin secretions, to stimulate the circulation and to moisturise and tighten the skin. Although they can be applied after ordinary cleansing, it is far better to apply them after an aromatic bath, facial steam or warm compress while the skin is still moist and warm, therefore more receptive to whatever you put on it. Afterwards, allow your skin to settle down for at least half an hour before applying your usual moisturiser or nourishing facial oil.

FOR MOST SKIN TYPES

Yoghurt Mask

Unless you are allergic to dairy products, one of the most beneficial substances to use as a face pack is yoghurt (live, natural yoghurt, full fat if possible). Fresh, live yoghurt without additives can help all skin types, particularly excessively dry or oily skin. The lactic acid of yoghurt (due to its fermentation) is similar to that of the skin acid mantle, and appears to exert a balancing action on the secretion of skin fluids.

You will need about two teaspoonfuls of yoghurt which you then apply to face and neck and leave on for ten to fifteen minutes. Rinse off with plenty of cool water.

Honey Mask

Raw honey, that which has not been pasteurised, pressure filtered or blended with other honeys, is one of nature's finest moisturising agents. It draws moisture from the air and imparts a soft dewy glow to the complexion. For best results, apply to the face and neck just before you get into an aromatic bath. Leave on for at least ten minutes. Rinse off with warm water, followed by a splashing of cool water to close the pores. Now admire the healthy glow!

Fruit Mask

The latest 'anti-wrinkle' agents being promoted by the beauty industry are alpha hydroxy acids (AHAs). AHAs are found in sugar cane and in fruits, especially papaya and apple. They work by exfoliating the skin and enhancing its ability to retain water, thus facial lines are softened.

However, if you have sensitive skin, it is advisable to carry out a patch test before trying any of the fruit masks suggested here.

Apricot Facial Mash to a pulp a fresh, raw apricot and sieve it into a bowl. Pat into clean skin and leave on for ten to fifteen minutes. Rinse off with warm and then cool water. Suitable for all skin types.

Papaya Facial Mash to a pulp half a fresh papaya and sieve it into a small bowl. Apply to clean skin, leaving on for ten to fifteen minutes before rinsing off with warm and then cool water. Suitable for all skin types.

Apple facial Simply rub a slice of raw apple into your skin immediately after cleansing, leave on for ten to fifteen minutes, then rinse off with warm and then cold water. Suitable for normal to oily skin.

Clay Mask

For generations clay has been popular with European Nature Cure therapists for treating skin. Applied as a face or body pack, clay draws out impurities and promotes rapid healing of inflamed tissues. However, clay treatments can be very drying and so they should only be used on oily and acneous skins. Green clay is the finest and is available from shops specialising in natural remedies and home-made cosmetic materials. The next best is fuller's earth, which can be obtained from most chemists.

Mix one teaspoonful of green clay or fuller's earth with one teaspoonful of bottled spring water to make a paste. Apply to clean skin, avoiding the delicate eye area, and leave on for ten minutes. Rinse off in warm then cool water.

SKIN TONICS

Skin tonics, which can also be used as gentle aftershave, are easy to make for they are simply a mixture of distilled water (or floral water), cider vinegar and a few drops of essential oil. Cider vinegar is included because it helps to restore the skin's natural acid mantle. If you wish to include rosewater or orange flower water in the blend, do ensure that it is the genuine product (synthetic substitutes abound) by purchasing from an essential oil supplier (see Useful Addresses, page 289).

Apply skin tonic after washing or shaving to leave your skin feeling fresh and invigorated. Skin tonics are also helpful if you live in a hard water area. Lime scale deposits in hard water can disrupt the skin's acid mantle causing dryness and irritation. A slightly acidic skin tonic will help to restore the balance.

METHOD

Put one teaspoonful of cider vinegar into a 100 ml dark glass bottle. Then add up to six drops of an appropriate essential oil, or a blend of essences amounting to no more than six drops altogether, suitable for your skin type (see the Skin Care charts on pages 218–21). Top up with distilled water, rosewater or orange flower water and shake well to disperse the oil droplets. For very oily skin or acne, you could use a more astringent base such as witch-hazel. This could be made slightly less astringent by mixing with an equal quantity of distilled water.

The blend should then be allowed to infuse for 24 hours. When it is ready, pour it through a coffee filter paper into a small jug, and then funnel it back into the bottle. The tonic is then ready to use. Keep in a cool dark place and use up within a few weeks (the aroma will gradually diminish the more often you open the bottle).

> **IMPORTANT** *If you do not mind shaking the bottle each time before use to disperse the oil droplets, then there is no need to filter the mixture. If this is the case, because no essential oil will be left behind on the filter paper, you can reduce the quantity to three drops.*

HAIR AND SCALP

Healthy hair is a reflection of a balanced diet and lifestyle and gentle treatment. However, present day practices such as bleaching, perming, blow drying and the excessive use of harsh hair products result in much time and money being spent on repairing the damage. Like skin, hair is naturally acidic; frequent washing with an alkaline shampoo, for instance, disrupts this acid balance, and can be damaging to healthy hair. So the first step in treating hair is to use a mild pH balanced shampoo (easy to obtain nowadays) and to wash as infrequently as you dare. Once every seven to ten days would be ideal, though if your hair is oily, or if you live or work in a polluted environment, you will have to shampoo more often.

AROMATIC SHAMPOO

You could add essential oils to an unperfumed pH balanced shampoo if you wish. Add up to six drops of an appropriate essential oil for your hair type (refer to the chart on page 224) to every 50 ml of shampoo. However, not all essential oils are stable in soap or detergent. These include cedarwood, cypress, juniper, lemon, lime, mandarin, orange, pine and ylang ylang. The oils which *are* stable in shampoo include bergamot FCF, chamomile (German and Roman), eucalyptus, geranium, lavender, neroli, patchouli, petitgrain, rosemary, sandalwood and tea tree.

For damaged hair, or for those times when your hair needs a conditioning treatment, one of the finest substances to apply is extra virgin olive oil. It is known to strengthen the hair shafts, thus promoting body and shine. Castor oil was frequently used by the ancients as a hair thickener. It is a wonderful hair shiner and, despite being very sticky, is surprisingly easy to wash out. Other excellent hair and scalp oils include jojoba, peachnut and sunflower seed. Being finely textured, they are suitable for most hair and scalp conditions, except the very oily. In this instance, a hair tonic would be preferable.

Recipes for aromatic hair oils and tonics are given in the Hair and Scalp charts on pages 224 and 225. Further advice and treatments for conditions such as dandruff and falling hair are given on the Hair and Scalp Problems chart on page 226.

PREPARING AND USING HAIR AND SCALP OILS

First choose the essential oil(s) most suitable for your hair and scalp condition, taking into account your aroma preference. Add up to 20 drops to a 50 ml bottle of base oil and shake well. Start with wet hair (otherwise it will be much more difficult to shampoo out the oil). Massage your scalp with the aromatic blend, working the oil into the hair, paying special attention to the ends which are prone to dryness and splitting. Cover your head with a towel and leave for up to an hour before shampooing. Use your essential oil blend as a weekly conditioning treatment.

HAIR AND SCALP OILS AND FORMULAS

HAIR TYPE NORMAL

Recommended Essential Oils	Recommended Base Oils	Suggested formula
Chamomile (Roman), geranium, lavender, mandarin, neroli, petitgrain, rose otto.	Jojoba, peachnut, sunflower seed.	3 drops geranium 5 drops neroli 8 drops lavender 50 ml peachnut

HAIR TYPE DRY

Recommended Essential Oils	Recommended Base Oils	Suggested formula
Chamomile (Roman), lavender, rose otto, sandalwood, ylang ylang.	Extra virgin olive, jojoba, peachnut, sunflower seed, wheatgerm (5 ml to every 45 ml of another base oil).	12 drops sandalwood 5 drops ylang ylang 50 ml extra virgin olive oil

HAIR TYPE SPARSE AND/OR FRAGILE

Recommended Essential Oils	Recommended Base Oils	Suggested formula
Lavender, patchouli, rosemary, ylang ylang.	Extra virgin olive, castor, wheatgerm (10 ml to every 30 ml of another base oil).	12 drops rosemary 5 drops patchouli 10 ml castor oil 30 ml extra virgin olive oil 10 ml wheatgerm oil

PREPARING AND USING HAIR AND SCALP TONICS

These are made in the same way as skin tonics, except that there is no need to filter the mixture. But do remember to shake the bottle each time before use to disperse the oil droplets.

Pour a little hair tonic into the palm of your hand and massage into the scalp and through the hair. If used regularly (several times a week), an essential oil hair tonic will improve the condition of your hair as well as making it smell good. Since hair tonics are aqueous rather than oily, there is no need to wet your hair before applying. Moreover, if you have oily hair, you may find that regular use of a hair tonic reduces over-secretion of sebum, and thus the need to shampoo quite so often.

HAIR AND SCALP TONICS

HAIR TYPE NORMAL

Recommended Essential Oils

Chamomile (Roman), geranium, lavender, mandarin, neroli, petitgrain, rose otto.

Tonic Base

Distilled water, rosewater or a 50/50 mixture of distilled water and orange flower water, cider vinegar.

Suggested formula

3 drops geranium
4 drops mandarin
5 drops lavender
3 drops petitgrain
300 ml orange flower water
2 teaspoonfuls cider vinegar

HAIR TYPE DRY

Recommended Essential Oils

Chamomile (Roman), lavender, rose otto, sandalwood, ylang ylang.

Tonic Base

Distilled water, rosewater or a 50/50 mixture of distilled water and rosewater, cider vinegar.

Suggested formula

8 drops sandalwood
1 drop rose otto
4 drops ylang ylang
300 ml rosewater
2 teaspoonfuls cider vinegar

HAIR TYPE OILY

Recommended Essential Oils

Bergamot FCF, cedarwood, cypress, eucalyptus, frankincense, grapefruit, juniper berry, lavender, lemon, patchouli, rosemary, tea tree.

Tonic Base

Distilled water, or a 50/50 mixture of distilled water and witch-hazel, or orange flower water, or a 50/50 mixture of orange flower water and rosewater, cider vinegar

Suggested formula

4 drops bergamot FCF
3 drops frankincense
4 drops grapefruit
4 drops rosemary
150 ml orange flower water
150 ml rosewater
2 teaspoonfuls cider vinegar

HAIR TYPE SPARSE AND/OR FRAGILE

Recommended Essential Oils

Lavender, patchouli, rosemary, ylang ylang.

Tonic Base

Distilled water, rosewater, orange flower water, cider vinegar.

Suggested formula

Normal to oily
6 drops rosemary
6 drops patchouli
300 ml rosewater
2 teaspoonfuls cider vinegar
Normal to dry
8 drops ylang ylang
5 drops patchouli
300 ml distilled water
2 teaspoonfuls cider vinegar

HAIR AND SCALP TREATMENTS FOR SPECIAL PROBLEMS

To find out how to treat an infestation of headlice, refer to the therapeutic chart on page 57 and the Aromatic Prescriptions and Procedures to be found at the end of the same chapter.

DANDRUFF, SIMPLE (PITYRIASIS)

Description

This type is known as simple dandruff which is just dry flaking of the superficial skin cells of the scalp.

Possible Causes

Too little brushing, poor scalp circulation, use of harsh hair cosmetics and insufficient rinsing out after shampooing.

Aggravated by

Medicated shampoos, which should be avoided; they tend to clear up the condition for a day or two, but the dandruff often returns with a vengeance, especially if you are allergic to common ingredients such as coal tar derivatives, salicylic acid, sulphur solutions and rescorcinol.

Recommended Essential Oils

Oily hair cedarwood, cypress, lavender, patchouli, rosemary, tea tree.
Normal/dry hair chamomile (German and Roman), geranium, lavender.

Suggested formulas

Tonic (for oily hair)
300 ml distilled water
3 teaspoonfuls cider vinegar
5 drops cedarwood
10 drops rosemary

Oil (for normal to dry hair)
45 ml extra virgin olive oil
5 ml wheatgerm oil
5 drops chamomile (Roman)
5 drops lavender
5 drops geranium

DANDRUFF, GREASY (SEBORRHEIC DERMATITIS)

Description

This is much more severe than simple dandruff and appears as thick greasy patches which can easily become infected resulting in scabbing and inflammation.

Possible Causes

Almost certainly the result of a faulty diet or food allergy.

Aggravated by

Prolonged stress and/or excessive consumption of dairy products and 'junk foods' are cited as the main offenders.

Recommended Essential Oils

Cedarwood, chamomile (German and Roman), eucalyptus, lavender, rosemary, tea tree.

Suggested formulas

Even if your hair is oily, an oily formula is the best external treatment. Leave on for about one hour before shampooing out.

Oil
50 ml extra virgin olive oil
5 drops chamomile (German)
8 drops lavender
contents of 2 vitamin E capsules *or*
2 evening primrose oil capsules

Nutritional Supplements

It may be worth while taking 4 x 500 mg of evening primrose oil every day; it has been shown to help many skin disorders including eczema and dermatitis which are similar to seborrheic dermatitis.

Further Advice

It is advisable to have a food allergy test and/or consult a medical herbalist or homoeopath for constitutional treatment.

FALLING HAIR (ALOPECIA)

Description

Hair may fall out in patches or become gradually thinner. It should be pointed out that it is virtually impossible to restore a full head of hair to a man suffering from male pattern baldness, at least not without the use of risky hormone treatments.

Possible Causes

There are numerous possible causes, including illness, drugs, poor nutrition, harsh chemical treatments, menopause, prolonged stress, emotional shock, the influence of the male hormone testosterone.

Aggravated by

Faulty nutrition, prolonged stress, poor scalp circulation.

Recommended Essential Oils

Lavender, patchouli, rosemary.

Suggested formulas

Tonic (oily)
300 ml distilled water
3 teaspoonfuls cider vinegar
10 drops lavender
5 drops patchouli
5 drops rosemary

Oil (normal to dry)
30 ml extra virgin olive oil
20 ml castor oil
contents of 2 vitamin E capsules
10 drops lavender
5 drops patchouli

Nutritional Supplements

During the healing period, take a good multi-vitamin and mineral supplement containing the full B-complex range of nutrients and 4 x 500 mg evening primrose oil capsules.

Further Advice

Take steps to improve your diet and lifestyle, To increase scalp circulation, regular massage to head, neck and shoulders helps. Yoga, especially the inverted positions, also helps to stimulate scalp circulation. If you suspect a serious underlying health problem, do seek medical advice. It may also be advisable to consult an holistic nutritionist, herbalist or homoeopath for constitutional treatment.

OTHER BODY TREATS

MAKING SKIN CREAMS

Home-made skin creams are richer and heavier than the super-light commercial formulas, but they are extremely effective and economical. The following recipe makes a fairly soft cream which will harden slightly if kept in the fridge (to slow down the formation of mould). However, it should be used up within two months. You will find that a tiny amount goes a long way, so do not be tempted to make too much. Use it as a hand cream, aftersun body soother, or as a face cream for drier skin.

Although the recipe specifies almond oil, you can experiment with other vegetable oils as long as they add up to 120 ml in all. Beeswax is a marvellous skin softener and does not clog the pores. However, if you have sensitive skin it is essential to carry out a patch test before using. Beeswax is obtainable from shops specialising in natural remedies and home-made cosmetic materials, or it can be obtained directly from some beekeepers.

15 g yellow beeswax
120 ml almond oil
50 ml distilled water or rosewater or orange flower water
4–6 drops essential oil (refer to the Skin Care chart
on page 218)

Melt the beeswax with the oil in a heat-resistant basin over a pan of simmering water. Meanwhile, heat the distilled water (or floral water) in another basin over a pan of simmering water until it has warmed. Begin to add the warm water, drop by drop at first, to the oil and wax, beating with a rotary whisk, balloon whisk or an electric food mixer set at the lowest speed. After you have mixed about two teaspoonfuls of the water into the oil and wax, remove from the heat and continue adding the water a little at a time until you have incorporated it all. As soon as the mixture begins to set, stir in the essences. Divide the mixture into little sterilised glass pots, cover tightly and label.

BODY PACKS

You could give yourself a body pack with the same ingredients as you would use on your face. It helps to have someone else around to apply the mixture to your back, though you should manage reasonably well on your own. Begin with dry skin brushing, followed by a hot bath or shower to open the pores. It should be easy enough to apply any of the ingredients suggested for face packs (see page 222), increasing the quantities accordingly. Unless you decide to apply the pack to just one problem area, say, a spotty back, you will have to remain standing for fifteen to twenty minutes to allow the body pack to do its good work. What you should do to amuse yourself while this is happening is entirely up to you! Afterwards, rinse the pack off with lukewarm water (much easier in the shower), or with cold water if you are brave enough, and pat dry.

NATURAL DEODORANTS

If you are healthy, fresh perspiration is not at all offensive. It is only when the resident skin bacteria start to break it down, producing an excess of lactic acid, that it becomes malodorous. The most obvious solution to the problem of body odour is to wash frequently and to avoid synthetic fibres against your skin. Fabrics such as polyester and lycra create an airless environment, and thus hinder the evaporation of sweat. Excessive perspiration is often caused by stress and anxiety, so worrying about body odour only serves to exacerbate the problem.

Aluminium-based commercial deodorants can irritate the sensitive underarm area and may even promote widespread allergic reactions in susceptible individuals. Gentle deodorants containing chlorophyll (the green colouring matter of leaves) is available from health shops. Chlorophyll destroys the bacteria which causes perspiration odour.

REFRESHING TIRED EYES

The most effective way to soothe and refresh tired eyes is to lie down in a quiet darkened room, with your feet raised above the level of your head. Apply one of the following to your eyelids and leave on for at least fifteen mintues:

Witch-hazel compress Sterile gauze or cotton wool pads soaked in an equal quantity of witch-hazel and cooled, boiled water.
Flower water compress Sterile gauze or cotton wool pads soaked in rosewater or cornflower water. Distilled cornflower water is not widely available, though it can be obtained by mail order from a few essential oil suppliers. If, however, you can obtain the fresh flowers, make a tea from a handful of flower heads and about 300 ml of boiling water. Leave to infuse for fifteen minutes, strain and allow to cool before using as a compress.
Indian Tea Bags Having made a pot of ordinary tea and allowed it to cool, squeeze out the excess moisture from two tea bags and apply.
Herbal Tea Bags Using the same method as for Indian tea, apply peppermint or chamomile tea bags.

27
CREATE YOUR OWN PERFUMES

To the highly trained nose of the perfume scientist, fragrances composed entirely of organic essences are little more than primitive offerings to the Goat God Pan. Indeed, they would argue, such 'crude' mixtures of essences may have tantalised and seduced the senses in former times, but the modern nose is much more discerning and sophisticated.

If the truth be known, most people would be surprised if they knew exactly what went into some of the big name perfumes. The beautiful bottles contain exotic cocktails of aroma chemicals with unromantic names like trimethylundecylenic aldehyde, isoamyl salicylate and terpineol extra. Unmodified essential oils hardly get a look in. Yet even though you may be intoxicated by 'Opium', beguiled by 'Charlie' and distracted by 'Obsession' this does not mean that you cannot rediscover the mystery and allure of perfumes in their natural state. But be warned: once weaned on to naturals, your senses will never be the same again. An expensive big name perfume whose aura once held you spellbound may now cause your nose to twitch in disbelief, or in defence from chemical warfare!

If you are already enamoured of aromatherapy, creating perfumes using essential oils is a natural progression in your alchemical apprenticeship. You will be ready to delve a little deeper into the mysteries of creative blending, and to indulge in the scentsational art of seduction.

APPRENTICED TO ALCHEMY

PERFUME NOTES

It was the nineteenth-century French perfumer Charles Piesse who categorised aromatic oils according to a scale of top, middle and base notes, corresponding to the notes on the musical stave. The top note of a blend is what you smell as soon as the fragrance begins to vaporise on your skin. It awakens and stimulates the senses. This quickly disappears to reveal the longer-lasting middle note. The base note is what you smell sometimes hours after the first application, when the top and middle notes have faded.

Some of the most popular top notes (also called 'head' notes) are bergamot, and lemon. These highly volatile essences add brightness and clarity to a blend, much like a flute adds high-pitched purity to an orchestra. The middle notes (sometimes called 'heart' notes) such as rose, vanilla and ylang ylang, impart warmth and fullness to the fragrant composition, rather like the mellow tone of the oboe. Then there are the heavy lingering base notes (also known as 'bottom' notes or the 'dry out'). These include patchouli, frankincense, sandalwood and vetiver. Just like the haunting voice of the cello, they have a profound influence on the blend as a whole. They are also good 'fixatives', which means they slow down the evaporation rate of the top and middle notes, thus improving the 'staying power' of the blend. Sandalwood is the base note which is regarded as one of the finest natural fixatives because its soft aroma harmonises as a background note to a wide variety of fragrant compositions.

However, as nature would have it, few essential oils resonate entirely from one of the three ranges; a reflection of their complex chemical nature. Most reach up or down to an adjacent level (see the Perfume Notes chart on page 231). Thus they are able to link hands with the similarly friendly molecules of other essences. Oils which are especially good at linking with others are called 'bridges'; they connect many individual components and allow them to merge into perfect accord. Rose otto could be described as the bridging note supreme, for although resonating mainly from the heart, it also embraces both head and base. Indeed, at one time no perfume (whether regarded as a feminine or masculine fragrance) was deemed complete without the addition of rose.

NOTES WITHIN NOTES

You may find it interesting to see if you can perceive 'notes within notes'. Put a drop of essential oil on a piece of blotting paper or a purpose-designed smelling strip and try to experience the emerging nuances of aroma. Take geranium, for example; initially the scent is intensely sweet (almost honey-like), but stay with it a little longer and you may perceive an unexpected hint of mint, which gives way to a peppery rosy note and a sensation of 'cold'. To take another example, the first hint of ylang ylang reveals a richly floral fragrance, but with a disconcerting tinge reminiscent of nail polish. Thankfully, the harsh element soon gives way to the pleasure of cream soda and almonds, drying out to reveal a jasmine-like undertone.

ADAPTING PERFUMES

Although the blending of essences for aesthetic purposes may seem more complicated than therapeutic blending, in practice your developing sense of smell will be your guide. Just as a good cook will check the flavour of a dish by tasting every so often and adjusting the seasoning accordingly, the kitchen alchemist builds a perfume step by step.

For example: should an aromatic concoction smell too garish, the top note being far removed from the middle note, the formula can be toned down by adding a tiny amount of an essence with a softer quality, yet at the same time one that vibrates from the middle towards the upper range. Lavender or clary sage would be a good choice. If, on the other hand, the base note has taken over, simply lift the aroma by adding an oil that smells a little brighter, resonating from middle to base: ylang ylang may suit. Should the base note still be predominant, try adding a single drop of a lighter, fresher-smelling oil, one that will connect with the higher notes of ylang ylang. Bergamot may well be the essence required to bind the spell.

But your blends need not be so complex: cedarwood (base), clary sage (middle) and petitgrain (top) make an interesting 'woodland' blend. Or you may find that a certain aromatic oil smells wonderful just as it is. Oils such as carnation, jasmine, rose, ylang ylang, patchouli and sandalwood are often used as loners.

Yet not all perfumes conform to the traditional top, middle and base note pattern. Light, refreshing fragrances like classic eau-de-Cologne never contain heavy base notes, but are composed mainly of top notes. However, they are skilfully blended taking into account the 'notes within notes' theme. The highly volatile bergamot is the principal component of such blends; its pur-

pose is to temper the evaporation rate of the even flightier essences of grapefruit, lemon, lime, orange or mandarin. Neroli, another popular ingredient of the highest quality eau-de-Cologne, has the same slight tempering effect on bergamot and other citrus essences. Add a touch of rosemary, which resonates within the middle range, and this acts to slow down the volatility rate of neroli as well as the citrus element of the blend.

But no matter how skilfully blended, a light-hearted eau-de-Cologne formula can never be more than a fleeting encounter, even when held in check with the addition of relatively powerful chemical fixatives (as is the case with commercial eaux-de-Cologne). Unless a blend contains one of the heavy lingerers like jasmine, patchouli or sandalwood (or a similarly heavy chemical fixative), once applied to the skin it will rarely last for more than a couple of hours. On the other hand a rich blend featuring the deeply resonating patchouli will waft its earthy fragrance for many hours; and when used to perfume clothing, for instance a heavy woollen coat, will continue to broadcast its presence for some months.

A WORD ABOUT ABSOLUTES

Although some aromatherapists prefer not to use solvent-extracted absolutes for aromatherapy treatments, for perfumery purposes it is difficult not to concede; many of these oils smell exquisite. With the exception of oakmoss, however, absolutes are very pricey. But there is a choice of perfumery materials for the blends suggested in this chapter, so you can avoid using solvent-extracted oils if you wish. Alternatively, if you can obtain oils extracted by the Phytonics Process, these are preferable for aromatherapy perfumes because the amount of toxic residue is negligible.

PERFUME NOTES CHART

As far as aromatherapy perfumes are concerned, harmonious blends can be composed entirely of middle notes or of base notes, or whatever permutation you can think of. But should you be determined to compose according to the rules, the following information will help. Instructions for mixing perfumes are to be found on pages 233–6.

Top Notes

(also known as 'head' notes)
Angelica
Basil
Bergamot
Cardamom
Coriander
Eucalyptus**
Fennel
Grapefruit
Lavender
Lemon
Lemongrass
Lime
Mandarin
Melissa (true)
Orange
Peppermint
Petitgrain
Tea tree**

Top to Middle

Angelica
Basil
Bergamot
Cajeput**
Cardamom
Fennel*
Geranium
Lavender
Lemongrass
Melissa (true)
Neroli
Petitgrain
Tagetes*

Middle to Top

Black pepper
Chamomile (Roman)*
Chamomile (German)**
Clary sage
Clove (room scent)
Galbanum*
Geranium
Juniper berry
Lavender
Neroli
Myrtle*
Nutmeg
Palmarosa
Pine**
Rose absolute
Rose otto
Rose phytol
Rosemary

Middle Notes

(also known as 'heart' notes)
Black pepper
Cinnamon bark (room scent)
Clary sage
Clove (room scent)
Galbanum*
Geranium
Ginger
Juniper berry
Lavender
Marjoram*
Mimosa absolute
Neroli
Nutmeg
Palmarosa
Pine
Rose absolute
Rose otto
Rose phytol
Rosemary
Vanilla absolute (also infused oil of vanilla)
Ylang ylang

Middle to Base

Carnation absolute
Cypress**
Elemi
Galbanum*
Jasmine absolute
Myrrh**
Rose otto
Rose phytol
Vanilla absolute (also infused oil of vanilla)
Ylang ylang

Base to Middle

Cedarwood
Frankincense
Jasmine absolute
Myrrh**
Oakmoss
Sandalwood

Base Notes

(also known as 'bottom' notes or 'dry out')
Cedarwood
Frankincense
Oakmoss
Patchouli
Sandalwood
Vetiver

ESSENCES OF DESIRE

The most fascinating aromatics of all must surely be those that have been used for centuries as charms and love potions. Yet putting plant secretions on the human body to capture an erotic allure seems an odd thing to do. Is there any truth in the ancient belief that such sweet-smelling elixirs really can work such magic? We do know that many aromatic plants exude enticing substances with a similar chemical make-up to our own sexual secretions. But before setting out in search of the aphrodisiac qualities of aromatic oils, we need to learn something about our own natural essences of desire, collectively known as pheromones.

PHEROMONES

Just like plants, insects and animals, people secrete subtly fragrant hormone-like chemicals called pheromones. The word pheromone was coined by researchers in 1959 and is derived from the Greek *pherin*, to transfer, and *hormone*, to excite. While hormones are broadly classified as internal messengers, secreted into the bloodstream to influence the activity of target cells, the closely-related pheromones are external messengers: they are radiated by the skin to evoke a response in other people.

However, not all human pheromones are erogenic. Some contribute to our characteristic body scent. While no two people smell exactly alike (we each have our own 'fingerprint' odour), there are similarities between races. There are also recognisable 'male' and 'female' odours to be found within any ethnic group. Body scent is also influenced by the type of food eaten, the odours of which appear in our body fluids, most noticeably in sweat.

The 'fingerprint' odour apart, the ebb and flow of emotion, illness, the pill (and other drugs), as well as hormonal changes such as puberty, pregnancy, menstruation and menopause, also influence our body odour. It is also interesting to note that body odour influences our choice of perfume. When the fragrance is applied to the skin it intermingles with our own body chemistry. This explains why the same scent smells different on each person, and why we go off certain fragrances from time to time and begin to enjoy those which we previously found distasteful.

EROGENIC PHEROMONES

But what of the erogenic pheromones? To discuss human sexuality in terms of volatile secretions can be something of a 'turn off'. After all, we relate with one another in a great number of sophisticated, emotionally complex and imaginative ways. Indeed, unlike animals, whose sexual cycles are governed by the release of pheromones, the prefrontal lobe of the human brain acts to filter instinct. This means we can maintain a measure of control over our basic instincts. As the American biophysiologist Avery Gilbert puts it: 'If you had a bottle full of fluids generated by the female genital glands during copulation, and you put it on a guy's desk, and if he recognised the odor, he'd be *embarrassed*. Because it's out of context, and that's what makes the difference.'

Even so, more and more evidence is accumulating to suggest that human social and sexual behaviour is at least partly influenced by the scent of others in our sphere. Just like a flower whose fragrance declares to the world that it is both fertile and desirable, during sexual excitement we humans produce a cascade of enticing essences. These pheromones are radiated by the apocrine glands in the skin, found mainly in the armpits, pubic area, face and nipples. Hair, especially pubic hair, facilitates the radiation of these sexual odours. Pheromones are also found in the vaginal secretions, semen and saliva. During a passionate kiss, the apocrine glands in the face are especially active, which is part of the reason why kissing is so enjoyable.

Of the 200 separate components distinguishable in normal body odours, the female pheromones or copulins are reported to have a faint 'fishy' odour. However, the musky androstenone is believed to be the principle chemical of attraction. It is a biochemical cousin of the male sex hormone testosterone, which is produced in the female body too, albeit in miniscule amounts. Similarly, a tiny amount of the female hormone oestrogen is produced in the male body. Testosterone and androstenone are thought to play a major part in driving the libido in both sexes.

The quantity of pheromones produced by individuals can vary enormously. This may be one reason why an ordinary looking man or woman can sometimes possess an amazingly sexy aura, and why a perfect Adonis or Aphrodite may come over as somewhat bland. The writer Somerset Maugham, curious to know the secret of H.G. Wells's success with women, reported, 'He was fat and homely. I once asked one of his mistresses what attracted her to him. I expected her to say his acute mind and sense of fun: not at all; she said that his body smelt of honey.'

And women who produce higher than average amounts of androstenone are reputed to be extremely attractive; they also have a strong libido. All things being equal, there may be a grain of truth in this claim. Although far from being 'fat and homely', it has been revealed that Brigitte Bardot radiates a musky aroma, not from a bottle of costly French perfume, but from her own enticing essence!

TRADITIONAL APHRODISIAC PERFUMES

Traditionalists in the perfumery world insist that the most successful aphrodisiac formulas contain odour nuances which are *subliminally* reminiscent of the secretions, even excretions, of the human body. But if the 'animal' note is consciously recognised, the blend becomes objectionable. But it is not just the 'animal' note which gives the blend its erotic charge. The seductive mood of the whole can only be achieved by an interaction of four types of odour effect:

- **Erogenic** (aromatics which contain subthreshold faecal, urinous or sweaty odour nuances). Good examples include clary sage, jasmine, neroli, rose absolute, rose otto, rose phytol, sandalwood.
- **Narcotic** (those which have a heady, sweet, mellow overtone or undertone). These include carnation, cedarwood, chamomile (Roman), clary sage, frankincense, neroli, mimosa, nutmeg, patchouli, rose absolute, rose otto, rose phytol, sandalwood, vanilla, vetiver, ylang ylang.
- **Anti-erogenic** (essences with refreshing, uplifting or cooling fragrances). Good examples include bergamot, geranium, grapefruit, lavender, lemon, lime, mandarin, orange, peppermint, petitgrain, pine.
- **Stimulating** (essences with activating or warming aromas). Good examples being angelica, basil, black pepper, cardamom, carnation, coriander, elemi, fennel, ginger, juniper, oakmoss, rosemary.

As you can see, a few aromatic oils embrace more than one odour group; a reflection of their multifarious nature. This means that a blend of two or three essences is often enough to create a sensual massage oil, skin perfume, room scent or whatever you have in mind. A good example is rose absolute (erogenic and narcotic) with bergamot (anti-erogenic) and coriander (stimulating). However, there are no base notes in this blend. So if you would prefer a longer-lasting embrace, you could perhaps incorporate a touch of sandalwood or patchouli. So far so good, but what is the reasoning behind this pattern of blending?

HOW APHRODISIAC BLENDS WORK

Although an aphrodisiac perfume is worn as a means of attraction, it should also enhance the mood of the wearer. Unlike mind-bending drugs, essential oils can only work their special magic if both partners are open and receptive to the charm of the blend. This being the case, the first nuance of an erogenic perfume reveals the fresh, anti-erogenic top note. This gently awakens interest, rendering you more receptive to the heavier, narcotic element of the blend. The narcotic odour cannot act as an aphrodisiac by itself, but it does increase receptivity to erotic sensations such as pleasant surroundings, soft music, wonderful food and the company of your lover. The stimulating notes have a preparatory function similar to the narcotic notes: they stimulate your sense of smell, so that it reacts to the faint underlying erogenic or 'animal' nuance in the formula. This increased receptivity to erogenic odours, triggered by the combination of fresh, narcotic and stimulating notes, results in the activation of erotic feelings and images.

ANDROGYNOUS SCENTS

Generally speaking, the odour effect of an erogenic essential oil is fundamentally androgynous and can be used in both 'masculine' and 'feminine' blends. Likewise, our sex hormones (and their related pheromones) could also be described as androgynous. For, as mentioned earlier, both men and women secrete male and female hormones, albeit in differing amounts.

When blending, the secret is to mix the oils in the correct proportions. A traditional feminine blend is likely to emphasise flowers and sweet spices, because these scents are especially harmonious with the feminine body scent. A masculine blend will tend towards woods, earthy scents or pungent spices, for such aromas enhance the natural odour of man. It is also worth remembering that both feminine and masculine blends can be enhanced with a tinge of citrus.

However, if you are a woman who prefers a deeply resonating blend of woods and resins, or if you are a man with a penchant for a predominantly rose scented brew, then so be it. In this book, rules are meant to be broken! Always allow your aroma preference to be your guide. The aromas we like best tend to reflect our own body scent as well as our emotional needs.

BASIC PROCEDURES FOR PERFUME MAKING

Most commercial perfumes and colognes are suspended in alcohol, usually ethanol. Essential oils can be partially suspended in distilled water or in rosewater or orange flower water. The aromatic material will float on the surface so the mixture will need to be poured through a coffee filter paper before use: that is, unless you don't mind shaking the mixture each time before use.

Aromatherapists tend to favour oil-based perfumes which are much kinder to the skin (alcohol can be very drying for some skins). Oil-based perfumes also have the advantage of lingering on the skin for much longer. But they do smell a little different to alcoholic or aqueous mixtures, even when they are composed of exactly the same essential oils. Apart from the greater tenacity of oil-based perfumes, the oil itself imparts its own odour to the blend, no matter how bland the oil may seem to be. Strangely, the odour of the base intensifies when essential oils are added. This is an example of synergy, albeit not especially welcome in this instance.

The best base oil for aromatherapy perfumes is jojoba because it is only faintly odoriferous with excellent keeping qualities. Alternatively, you could use fractionated coconut oil, usually labelled 'Light Coconut', which is a highly refined oil (thus with a long shelf-life) and, unlike whole coconut oil, is not solid at room temperature. It also has very little odour of its own. Light coconut oil is obtainable by mail order from essential oil suppliers. Tiny amber bottles suitable for mixing and storing oil-based perfumes are also available from essential oil suppliers.

> **CAUTION** *The concentration of essential oil in perfume-strength blends is very high. Therefore, it may be advisable to carry out a skin test before use (see Essential Oil Safety, page 22).*

OIL-BASED PERFUME

Fill a 10 ml dark glass bottle almost to the top with jojoba or light coconut oil. Build your perfume slowly drop by drop, shaking the bottle well after each drop and smelling as you go. You will need 14 to 20 drops of essential oil altogether. Begin with the base note (if included) or with deepest resonating oil in your chosen repertoire, then develop the heart of the perfume and finally the top note. Label the bottle with the blend and date.

Once mixed, your perfume needs to be left for one or two weeks to mature. Keep in a cool dark place, but remember to shake the bottle once a day to facilitate the process. At the end of the maturation period, the blend will have lost its 'raw' overtones and will smell much more rounded. Oil-based perfume blends will keep for up to six months if stored in a cool dark place, in a drawer, for example, rather than displayed in a sunny spot on the dressing table.

How To Apply Perfume

Perfume is usually applied to the pulse points, behind the ears, the sides of the neck, the inside of the wrists, the elbow creases, behind the knees and around the ankles, as these points are fractionally warmer than the rest of the body and help to radiate the fragrance. However, don't overdo it. When it comes to perfume, less is definitely more.

AROMATIC WATER

Fill a 100 ml dark glass bottle with distilled water. Never use tap water as this does not keep very well; it also imparts a chemicalised odour to blends, intensified by the phenomenon of synergy. Bottled spring water is also unsuitable because it harbours bacteria. Distilled water, on the other hand, is relatively inert and so has excellent keeping qualities. Alternatively, use genuine orange flower water or rosewater, or a 50/50 mixture of the two.

Build the fragrance gradually by adding a few drops of essential oil at a time, shaking the bottle and smelling the water as you go. Add up to 100 drops of essential oil in all (the average strength for most colognes). However, you may find that a weaker solution of 55 to 60 drops of essential oil to 100 ml of water is potent enough. Allow the mixture to ripen for one or two weeks before use. Keep in a cool dark place, but remember to shake well each day to facilitate the infusion process. When ready, pour through a *damp* coffee filter paper (a dry filter paper will absorb too much of the liquid). This will clarify the mixture as a number of unmodified essential oils cause water or alcohol to turn cloudy. Filtering also drastically reduces the problem of separation of oil and water. Rebottle the mixture and label with the blend and date. Store in a cool dark place and use up within four months.

How to Apply Aromatic Waters

These can be used in the same way as commercial products, that is splashed on after a bath or shower, brushed through the hair or sprinkled over clothes. However, the best way to apply an aromatic water is to funnel it into a perfume atomiser and use as a spray. These can be purchased from a good chemist or the perfume counter of a department store.

HAIR PERFUME

Hair is a marvellous fixative for perfume. As well as increasing the staying power of the blend, it imparts its own faintly musky fragrance. Moreover, the odour of hair intensifies the perfume by means of the magical power of synergy. Lighthearted citrus or lavender-based aromatic waters are especially enhanced by the subtle odour of hair. If you have an atomiser (and enough hair!) spray a little aromatic water over your crowning glory. Otherwise, pour a little into the palm of your hand, dip your hair brush into this and brush it through. But do try to avoid getting too much of the blend on your scalp as the skin is sensitive there.

Unless your hair is thick and heavy, an oil-based perfume may leave a greasy feel. For this reason, it may be preferable to use neat essential oil and to apply this to the ends of your hair. The oil will not damage your hair, nor will it leave a greasy film. A few neat essences could be blended in a bottle to make a complex perfume, or you could use a favourite single essence such as neroli, rose, jasmine, or ylang ylang.

Incidentally, if you are a man with a goodly growth of beard, then you could perfume the ends of those whiskers! Essences that are especially popular with men include sandalwood, patchouli and cedarwood.

THE JOY OF VANILLA

It was the sixteenth-century Spanish explorer Cortez who introduced vanilla to Europe. He discovered it in Mexico, where the Aztecs used it to flavour their chocolate drinks. The combination of chocolate and vanilla was deemed so erogenic (especially to females) that Aztec women were forbidden the pleasure!

Unfortunately, vanilla absolute is not only difficult to come by, it is terrifically expensive when it is available. So if you delight in this soulful aroma, it makes sense to concoct your own version, albeit a very much weaker mixture than the solvent-extracted substance. The recipe given below makes a beautifully sensual base for a love potion or erotic massage oil. However, it is advisable to carry out a patch test beforehand (see page 23) because some people are sensitive to vanilla.

INFUSED OIL OF VANILLA

You will need 50 ml of jojoba or light coconut oil, two vanilla pods and a clear glass jar with a tight-fitting lid. Simply split the vanilla pods down the middle, then cut them into little pieces and put them in the jar. Cover the vanilla with the oil, then leave the tightly sealed jar outside in the sun (or on a warm radiator or boiler) for about five weeks, bringing the jar indoors at night. Give the jar a good shake every time you pass by to facilitate the process of infusion. After five weeks, or when the oil smells fragrant enough for your taste, strain the mixture through muslin and store in a dark glass bottle. The oil will keep for about a year.

AROMATIC FORMULAS

Most of the fragrant compositions suggested on the Aromatic Formulas charts can be transposed into massage oil blends or room perfumes. Simply adjust the number of drops accordingly. For example, up to 10 drops per 25 ml of base oil for a massage blend, and about 6 drops per 30 ml of water for the vaporiser.

OIL-BASED LOVE POTIONS

Each of the potions below specifies the number of drops per 10 ml of base oil. Where infused oil of vanilla is suggested as a base, you could use plain jojoba or light coconut oil if preferred.

FOR WOMEN

Sweet Mystery

4 drops coriander
8 drops bergamot
3 drops neroli
3 drops jasmine absolute or
1 drop rose otto
10 ml infused oil of vanilla

Forever Sheba

5 drops bergamot
3 drops mandarin
3 drops black pepper
4 drops rose absolute or
1 drop rose otto
2 drops patchouli
10 ml jojoba or light coconut oil

Love-in-a-Wood

3 drops neroli
4 drops lavender
2 drops mimosa absolute
1 drop oakmoss absolute
3 drops cedarwood
10 ml jojoba or light coconut oil

FOR MEN

Enigma

3 drops lavender
3 drops coriander
5 drops sandalwood
5 drops cedarwood
10 ml jojoba or light coconut oil

Song of Solomon

4 drops coriander
2 drops mandarin
1 drop ginger
1 drop frankincense
6 drops sandalwood
10 ml infused oil of vanilla

Wildwood Magic

3 drops clary sage
2 drops lavender
3 drops petitgrain
5 drops cedarwood
1 drop oakmoss absolute
10 ml jojoba or light coconut oil

AROMATIC WATERS

Each blend below specifies a number of drops per 100 ml of distilled water or floral water.

Traditional Eau-de-Cologne

30 drops bergamot
10 drops petitgrain
10 drops orange
10 drops lemon
5 drops lavender
5 drops neroli
5 drops rosemary
50 ml rosewater *and*
50 ml orange flower water *or*
100 ml distilled water

Mint and Rosemary Cologne

8 drops peppermint
10 drops rosemary
15 drops orange
15 drops lemon
10 drops petitgrain
5 drops geranium
100 ml distilled water *or* rosewater

Old-fashioned Lavender Water

50 drops lavender
10 drops bergamot
5 drops rose absolute *or*
1 drop rose otto
100 ml rosewater

Green Sleeves

20 drops bergamot
8 drops clary sage
10 drops lavender
3 drops mimosa absolute (optional)
6 drops rose absolute *or*
2 drops rose otto
8 drops cedarwood
100 ml rosewater *or* distilled water

Forest

12 drops bergamot
12 drops petitgrain
8 drops clary sage
2 drops oakmoss absolute (optional)
10 drops sandalwood
10 drops cedarwood
100 ml orange flower water *or* distilled water

Eastern Promise

12 drops orange
5 drops lime
12 drops lemon
8 drops geranium
12 drops coriander
1 drop cardamon
5 drops rose absolute *or*
2 drops rose otto
100 ml rosewater *or* distilled water

MOCK TURTLES

Many of the essences and absolutes used for perfumery work are very expensive and/or difficult to obtain. However, certain cheaper essential oils when blended together take on a similar aroma to some of the luxury oils. The following combinations are worth trying:

- **Mock Carnation** Equal quantities of black pepper and ylang ylang with a touch of geranium in a base of infused oil of vanilla.
- **Mock Jasmine** One part patchouli with two parts ylang ylang in a base of infused oil of vanilla.
- **Mock Neroli** Equal quantities of mandarin and petitgrain.
- **Mock Oakmoss** Equal quantities of cedarwood, petitgrain and clary sage.

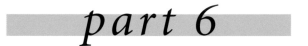

part 6

HOME AND GARDEN

…take 12 spoonfulls of bright red rosewater, the weight of sixpence in fine powder of sugar, and boyle it on hot Embers and coals softly and the house will smell as though it were full of Roses: but you must burn sweet Cypress wood before, to take away the gross air.

FROM THE QUEEN'S CLOSET
OPENED
BY W.M. COOK TO
QUEEN HENRIETTA MARIA, 1665

28
HOME SWEET HOME

Although essential oils are potent antiseptics, most are too expensive for the average homemaker to use freely for such purposes as one would normally use household disinfectant, so the best way to ensure that your home is fragrant and germ free is to make good use of the vaporiser. However, there are several other ways to enjoy ambience in the making, as you are about to discover.

MIST SPRAYS

Although the effect is short-lived compared to that achieved by using an electric diffuser or nightlight vaporiser, the mobile aromatic spray is especially convenient should you wish to freshen the house from top to bottom in a thrice.

The method is simple; fill a small house plant mister with water, then add the essential oil. Exact quantities are not at all crucial, but as a rough guide, add up to 18 drops of essential oil to 125 ml of water (tap water is fine for this purpose). Remember to shake well each time before use to disperse the oil droplets. Just in case you are stuck for blending ideas, here are a few possibilities to inspire you.

ROOM FRESHENERS

For imparting a light and airy fragrance to the whole house.

Sunbeam

5 drops lemon
5 drops bergamot
3 drops petitgrain
3 drops geranium

Mountain Breeze

4 drops peppermint
6 drops lavender
5 drops clary sage

Wood Nymph

5 drops cedarwood
5 drops juniper
8 drops pine

STENCH BUSTERS

The following extra-strength blends will help break down stale cooking odours as well as the lingering smell of cigarette smoke. Spray several times within two hours or, better still, use the same combination of oils in the vaporiser, in which case, you will need to halve the quantity of essential oil.

Vamoosh

10 drops eucalyptus
8 drops lavender
5 drops lemongrass

Blitz

5 drops thyme
12 drops rosemary
8 drops pine

DRIVE EASY

Any of the following sprays will help keep you alert whilst driving. Incidentally, the same combination of essences can be used in the vaporiser for study purposes (see also the recipes on page 236).

Top Gear

8 drops rosemary
5 drops pine
2 drops peppermint

Sun Roof

6 drops bergamot
5 drops lemon
4 drops coriander

Flywheel

5 drops rosemary
4 drops lime
6 drops bergamot

TRAVELLER'S JOY

For spraying around a hotel bedroom, for example.

Luxury Suite

3 drops rose otto
4 drops clary sage
4 drops neroli

Standard Suite

4 drops geranium
8 drops lavender
5 drops petitgrain

Sweet Dreams

4 drops chamomile (Roman)
4 drops clary sage
6 drops lavender

LIGHT-BULB PERFUMERY

It is said that women of the night perfume their light bulbs with patchouli essence! However, there is no need to be engaged in the oldest profession to enjoy the delights of light-bulb perfumery, for it has become quite a respectable practice. You may be able to obtain a fragrance ring which is usually a ceramic, robust plastic or heavy cardboard disk that balances over the top of the light bulb. The essences are dropped on the ring and the warmth from the bulb releases the aromatic vapour. Alternatively, simply rub a few drops of essential oil on to a cold light bulb (a desk or table lamp with a fairly low wattage bulb works well), then turn on the light. Voila! A scented room.

The only drawback with these methods is that the fragrance ring or light bulb will eventually become very sticky. Plastic or ceramic fragrance rings can be wiped with an alcohol-based substance such as surgical spirit which will dissolve the essential oil residue. It is important to wash the ring with hot soapy water afterwards to remove every trace or surgical spirit whose harsh odour will intermingle with the essential oils. But do ensure that the ring is thoroughly dry before replacing it over the light fitting, otherwise you could get an electric shock. As for sticky light bulbs, it is safer to leave well alone. It should also be mentioned that essential oil is highly flammable. Even though I am unaware of a single recorded case of a fire having started as a result of light-bulb perfumery or the use of fragrance rings, it is as well to be cautious.

SCENTED PINE CONES

A delightful way to perfume a room is to drape over radiators bunches of scented pine cones tied together with cotton thread. They could also be hung on doors and walls, suspended from ceiling beams, or secured so that they hang over the edge of the mantelpiece. However, do remember to keep the cones a safe distance from the fire itself, whether gas, electric or solid fuel, as essential oils are highly flammable.

The cones need to be soaked for at least one hour, preferably overnight, in 150 ml of water with up to 25 drops of essential oil. Choose highly odoriferous essences such as ginger, clove, cinnamon, geranium or patchouli. Another good choice is cedarwood, which is long lasting, but less odoriferous. To keep the cones redolent with fragrance, you will need to soak them again every seven to twelve days. Any leftover aromatic soak-water can be used in the nightlight vaporiser. It will probably contain debris from the pine cones, but this will not affect the fragrance.

KEEPING MOTHS AT BAY

Bunches of fragrant cones can be hung in the wardrobe as a moth repellent. Choose from the following essences: cedarwood, clove, lavender, lemongrass, patchouli, rosemary. Alternatively, you could place on the bottom of the wardrobe a little dish of essential oil impregnated dried flowers or woodshavings. Dried plant material suitable for this purpose (not that which is already perfumed with synthetic pot pourri oil) can be purchased from good herbal suppliers. Wood shavings can usually be obtained free from any carpenter's workshop.

Simply put a handful of dried flowers or woodshavings into a polythene bag, then sprinkle with about 20 drops of essential oil and mix well. Seal the bag tightly and allow the aroma to permeate the base material for at least 24 hours before use.

AROMATHERAPY FOR YOUR CARPET

Carpet Fresheners

8 oz bicarbonate of soda
35-45 drops essential oil

Put the bicarbonate of soda into a polythene bag, then sprinkle with the essential oil and mix well. Seal the bag tightly and allow the aroma to permeate the soda for at least 24 hours. Sprinkle over the carpet, leave for at least half an hour before vacuuming. As a bonus, if the dust bag does not need changing immediately, fragrance will waft from the air vent each time you use the vacuum cleaner; aromatherapy while you work! Here are a few fragrant possibilities to transport you from the mundane.

Magic Carpet

10 drops clove
15 drops orange
15 drops lavender

Bazaar

10 drops patchouli
10 drops vetiver
20 drops lime

Persian Dream

25 drops cedarwood
10 drops coriander
10 drops lemon

SCENTED LINEN

In the past, aromatic plants such as lavender and woodruff were placed between freshly laundered linen sheets and clothing to impart their sweet fragrances and to deter fleas and moths. Another way is to make an aromatic spray using refreshing essences such as lavender, lemon, bergamot, geranium and rosemary. You will need about 15 drops of essential oil to 125 ml of water. Spray a fine mist over cotton and linen fabrics (synthetic fibres may become stained by the oils). Put in the airing cupboard to dry. You may also discover that the rest of your laundry has become faintly aromatic too.

SCENTED DRAWER LINERS

To keep musty drawers fresh, line with essential oil impregnated wallpaper. Cut the wallpaper to size, then spray the underside of the wallpaper (to avoid possible staining of clothes) with a strong aromatic solution: up to 40 drops of essential oil to 50 ml of water in a house plant mister.

The longer lasting essences are those in the base note range such as patchouli, cedarwood and vetiver. But if these are too earthy-smelling for your own aromatic good taste, choose lighter essences such as coriander, geranium, lavender and citrus oils. The drawer liner will need a refresher spray every three months or so, depending on the odour intensity of the oils.

AROMATHERAPY FOR YOUR FURNITURE

Beeswax, linseed oil and plant essences blended together make a superb furniture polish, imparting a lovely scent and a satiny finish. Blocks of natural yellow beeswax can be obtained from antique furniture dealers, beekeepers, herbal suppliers and craft shops. Real turpentine (as used in the second recipe) and linseed oil can be obtained from most hardware shops.

Beewitched Furniture Pomade

30 g yellow beeswax
125 ml linseed oil
8 drops cedarwood
6 drops rosemary or sandalwood

Grate the beeswax, then heat with the oil in a heat-proof basin over a pan of simmering water. Stir well, then remove from the heat. As soon as the mixture begins to thicken, stir in the essential oils then spoon into a glass pot. Use like ordinary wax polish, rubbing it on with one duster and buffing it with another.

Traditional Lavender Furniture Cream

30 g yellow beeswax
125 ml turpentine
15 drops lavender

Grate the beeswax, then heat in a basin over a pan of simmering water until completely melted. Remove from the heat and immediately stir in the turpentine, before the wax begins to set, ensuring that it is thoroughly mixed.

(Turpentine can easily burst into flames, so never add this to the basin whilst on the stove.) Pour the polish into a glass pot. Use like ordinary wax polish.

AROMATIC WOOD FIRES

In rural areas, the old practice of fumigating rooms by burning aromatic plant material on the hearth fire continued right up to the early part of the twentieth century. Most of these aromatics were obtained from the countryside at little or no cost. Dried aromatic herbs, roots and seeds were found to perfume a room if placed directly on an open fire when the flames were low.

If you are fortunate enough to have an open fire and a garden full of herbs, then you too can indulge in the delights of fireside perfumery. A wood fire is best, as wood imparts its own scents to those of the herbs. However, if you are able to collect fallen branches or thinnings of aromatic woods such as apple, pear, cherry and laurel, savour these for their own sake. Once seasoned, they burn bright and clear and their scents are truly divine.

Here is a partial list of suitable aromatic plants which smell delightful when burned on a low fire, though do remember to use dried plant material, otherwise it will not burn properly.

- Angelica (seed heads)
- Elecampane (roots)
- Lavender (flower spikes)
- Inula conyza (roots)
- Juniper (twigs and branches)
- Lovage (seed heads)
- Pine cones
- Rosemary (leaves and twigs)
- Sage (leaves and twigs)
- Southernwood

SCENTED CANDLES

Most of the 'aromatherapy' candles available in gift shops are perfumed with harsh synthetic scents. Unlike natural essences, aroma chemicals are much more likely to trigger allergic reactions such as wheezing and sneezing. Even when genuine essential oil candles are available, the choice is usually limited to a handful of modestly priced essences such as lavender, rosemary, geranium or pine.

While candle-making kits can be obtained from craft outlets, it is much easier to buy one very fat candle and a few of your favourite essential oils. Before we consider the method for scenting candles, it should be mentioned that most are made from paraffin wax, though beeswax candles are also available. Beeswax candles are much more expensive than the usual kind, but for special occasions they are well worth considering. The beeswax imparts its own delicious honey scent into the room. Nonetheless, the aroma can be enhanced by adding a few drops of a floral or woody essence such as rose, sandalwood or ylang ylang.

The method for scenting candles is simple. First light the candle, wait a few moments for the wax to melt around the wick, then blow it out and immediately add a few drops of essential oil to the molten wax (the fatter the candle, the bigger the pool of wax) before re-lighting.

> **IMPORTANT** *Essential oil is highly flammable, so never try to add this whilst the candle is still burning, as it will flare up, leaving in its wake a puff of black smoke. It is also important to keep the wick trimmed very short, otherwise the flame will be too big and the aromatic vapour relatively short lived. If the pool of wax is big enough and the flame low enough, the aroma will continue to diffuse for at least an hour. Once all the oil has evaporated, you may wish to ring the changes by adding a different essence or a blend of two or three (extinguishing the flame first).*

VAPORISING WHOLE SPICES

If you own a nightlight candle vaporiser with a good sized reservoir, you can perfume a room using dried whole spices such as cloves, ginger, black pepper, juniper berries, lemongrass, coriander seed, pieces of cinnamon stick or snips of vanilla pod. Simply add about one teaspoonful of plant material to the water-filled reservoir (tap water is fine for this purpose). The aroma will gradually develop, reaching maximum intensity after about one hour.

The aroma can be made more aromatic and interesting with the addition of a few drops of essential oil. For special occasions, instead of vaporising the spices in plain water, you could use orange flower water or rosewater, or perhaps an equal quantity of each. A touch of citrus peel imparts an interesting note to most spicy blends. A little sugar (about half a teaspoonful) added to almost any blend seems to enhance the aroma; try it and see.

ROOM SCENTS USING WHOLE SPICES

Here are some aromatic suggestions for the night-light vaporiser just to inspire your creative instinct. Exact quantities are not at all crucial, so just follow your nose.

- Whole cloves, cinnamon stick, orange peel.
- Vanilla pod, lime peel.
- Coriander seed, juniper berries, black peppercorns.
- Ginger root, cinnamon stick, dried lemongrass.
- Rosewater, vanilla pod.
- Orange flower water, coriander seed, dried lemongrass.
- Orange flower water, rosewater, cinnamon stick.
- Orange flower water, whole cloves, lavender essence.
- Vanilla pod, lime peel, ylang ylang essence.
- Rosewater, coriander seed, sandalwood essence.

29
THE AROMATIC PET

In Elizabethan times, the best perfumes would make one smell 'as sweet as any lady's dog'. Contrary to what you may be thinking, this was never said in jest. Indeed, the animal would have costly aromatics rubbed into its coat before being carried around by its owner when making social calls. Judging by the soporific scents used, which included labdanum, benzoin and ambergris, the poor creature must have been stupefied.

Similarly, the unsupervised use of aromatic oils for veterinary purposes is potentially harmful. Even though essential oils are wonderful healing agents, they can be toxic if misused, for example, if administered without a clear understanding of the underlying nature of the presenting symptoms and with scant knowledge regarding the pharmacological effects of the oils used. It also takes great skill to ascertain exactly how much essential oil to administer for individual animals within a given species. The physiology of a parrot, for example, is very different from that of a cat. And while the physiology of a cat is somewhat different from that of a dog, a horse presents yet another variation on the mammalian theme, and so it goes on.

Yet there is a growing number of popular aromatherapy books promoting the home use of essential oils for pet care, including the treatment of chronic conditions such as anaemia, emphysema, severe eczema and mange. Some authors do not even balk at advocating oral dosage. True, essential oils have proved efficacious in many serious cases, but they should always be administered under the supervision of a qualified holistic vet. As well as offering nutritional advice, most holistic vets employ a variety of therapeutic measures which may include homoeopathy, essential oils and conventional drugs if need be.

Despite the above cautions about the unsupervised use of plant essences for animals, there are a few ailments in cats and dogs which can be helped at home using simple aromatic remedies. Since my own experience of the veterinary uses of plant essences is somewhat limited, nearly all of the following aromatic treatments (excepting the flea collar recipes) have been contributed by Tim Couzens, an holistic veterinary practitioner who runs a busy practice in Sussex (England).

IMPORTANT *I feel obliged to point out that some of Tim's formulas are much more concentrated than I would normally recommend. There are great differences in human skin which is 6-8 cells thick, and that of most other animals, which is 2-3 cells thick. There are also differences between absorption, metabolism and elimination of essential oils in animals. Therefore, such functions cannot be compared with those of humans. My advice regarding the veterinary use of essential oils is to use them with great care, taking note of the cautions and procedures given with the recipes.*

ARTHRITIS OIL

To ease arthritic joints in dogs, the following combination has proved very successful. However, if the joint is swollen or inflamed (which can occur periodically with arthritis) do not apply firm massage as this will cause further pain and tissue damage; you may even get a nasty bite from your dog! Do not use this formula continuously for more than six weeks without a three-week break before resuming. Treatment for arthritis needs to be supported with good nutrition and perhaps also homoeopathic remedies, but do seek professional advice.

9 ml grapeseed oil
1 ml sesame oil
5 drops lavender
2 drops rosemary
1 drop German chamomile
1 drop ginger

Mix the grapeseed oil and sesame oil together well. Then add the essential oils. Using your fingertips, gently massage 1 or 2 drops of the blend into the joint until all the oil seems to have disappeared. Part the animal's hair if necessary to ensure that the oil reaches the skin and can penetrate into the joint.

Other helpful essences include black pepper, cajeput, coriander, eucalyptus, juniper, marjoram and vetiver.

FLEAS

Fleas are a continual problem, but you can use essential oils to help make dogs and cats less acceptable as hosts. Fleas definitely do not like aromatic oils! Moreover, dried aromatic herbs packed into small cotton sachets (perhaps made from a folded handkerchief sewn up each side and across the top) can help repel fleas from pet bedding. Try mixing together any combination of the following herbs: feverfew, lavender, rosemary, rue, sage, southernwood, tansy, wormwood.

Vegetable Oil Flea Repellent

10 ml sweet almond oil
10 drops lavender
5 drops cedar wood

Mix together the almond oil and essential oils. Use the oil sparingly, massaging a drop or two over the coat and into the skin twice weekly, more often if fleas are a real problem. You can replace the cedarwood with geranium if you wish.

FLEA COLLAR FOR CATS AND DOGS

Since fleas breed around the neck, a flea collar is a good deterrent. Moreover, the animal cannot easily reach the area with its tongue (cats are especially likely to lick off the essential oil), so this reduces the amount of oil ingested. Although a certain amount will be absorbed through the skin, this is generally regarded as a safer route. Excessive quantities of essential oil taken orally may damage delicate mucous membranes in the mouth and digestive tract.

Conventional flea collars reek of powerful chemicals which usually make the animal feel unwell for a few days until the fumes have waned. Essential oil collars, on the other hand, not only smell pleasant, but are infinitely less toxic. Even though they need to be replaced more often than conventional flea collars, this would seem a small price to pay for the long-term health and comfort of your pet.

Inexpensive, non-medicated fabric collars are widely available from pet shops and markets. The easiest way to permeate the fabric with essential oils is to dip the collar in a mixture of essences and cider vinegar, then to keep the collar in a sealed polythene bag for 24 hours to encourage maximum diffusion. Once in use, the collar will need to be replenished with the oil and vinegar mix every two or three weeks. It may be wise to alternate between two or three different formulas as animals may have an idiosyncratic sensitivity to a certain essential oil. If symptoms such as sneezing or a skin rash occur you should remove the collar immediately. Citronella is the essential oil most likely to cause allergic reactions (it is not recommended in this chapter).

Here are three suitable blends using low to medium priced essences:

Recipe 1

1 teaspoonful cider vinegar
5 drops cedarwood
5 drops eucalyptus
5 drops lavender

Recipe 2

1 teaspoonful cider vinegar
8 drops tea tree
6 drops geranium

Recipe 3

1 teaspoonful cider vinegar
5 drops rosemary
5 drops red thyme
5 drops cypress

Other essences with flea repellent properties include: bergamot, lemongrass, patchouli, pine and galbanum.

TICKS

Ticks (blood-sucking parasites) are an occasional problem which can be picked up in long grass. A drop or two of eucalyptus oil directly on the body of the tick will cause it to drop off.

SKIN CREAM

The following cream is useful for treating minor rashes, sores and wounds. However, severe skin problems like widespread eczema, scabies, mange and suppurating wounds must be treated by a qualified vet. In all cases, if there is no improvement after two or three weeks of home treatment, do seek professional advice.

100 g unperfumed base cream
20 drops lavender
10 drops geranium
20 drops chamomile (Roman)
1/2 teaspoonful calendular tincture (optional)

To the unperfumed base cream (available from most essential oil suppliers), add the lavender, geranium and Roman chamomile. You could also add $\frac{1}{2}$ teaspoonful of calendula tincture (available from herbal suppliers). Other oils can be used instead of chamomile, for instance 10 drops of cedarwood if the skin is greasy, or frankincense if there are weepy or sticky areas. Mix the base cream and essential oils well with the handle of a teaspoon and store in a suitable dark glass, airtight jar. Apply the cream twice daily.

(For more information about holistic pet care, see Recommended Reading).

30
THE AROMATHERAPEUTIC GARDEN

THE AROMATHERAPEUTIC GARDEN

What better way to receive the aromatherapeutic effects of herbs, flowers, trees and grasses than directly as nature intended? Even moist earth smells wonderful, especially during hot weather, when the first summer rains fall on the parched meadows causing the soil to release its enigmatic fragrance. Then there is the scent of honeysuckle heavy on the air of a sultry summer's evening, the velvety perfume of the old fashioned crimson rose, and the cooling fragrances of pine, cedar and cypress after rain. At such times we instinctively breathe more deeply in order to experience the scent fully – and the more deeply we breathe, the more relaxed and in harmony we feel.

If you have a garden, you may wish to take up the art of garden perfumery. Just as you learned to create a mood-enhancing perfume composed of essences resonating from the three spheres – top, middle and base – you can create an ethereal garden whose individual scents merge into a veritable symphony of fragrance.

The top notes are those that you can smell from a distance, such as the mock orange blossom (*Philadelphus*) whose sweet scent is reminiscent of the essential oil of neroli. Then there is the beautiful fragrance of wisteria, and the opulent scent of alyssum. The middle notes are those flowers whose fragrances smell the same close up as from a short distance. These include lavender, lily-of-the-valley, roses and bluebells. The base notes are the resinous, earthy, woody or musky aromas, which are present in the wood and needles of conifer trees such as pine and cedar, and in aromatic leaves such as the musky angelica, or in fading lilac blooms.

A few flowers are possessed of a certain enchantment, for their multifaceted scents shape-shift according to the time of day. Good examples are summer jasmine whose fragrance is softly sensuous in the afternoon, becoming warm, erogenic and intoxicating by dusk, and honeysuckle, especially the wild version whose country name is woodbine. Then there are those flowers whose complex scents smell quite differently close up than when caught as a faint whiff on the breeze. The mock orange blossom is one, but especially the tiny mignonette whose modest appearance belies her voluptuous aura.

Even if you do not have a garden, there is no need to forego the delights of living fragrance. Quite a few scented plants are suitable for growing outside in window boxes, or as house plants. Sweet allyssum, candytuft, jonquil, virginia stock and wallflower plants, for example, can be grown successfully in window boxes. Brunfelsia, gardenia, heliotrope, hyacinth, jasmine, easter lily and miniature rose plants are suitable for the house. Most are easily raised from seeds or bulbs, or can be obtained as young plants from nurseries and garden centres.

If this has stirred your imagination, the following tips may help in creating an aromatherapeutic garden with two distinctly different themes: a secluded garden of tranquillity and an open garden of frivolity.

GARDEN OF TRANQUILLITY

Create this in a secluded spot in a quiet corner of the garden, perhaps with a seat surrounded by soft foliage plants and gently arching branches. A semi-shaded place in which to escape from the hurly burly pace of life – a place where you can simply sit and stare and restore a sense of harmony to body and soul.

Even though many fragrant plants need to be grown in full sun, there are some exceptions, one spectacular example being the lovely nicotiana or tobacco plant which will emanate a heavenly scent if grown in semi-shade. If you wish to experience a wider variety of fragrance, ensure that the garden seat is positioned in such a way as to allow you to see and smell other scented plants growing in a sunny spot nearby.

When choosing fragrant plants, it is necessary to 'play it by nose'. While some people find the lingering scents of honeysuckle, jasmine and white lilies sedating, others find such perfumes overpowering and even nauseating if inhaled for too long. Even if you are relaxed by richly scented blooms, you could perhaps compromise to enable others of a weaker constitution to enjoy the area as well. In which case, opt for light, airy fragrances such as lavender, bluebells and softly scented rambling roses. But what about colour?

Colour therapists tell us that green is the colour that flows through the solar plexus. It helps to allay anxiety and brings about peace and well-being. Since green is the predominant colour of nature, no wonder communing with plants can bestow tranquillity to the frenzied and uplift the spirits of the downhearted.

Gardeners have always been aware of the healing powers of nature, the freeing sensation of coming close to the earth. When seeking to capture serenity, the creative gar-dener is drawn to plants whose colours, shapes and scents whisper but never shout. So the planting scheme most conducive to relaxation is one which emphasises cooling blues and purples, perhaps with a tinge of rose-pink to warm the heart, and a drift of white or cream to lift mood. unscented foliage plants such as ferns and ivy and also delicately painted flowers like larkspur, campanula, love-in-a-mist and columbine have a place too, as does the curiously beautiful passion flower. Any of these can be incorporated to enhance colour and form.

Of course, the flowers suggested here can only be a rough guide because you will need to discover which plants are suitable for your own garden with its idiosyncratic features, soil quality, climatic conditions and available space. A good gardening book is essential.

PLANTS FOR THE GARDEN OF TRANQUILLITY

Blue/Turquoise

Any shade of blue encourages inspiration and engenders tranquillity. It is also conducive to healing and meditation. If you are suffering from insomnia, tension or fear, it is a good colour to contemplate. Turquoise flowers are rare, though certain hybrid delphiniums, lobelia and forget-me-nots can almost capture the hue. Turquoise is said to boost the immune system.

Fragrant Flowers

Spring: hyacinth ('Queen of the Blues'), bluebell, lilac.
Summer: heliotrope ('Lord Roberts'), annual sweet pea ('Noel Sutton').
Autumn: buddleia ('Empire Blue'), sweet scabious ('Blue Moon').

Unscented Flowers

Spring: crocus ('Blue Pearl'), ceonothus (*C. impressus*), forget-me-not (the variety 'Ultramarine' has a turquoise hue), anemone (*A. blanda*).
Summer: delphinium (the variety 'Mullion' has a turquoise hue), morning glory ('Heavenly Blue'), lobelia (the variety 'Cambridge Blue' has a turquoise hue), larkspur.
Autumn: hebe ('Autumn Glory'), ceonothus ('Autumnal Blue'), love-in-a-mist ('Miss Jekyll').
Winter: iris (*I. stylosa*).

Lilac/Lavender

Although it can be hard to distinguish between the colours we call lilac and lavender, think of lilac as being pinkish-blue and lavender as bluish-purple. These colours soothe a tired nervous system and induce sleep.Fragrant Flowers
Spring: lilac.
Summer: lavender, wisteria, sweet pea ('Leamington'), sweet rocket, night-scented stock.
Autumn: rose (floribunda type 'Escapade').
Winter: daphne (*D. odora*).

Unscented Flowers

Spring: crocus ('Little Dorrit'), bergenia (*B. cordifolia*), columbine (also known as aquilegia), pasque flower.
Summer: corn cockle ('Milas'), hosta (*H. ventricosa*), viola (*V. cornuta*), lupin ('Lilac Time').
Autumn: hebe (*H. x andersonii*).
Winter: hellebore (*Helleborus atrorubens*).

Rose Pink

Colour healers associate pink with spiritual love, a colour which is especially helpful to those suffering from grief. It bridges the two states of relaxation and vivacity, and thus has an uplifting yet calming effect.

Fragrant Flowers

Spring: flowering currant (*Ribes sanguineum*), lilac ('Esther Staley').
Summer: verbena ('Delight'), sweet pea ('Geranium Pink'), dianthus ('Doris'), everlasting sweet pea (*Lathyrus rotundifolius*), clematis ('Elizabeth'), candytuft.
Autumn: roses (floribunda type 'English Miss'; rambling type 'Aloha').
Winter: viburnum (*V. grandiflorum*).

Unscented Flowers

Spring: rhododendron (*R. racemosum*).
Summer: spiraea ('Anthony Waterer'), thrift (also known as sea pink), larkspur.
Autumn: sedum (*S. spectabile*).
Winter: cyclamen (*C. coum*).

Violet

Violet is regarded as the colour of spirituality. It is said to stimulate the pineal gland (the mystical 'third eye') and calm a jangled nervous system. It is a colour conducive to meditation.

Fragrant Flowers

Spring: hyacinth ('Amethyst'), sweet violet.
Summer: heliotrope ('Vilmorin's Variety'), phlox ('Harlequin').
Autumn: buddleia ('Black Knight').

Unscented Flowers

Spring: pansy ('Jersey Gem').
Summer: spiderwort ('Leonora'), columbine, campanula ('Brentwood').
Autumn: aster ('Ostrich Plume').

Cream

This could be seen as a variant of yellow or a softer form of white. Either way, it is regarded as the colour of spiritual attunement, a balancing hue.

Fragrant Flowers

Spring: daphne (*D. blagayana*), magnolia (*M. stellata*).
Summer: rose (hybrid tea 'Elizabeth Harkness'), freesia ('Fantasy').
Autumn: rose (floribunda type 'Chanelle').
Winter: lonicera (*L. fragrantissima*).

Unscented Flowers

Spring: iris ('Green Spot').
Summer: delphinium ('Butterball'), hydrangea (*H. petiolaris*).
Autumn: chrysanthemum ('Cream Bouquet').
Winter: crocus ('Cream Beauty').

White

Colour healers regard this as the colour for inspiring self-knowledge. For some people, however, it can induce a sense of isolation, so it may need to be toned down with softer hues to make it more relaxing.

Fragrant Flowers

Spring: lily-of-the-valley, viburnum (*V. x burkwoodii*), narcissus ('Polar Ice').
Summer: philadelphus, sweet alyssum, nicotiana (*N. alata*), datura (*D. ceratocaula*), water lily.
Autumn: buddleia ('White Cloud').
Winter: viburnum (*V. fragrans*), sarcococca (*S. confusa*).

Unscented Flowers

Spring: star-of-Bethlehem (also a Bach flower remedy for helping to release suppressed grief and the effects of emotional shock), snowdrop, camellia ('Alba Simplex').
Summer: white buttercup, rose (hybrid tea 'Polar Star').
Autumn: erica ('Springwood White', 'Silver Bells').
Winter: viburnum (*V. timus*).

GARDEN OF FRIVOLITY

This needs to be created in a sunny part of the garden, a riot of colour planted in a free-spirit style. A place to go when you need to be revitalised. Albeit a seasonal experience, the memory will remain with you, to be fleetingly recalled on some gloomy winter's day.

Choose brightly coloured flowers whose scents are spicy, citrus or sweet and light-hearted. A good choice is dianthus (the garden pink) whose colours range from pale pink to deep red. The blooms have a warm scent with a spicy nuance reminiscent of cloves. Other plants like lemon balm, lemon geranium and rose geranium have deliciously fragrant leaves which release their scent molecules in hot sunshine, or whenever you brush past

them. If you have enough space the golden flowered azalea is a must. Its exotic fragrance suggests the essential oil of ylang ylang, albeit more airy and less intensely sweet.

No garden of frivolity can be crowned resplendent without the company of a few raucous annuals. Even though most have little or no scent, they can impart a sense of abandoned rapture. The rampant nasturtium is one of my own favourites. If left unchecked, it will trailblaze through the garden and beyond, providing a cornucopia of orange-red blooms from early summer until late autumn. As a bonus, the leaves, flowers and seeds can be used in salads for novelty. Then there is the lovely pot marigold whose faint dry fragrance can be detected if the blooms are sniffed close-up. And if you have room, the 'dwarf' multi-headed sunflower (reaching up to 5 ft) will add a certain leonine charm

PLANTS FOR THE GARDEN OF FRIVOLITY

Red

This is the colour of strength and vitality, the great energiser, though very bright shades of red can be too stimulating for some people.

Fragrant Flowers

Spring: wallflower ('Ruby Gem').
Summer: dianthus ('Queen of Hearts'), rose (rambling type 'Crimson Glory'), sweet pea ('Air Warden'), rose (shrub type Rosa gallica), verbena ('Sparkle').
Summer to Autumn: nicotiana ('Red Devil').

Unscented Flowers

Spring: camellia ('Chandleri'), Japanese quince.
Summer to Autumn: geraniums (bedding types, 'Fire Brand', 'Josephine', 'Pandora', 'Fire Dragon', 'Paul Crampel'), petunias ('Red Satin', 'Dream Girl').

Deep Pink

Every shade of pink, from the softest to the deepest hue is the colour to contemplate when there is a need to engender unconditional love; that which demands nothing in return. For most people, deep pink is a more comfortable colour with which to attune than bright red.

Fragrant Flowers

Spring: candytuft ('Red Flush'), hyacinth ('Jan Bros').
Summer: rose (hybrid tea 'Pink Peace'), dianthus ('Joy', 'Diane', 'Bovey Belle'), sweet pea ('Mrs R. Boulton'), buddleia (B. colvillei).

Unscented Flowers

Spring: magnolia ('Rubra').
Summer: godetia.
Summer to Autumn: geraniums ('Elaine', 'Salmon Pink', 'Springtime'), begonias ('Rosanna', 'Rhapsody').
Autumn: sedum (S. spectabile).

Orange

Orange is revitalising and freeing to the emotions, imparting a sense of joyous rapture.

Fragrant Flowers

Spring to Summer: wallflower ('Orange Queen').
Summer to Autumn: rose (floribunda type 'Geraldine').

Unscented Flowers

Spring: tulip ('Dutch Princess').
Summer to Autumn: pot marigold ('Orange King'), nasturtium, black-eyed-Susan (Thunbergia), helichrysum (also known as straw flower).

Peach

A variant of orange, but whose influence is less exuberant. The colour is comforting and softening to the emotions.

Fragrant Flowers

Summer to Autumn: rose (hybrid tea 'Royal Romance'), verbena ('Peaches and Cream'), sweet pea ('Royal Flush').

Unscented Flowers

Summer to Autumn: dahlia ('Newby'), pelargonium (regal type 'Georgia Peach').

Golden Yellow

This colour is a mixture of orange and yellow and is said to enhance a sense of goodwill.

Fragrant Flowers

Spring: azalea, daffodil ('Golden Rapture'), wallflower ('cloth of Gold').
Summer: honeysuckle (also the Bach flower remedy for healing the pain of nostalgia and regret).
Summer to Autumn: rose (hybrid tea 'Pot o' Gold').

Unscented Flowers

Spring: berberis (*B. darwinii*).
Summer to Autumn: rose of Sharon, rudbeckia ('Marmalade'), giant sunflower.
Autumn: dwarf sunflower ('Autumn Beauty').

Yellow

An energetic hue which is said to be helpful for depression and loneliness, yellow is also a stimulant to the intellect.

Fragrant Flowers

Spring: azalea (*Rhododendron luteum*).
Summer: Spanish broom.
Summer to Autumn: roses (hybrid tea 'Diorama'; shrub type 'Canary Bird'; climbing type 'Mermaid').

Unscented Flowers

Summer to Autumn: coreopsis (*C. grandiflora*), African marigold ('Doubloon'), dahlia ('Esmond').

WINDOW BOXES AND POTTED PLANTS

Even if you do not have a garden, there is no need to forego the delights of living fragrance. The following charts will serve as a useful guide to some of the most popular scented plants which are suitable for growing outside in window boxes or as house plants. Most are easily raised from seeds or bulbs or can be obtained as young plants from nurseries and garden centres.

SCENTED PLANTS FOR THE WINDOW BOX

Plant	Colour and Form	Scent
Sweet Allyssum (*Allyssum minimum*) 'Carpet of Snow'	Dense clusters of small, white blooms which are borne in profusion	Strong, sensuous and honey-like
Position	**Flowering Season**	
Full sun	Midsummer to autumn	

Plant	Colour and Form	Scent
Candytuft (*Iberis sempervirens*) 'Fairy Mixed'	Clusters of lavender, red, rose-pink and white blooms. The plant is excellent for a town environment, as it is tolerant of smoke and grime	Delicately sweet and airy
	Position	**Flowering Season**
	Full sun	Spring to late summer

Plant	Colour and Form	Scent
Hyacinth (*Galtonia*) 'Amethyst'	Large, waxen, compact, bell-shaped and violet blooms; grown from bulbs	Rich, heady, jasmine-like
	Position	**Flowering Season**
	Full sun or semi-shade	Spring

Plant	Colour and Form	Scent
Jonquil (*Narcissus jonquilla*) 'Sweetness'	Small, yellow or white flowers of the daffodil family, grown from bulbs	Strong, sweet and cooling with a faint musky undertone
	Position	**Flowering Season**
	Full sun or dappled shade	Spring

Plant	Colour and Form	Scent
Mignonette (*Reseda odorata*)	Loose heads of small, yellowish-white flowers which are grown for fragrance rather than beauty of its blooms	Intensely sweet, rich and heady
	Position	**Flowering Season**
	Full sun	Midsummer to autumn

Plant	Colour and Form	Scent
Night-Scented Stock (*Matthiola bicornis*)	Spikes of four-petalled, lilac flowers	Intensely fragrant: sweet-spicy and heady, especially after dusk
	Position	**Flowering Season**
	Full sun or semi-shade	Late summer

Plant	Colour and Form	Scent
Virginia Stock (*Matthiola maritima*) 'Dwarf Mixed'	Densely flowered spikes of crimson, lavender, pink and white blooms	Strong, yet softly sweet, with a spicy nuance
	Position	**Flowering Season**
	Full sun or semi-shade	Midsummer to early autumn

Plant	Colour and Form	Scent
Wallflower (*Cheiranthus cheiri*) ' Dwarf Bedding Mixed'	Clusters of cross-shaped, crimson, orange, purple, scarlet, white or yellow	Strong, velvety smooth and sweet
	Position	**Flowering Season**
	Full sun	Early spring to early summer

FRAGRANT HOUSE PLANTS

Plant	Colour and Form	Scent
Brunfelsia (*B. calycina*)	A slow-growing, evergreen shrub whose attractive salver-shaped blooms start off deep purple, fading to almost white (therefore several shades of purple can occur on a single plant)	Delicately sweet

Growing Conditions		Flowering Season
The plant needs to be put in a fairly warm room, not less than 10°C (approximately 50°F) in winter, where there will be no sudden or drastic changes in temperature. During the summer months it requires a semi-shaded position and frequent watering. In winter, place in a well-lit spot but out of direct sunlight, and water sparingly. Mist the leaves frequently.		The flowers are borne nearly all year round, with just a short break in winter and early spring

Plant	Colour and Form	Scent
Gardenia or Cape Jasmine (*Gardenia jasminoides*)	A small, evergreen shrub with glossy, dark green leaves and large, white double blooms, with a waxen texture	Intense, musky-sweet and heady

Growing Conditions		Flowering Season
A beautiful plant which requires a great deal of attention – strictly for the dedicated indoor gardener. The developing buds require night-time temperatures of 15 to 18°C (approximately 60-65°F) and day temperatures of approximately 20 to 23°C (approximately 70-75°F), otherwise the buds will drop off. Place in a bright position, but avoid direct, midday sun during the summer months. Keep the compost moist at all times, but reduce watering in winter. Use soft, tepid water (rainwater warmed in the airing cupboard is ideal). Mist the leaves frequently.		Spring

Plant	**Colour and Form**	**Scent**
Heliotrope (*Heliotropium hybrids*)	Although the individual lavender, purple or white flowers are tiny, they are borne in large, highly fragrant clusters	Strong and sweet, reminiscent of cherry pie

Growing Conditions	**Flowering Season**
A good choice if you are looking for an easy-to-grow, flowering plant with a strong fragrance. Bright light is required, but not direct midday, summer sun. Water often during the summer, less frequently during the winter months. The plant will continue to thrive in cool temperatures of around 7 to 11°C (approximately 40-50°F) in winter. This plant is also excellent for the window box (position in full sun, avoiding the wind and cold).	Summer to autumn

Plant	**Colour and Form**	**Scent**
Jasmine (*Jasminum polyanthum*)	Pannicles of white star-shaped blooms	Strong, heady and sweet, with a musky undertone, becoming stronger after dusk. A single bloom can perfume a whole room

Growing Conditions	**Flowering Season**
A perennial climber, requiring support in the form of a wire hoop or small trellis work. Grow in good light, but not in direct, hot, summer sun. Keep the compost moist and mist the leaves regularly. Flourishes in cool to average temperatures: not less than 9°C (approximately 45°F) in winter.	Midwinter to early spring

Plant	**Colour and Form**	**Scent**
Easter Lily (*Lilium longiflorum*)	A bulb which produces tall stems up to 1 m in height (approximately 3 ft), with white, trumpet-shaped blooms borne at the top of the stem	Strong, heady and sensuous, with hints of vanilla and musk

Growing Conditions	**Flowering Season**
The plant requires bright light, but not direct sunlight. The compost should be kept moist during the growing season and the leaves misted occasionally. Keep the plant cool, but not less than 2°C (approximately 35°F).	Early summer

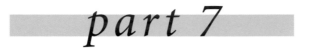

part 7

AROMATIC PROFILES

The Rose…Our own experiences have taught us that the rose has a considerable influence on the female sexual organs. Not by stimulus, but on the contrary, by cleansing and regulating their function…

Lemongrass…In the different pharmacopoeias one reads that this essence is eminently prophylactic and bactericidal…

Palmarosa…this essence favours the transmutation of the pathogenic agent into normal cells…

MARGUERITE MAURY,
THE SECRET OF LIFE AND YOUTH
(MACDONALD & CO), 1964

31
GUIDE TO THE AROMATIC PROFILES

There are hundreds of aromatic oils available to the perfume and flavour industries, but comparatively few are considered safe for aromatherapy or home use. The majority of the oils included in this section are commonly used by aromatherapists, the exceptions being carnation, oakmoss, mimosa and vanilla. Even though these aromatics are regarded as having minimal medicinal value, they do have pleasing aromas with psychotherapeutic potential (see 'Create Your Own Perfumes', Chapter 27).

Although botanical names are given for the essential oil-yielding plants, sometimes it can be difficult to ascertain the exact variety used. There are numerous sub-varieties and clones used commercially. Moreover, in the case of jasmine, for example, some plantations use one variety as a rootstock with another grafted on to the root for the superior quality of the oil-secreting blooms. So, unless the oil is obtained from a specific plantation and the exact plant variety is known, the botanical name on the label is likely to be nothing more than a trade term.

Of course, the exact botanical source may be of little interest to the home user, but for professional purposes it serves as a guide to the probable chemical composition or chemotype of the chosen oil. This information is necessary to assess the oil's pharmacological effect. Since very few aromatherapists have access to gas-liquid chromatography (GLC) testing equipment, they must rely on the integrity and knowledge of their suppliers to furnish them with a pure oil from a named botanical source, including the chemotype if possible. For example, when using tea tree essence for treating vaginal thrush, it is important to choose an oil with low cineol and high terpinene-4-ol content. Aromatherapy-grade oils should include this information on the label.

To make sense of the 'Medicinal Actions' section given in each profile below, refer to the 'Glossary of Medical Terms' on page 286. Instructions for preparing and using essential oils for therapy are found in Chapter 3. For more detailed information about treating specific ailments, see Part 3. Where an oil is described as 'widely available', this means that it can be obtained from most

health shops and retail outlets specialising in herbs and natural remedies. In case of difficulty, a number of reputable mail order suppliers of aromatic oils are listed in the 'Useful Addresses' section (see page 289). For further advice about the safe use of essential oils, including instructions for carrying out skin tests, see Chapter 4.

THE AROMATIC OILS

ANGELICA
(*Angelica archangelica*)

Plant Family
Apiaceae (Umbelliferae)

Synonyms
A. *Officinalis*, European angelica

Description and Distribution
A tall hairy perennial, reaching up to 6 feet (2 m). It has attractive ferny leaves and umbels of whitish-green flowers. This particular species is native to Europe and Siberia. Most of the oil-producing plants are cultivated in Belgium, Hungary and Germany.

Extraction Method
Steam distillation of the fruits or seeds. An essential oil is also distilled from the roots and rhizomes, but this is not recommended for aromatherapy (see 'Cautions').

Nature of the Oil
Angelica seed oil has the viscosity of alcohol and is virtually colourless. The aroma is earthy-herbaceous with a piquant top-note. The odour effect is warming, and stimulating; a reputed aphrodisiac. If used in excess, however, the aroma is soporific.

Main Constituents

Phellandrene, pinene, limonene, linalol, borneol.

Properties

Antispasmodic, bactericidal, carminative, depurative, digestive, diuretic, emmenagoguic, expectorant, febrifugal, fungicidal, nervine, stimulant, stomachic, sudorific, tonic.

Aromatherapeutic Uses

Psoriasis, arthritis, rheumatism, gout, respiratory disorders, flatulence, indigestion, fatigue, migraine, stress-related disorders.

Blends Well With

Citrus essences, clary sage, oakmoss, patchouli, vetiver. The oil is highly odoriferous, so use sparingly.

Price and Availability

High price range; obtainable from specialist mail order suppliers.

Cautions

Angelica *root* oil is highly phototoxic when applied to skin shortly before exposure to natural or simulated sunlight. It can also cause dermatitis in sensitive individuals. Angelica *seed* oil is the preferred oil for aromatherapy. Tests on humans indicate that the oil is non-phototoxic. However, it may cause skin irritation in some people. Never use the oil in concentrations above 1 per cent. Avoid during pregnancy.

BASIL, FRENCH
(*Ocimum basilicum var album*)

Plant Family

Labiatae or Lamiaceae

Synonyms

Common basil, sweet basil

Description and Distribution

A half-hardy or tender herb with highly aromatic leaves. It reaches a height of up to 3 feet (60 cms). Basil is native to tropical Asia and the Middle East, but is cultivated throughout Europe.

Extraction Method

Steam distillation of the flowering tops and leaves.

Nature of the Oil

A colourless or pale yellow liquid, having a light, fresh sweet–spicy scent with a balsamic undertone. Its odour effect is at first enlivening, giving way to a warm, comforting feeling.

Main Constituents

Linalol, methyl chavicol, eugenol, limonene, citronella.

Properties

Antidepressant, antiseptic, antispasmodic, carminative, cephalic, emmenagoguic, expectorant, febrifugal, galactagoguic, nervine, prophylactic, stimulant of adrenal cortex, stomachic, tonic.

Aromatherapeutic Uses

Muscular aches and pains, respiratory disorders, scanty menstruation, colds and 'flu, mental fatigue, anxiety, depression.

Blends Well With

Bergamot, clary sage, frankincense, geranium, neroli.

Price and Availability

Medium price range; widely available.

Cautions

Avoid during pregnancy. It is advisable to use the oil in low concentrations of around 1 per cent as it can be highly irritant to skin. Better still, avoid skin applications and use in the vaporiser to perfume rooms.

BERGAMOT
(*Citrus bergamia*)

Plant Family

Rutaceae

Description and Distribution

A small evergreen tree growing to a height of around 15 feet (4.5 m). The pear-shaped fruit ripen from green to yellow, rather like miniature oranges in appearance. Like other citrus trees, bergamot is native to tropical Asia. Most of the oil is produced in southern Italy.

Extraction Method

Cold expression of the rind of the fruit.

Nature of the Oil

A pale green liquid. The aroma is delightfully citrus with just a hint of spice. Its odour effect is uplifting and refreshing.

Main Constituents

Linalyl, acetate, linalol, sequiterpenes, terpenes, furocoumarins.

Properties

Antidepressant, antiseptic (pulmonary, genitourinary), antispasmodic, antitoxic, carminative, diuretic, deodorant, febrifugal, laxative, parasiticidal, rubefacient, stimulant, stomachic, tonic, vermifugal, vulnerary.

Aromatherapeutic Uses

Colds and 'flu, cystitis, fever, infectious illness, anxiety, depression, pre-menstrual syndrome.

Blends Well With

Other citrus oils, angelica, basil, cedarwood, chamomile (German and Roman), clary sage, lavender, neroli, cypress, elemi, geranium, jasmine, juniper, coriander, ginger, frankincense, oakmoss, rose, sandalwood, vetiver.

Price and Availability

Medium price range; widely available. However, bergamot FCF (see 'Cautions') is more easily obtained by mail order from specialist suppliers.

Cautions

Expressed bergamot oil is phototoxic because it contains high levels of furocoumarins. It should never be applied to skin shortly before exposure to natural or simulated sunlight. Aromatherapists are increasingly using the rectified version known as bergamot FCF (furocourmarin-free), which is non-phototoxic. It is also free of other non-volatile substances, such as waxes, which can irritate sensitive skin.

BLACK PEPPER
(*Piper nigrum*)

Plant Family

Piperaceae

Description and Distribution

Black pepper is a perennial vine reaching a height of 20 feet or more (5 m). The small white flowers are followed by red berries which become black when mature. Although the plant is native to south-west India, it is extensively cultivated in Malaysia, China and Madagascar. The oil is distilled in Europe and the USA from imported dried fruits.

Extraction Method

Steam distillation of the dried fruits (peppercorns).

Nature of the Oil

A pale, greenish-yellow liquid, with a hot, spicy, piquant aroma. Its odour effect is stimulating and warming; a reputed aphrodisiac.

Main Constituents

Thujene, pinene, camphene, sabinene, carene, myrcene, limonene, phellandrene, beta-caryophyllene.

Properties

Analgesic, antimicrobial, antiseptic, antispasmodic, antitoxic, appetite-stimulant, bactericidal, carminative, digestive, diuretic, febrifugal, laxative, rubefacient, stimulant (nervous, circulatory, digestive), stomachic, sudorific, tonic.

Aromatherapeutic Uses

Poor circulation, muscular aches and pains, loss of appetite, nausea, colds and 'flu, lethargy, mental fatigue.

Blends Well With

Other spices, citrus essences, frankincense, jasmine, lavender, geranium, rose, ylang ylang, rosemary, sandalwood.

Price and Availability

Medium price range; widely available.

Caution

Use in the lowest concentrations as it may irritate skin.

CAJEPUT
(*Melaleuca leucadendron*)

Plant Family

Myrtaceae

Synonyms

Cajuput, white tea tree

Description and Distribution

A tall evergreen tree native to Malaysia, the Philippines, Australia and south-eastern Asia. In the Philippines 'kajuputi' means 'white wood' which is indeed the colour of the timber. Cajeput is closely related to many other trees of the *Melaleuca* genus, notably eucalyptus and tea tree.

Extraction Method

Steam distillation of the leaves, buds and twigs.

Nature of the Oil

A pale yellow liquid. The aroma is camphoraceous with a peppery nuance. The odour effect is head-clearing and stimulating, followed by a sensation of cold.

Main Constituents

Cineol, terpineol, pinene, eucalyptol, nerolidol.

Properties

Analgesic, antimicrobial, antineuralgic, antispasmodic, antiseptic, expectorant, febrifugal, insecticidal, sudorific, vermifugal.

Aromatherapeutic Uses

Acne, arthritis, muscular aches and pains, rheumatism, stiff joints, respiratory ailments, cystitis, colds and 'flu.

Blends Well With

Bergamot, cypress, juniper berry, lemon, pine, rosemary. The oil is highly odoriferous, so use sparingly.

Price and Availability

Medium price range; more easily obtained by mail order from specialist suppliers.

Cautions

Cajeput oil has been reported to cause skin irritation. However, the chance of this occurring is greatly reduced if the rectified oil is used. Many of the problems associated with cajeput may also be due to the fact that it is often adulterated with substances such as turpentine (highly irritant) and synthetic colourant. It is essential to obtain the oil from a reputable supplier who can vouch for its purity.

CARDAMOM
(Elettaria cardomomum)

Plant Family

Zingiberaceae

Synonyms

Cardomon, cardamomi, cardomum, mysore cardomom

Description and Distribution

Cardamom, a member of the ginger family, is a perennial reed-like shrub rising from fleshy rhizomes. The small yellow flowers are followed by fruits, or seed capsules, containing several reddish-brown seeds. The plant is native to Asia and is extensively cultivated for the spice trade. The essential oil is produced mainly in India.

Extraction Method

Steam distillation of the dried fruit (seeds).

Nature of the Oil

A colourless to pale yellow liquid. The aroma is sweet and spicy with just a hint of eucalyptus. The odour effect is warming, head-clearing and stimulating; a reputed aphrodisiac.

Main Constituents

Terpinyl acetate, cineol, limonene, sabinene, linalol, linalyl acetate, pinene, zingiberene.

Properties

Antiseptic, antispasmodic, carminative, cephalic, digestive, diuretic, stimulant, stomachic, nerve tonic.

Aromatherapeutic Uses

Digestive disturbances, mental fatigue, nervous exhaustion.

Blends Well With

Cedarwood, frankincense, cinnamon, cloves, ginger, citrus essences, rose, jasmine, geranium, lavender, neroli, ylang ylang. The oil is highly odoriferous, so use sparingly.

Price and Availability

Medium to high price range; widely available.

Cautions

Generally regarded as non-irritant and non-sensitising. However, it is a powerful oil and must be used in low concentrations.

CARNATION ABSOLUTE
(Dianthus caryophyllus)

Plant Family

Caryophyllaceae

Synonyms

Gilliflower, clove pink

Description and Distribution

A perennial, low-growing shrub with bright greyish-green foliage and pinkish-purple flowers borne on high stems. The plant is native to the Mediterranean region, but extensively cultivated worldwide. Most of the oil is produced in Egypt and France.

Extraction Method

Solvent extraction of the fresh flowers.

Nature of the Oil

A slightly viscous, light amber liquid. The aroma is highly tenacious, rich and honey-like with a hint of clove. The odour effect is warming and intoxicating; a reputed aphrodisiac.

Main Constituents

Benzyl benzoate, eugenol, phenylethyl alcohol, benzyl salicylate, methyl salicylate.

Properties

Antidepressant, antifungal, antimicrobial.

Aromatherapeutic Uses

Not generally used in aromatherapy. However, the oil can be used as a room scent (or luxury fumigant!) or as a personal perfume.

Blends Well With

Cedarwood, citrus essences, clary sage, coriander, lavender, petitgrain, frankincense. The oil is extremely odoriferous, so use sparingly.

Price and Availability

Very high price range; obtainable by mail order from a few specialist suppliers.

Cautions

The oil may irritate sensitive skin. Always use in very low concentrations of 0.5 per cent or even less. It is also advisable to carry out a patch test before use.

Aromatherapeutic Uses

Acne, oily skin and hair, dandruff, eczema, fungal infections, arthritis, rheumatism, respiratory disorders, cystitis, pre-menstrual syndrome, loss of menstruation outside pregnancy, nervous tension, stress-related disorders.

Blends Well With

Bergamot, clary sage, cypress, frankincense, jasmine, juniper berry, neroli, mimosa, oakmoss, rose, rosemary, vetiver, ylang ylang.

Price and Availability

Medium price range; more easily obtained by mail order from specialist suppliers.

Cautions

Unlike the oil extracted from Virginian cedarwood, Atlas cedarwood oil is not known to be an abortifacient. None the less, the aromatherapy associations advise against the use of this essence during pregnancy. The oil may irritate sensitive skin.

CEDARWOOD, ATLAS
(Cedrus atlantica)

Plant Family

Pinaceae

Synonyms

Atlantic cedar, African cedar

Description and Distribution

An evergreen conifer tree native to the Atlas Mountains of Algeria and Morocco. Most specimens attain a height of around 120 feet (36 m). The oil is mainly produced in Morocco.

Extraction Method

Steam distillation of the wood, stumps and sawdust.

Nature of the Oil

A dark amber viscous liquid with a sweet woody aroma which improves as the oil ages. Its odour effect is calming; a reputed aphrodisiac.

Main Constituents

Atlantone, caryophyllene, cedrol, cadinene.

Properties

Antiseptic, antiputrescent, antiseborrheic, astringent, circulatory stimulant, diuretic, expectorant, fungicidal, sedative.

CEDARWOOD, VIRGINIAN
(Juniperus virginiana)

Plant Family

Cupressaceae

Synonyms

Eastern red cedar, pencil cedar, red cedar

Description and Distribution

An evergreen conifer tree native to eastern and central North America. Most specimens reach up to 50 feet (15 m), though occasionally they may grow to twice this height. However, this species and other American conifers used for producing 'cedarwood' essential oils are not true cedarwoods; their essences only have similar fragrances. True cedarwood oil is extracted from the Atlas and Himalayan varieties, *Cedrus atlantica* and *C. deodra*, respectively. Although Himalayan cedarwood has an exquisite aroma, it is extremely difficult to obtain as the tree is now a protected species.

Extraction Method

Steam distillation of the sawdust and wood shavings.

Nature of the Oil

A pale yellow or orange liquid. The aroma is distinctly woody with a camphoraceous tinge. The odour effect is warming and calming; a reputed aphrodisiac.

Main Constituents
Cedrene, cedrol, cedrenol

Properties
Abortifacient, antiseborrheic, antiseptic (pulmonary, genito-urinary), antispasmodic, astringent, diuretic, circulatory stimulant, emmenagoguic, expectorant, insecticidal, sedative.

Aromatherapeutic Uses
Acne, oily skin and hair, dandruff, eczema, psoriasis, arthritis, rheumatism, bronchitis, catarrh, coughs, sinusitis, cystitis, loss of menstruation outside pregnancy, premenstrual syndrome, stress-related disorders.

Blends Well With
Bergamot, clary sage, cypress, juniper berry, frankincense, neroli, petitgrain, rose, jasmine, oakmoss, rosemary, sandalwood, vetiver, ylang ylang.

Price and Availability
Low to medium price range; widely available.

Cautions
Not to be used during pregnancy. The oil may irritate sensitive skin.

CHAMOMILE, GERMAN
(*Matricaria recutica*)

Plant Family
Asteraceae (Compositae)

Synonyms
Blue chamomile (oil), Hungarian chamomile, scented mayweed, wild chamomile

Description and Distribution
A low-growing annual herb with sparse, finely divided leaves and daisy-like white flowers on single stems. The plant is native to Europe and northern Asia, but is extensively cultivated in Hungary and eastern Europe.

Extraction Method
Steam distillation of the flower heads.

Nature of the Oil
An inky-blue viscous liquid with a pungent aroma faintly reminiscent of seaweed. The odour effect is calming if liked, though most people prefer the sweeter scent of Roman chamomile.

Main Constituents
Chamazulene (not present in the fresh plant, but produced during the process of distillation), bisabolol oxide, enyndicycloether, farnesene.

Properties
Analgesic, anti-allergenic, anti-inflammatory, antispasmodic, bactericidal, carminative, cicatrisant, cholagogue, cytophylactic, digestive, emmenagoguic, febrifugal, fungicidal, hepatic, sedative, stomachic, sudorific, vermifugal, vulnerary.

Aromatherapeutic Uses
Skin care (most skin-types), acne, allergies, boils, burns, eczema, inflamed skin conditions, earache, wounds, menstrual pain, pre-menstrual syndrome, headache, insomnia, nervous tension and other stress-related disorders.

Blends Well With
Citrus essences, clary sage, lavender, marjoram, geranium, neroli, rose. The oil is highly odoriferous, so use sparingly.

Price and Availability
High price range; more easily obtained by mail order from specialist suppliers.

Cautions
Although the oil is recommended for skin and respiratory allergies, in some cases it can actually exacerbate an existing condition or provoke an allergic reaction. To prevent such problems, always use the lowest advocated concentration, around 0.5 per cent. If you are prone to allergies, carry out a patch test beforehand. Avoid during the first trimester of pregnancy.

CHAMOMILE, ROMAN
(*Chamaemelum nobile*)

Plant Family
Asteraceae (Compositae)

Synonyms
Athemis noblis, camomile, common chamomile, English chamomile, sweet chamomile, true chamomile

Description and Distribution
A low-growing trailing perennial with finely divided leaves which give the plant a soft feathery appearance. The white daisy-like flowers are borne on solitary stems. The plant is native to southern and western Europe and is cultivated mainly in Belgium, Britain, France, Hungary, Italy and the USA.

Extraction Method

Steam distillation of the flower heads.

Nature of the Oil

A pale yellow liquid. The aroma is sweet and dry with an apple-like tinge. The odour effect is warming and calming.

Main Constituents

Esters, pinene, fanesol, nerolidol, chamazulene, pinocarvone, cineol.

Properties

Analgesic, anti-anaemic, antineuralgic, anti-inflammatory, antiseptic, antispasmodic, bactericidal, carminative, cholagogue, cicatrisant, digestive, emmenagoguic, febrifugal, hepatic, hypnotic, sedative, stomachic, sudorific, tonic, vermifugal, vulnerary.

Aromatherapeutic Uses

Skin care (most skin-types), acne, allergies, burns, eczema, inflamed skin conditions, earache, wounds, menstrual pain, pre-menstrual syndrome, headache, insomnia, nervous tension and other stress-related disorders.

Blends Well With

Citrus essences, clary sage, lavender, geranium, jasmine, neroli, rose, ylang ylang. The oil is highly odoriferous, so use sparingly.

Price and Availability

High price range; widely available.

Cautions

Avoid during the first trimester of pregnancy. Can cause skin irritation or provoke wheezing in susceptible individuals. Always use in low concentrations (0.5 to 1 per cent). If you are prone to allergies, carry out a patch test beforehand.

Because of the high price of Roman chamomile essence, a growing number of suppliers promote Moroccan chamomile (*Ormenis multicaulis*) as a cheaper alternative. Although the plant is distantly related to Roman chamomile and has a similar aroma, its medicinal properties have not been thoroughly investigated, nor has the oil undergone formal safety testing procedures on humans.

CINNAMON
(*Cinnamomum zeylanicum*)

Plant Family

Lauraceae

Synonyms

Cinnamomum verum, Laurus cinnamomum, Ceylon cinnamon, true cinnamon.

Description and Distribution

A tropical evergreen tree reaching up to 60 feet (18 m), with a highly aromatic bark, shiny leaves and clusters of yellow flowers followed by bluish-white berries. It is a native of Sri Lanka, India and Madagascar and is also cultivated in Jamaica and Africa.

Extraction Method

Steam distillation of the bark chips. An oil is also distilled from the leaves and twigs.

Nature of the Oil

Cinnamon bark oil is light amber with a warm, sweet and spicy aroma. Cinnamon leaf oil is a yellowish liquid with a much less refined, hot and spicy aroma. The odour effect of cinnamon (especially cinnamon bark) is warming and stimulating; a reputed aphrodisiac.

Main Constituents

Cinnamon bark oil: cinnamaldehyde, eugenol (4–10 per cent), benzaldehyde, pinene, cineol, phellandrene, furfurol, cymene, linalol. Cinnamon leaf oil: eugenol (80–95 per cent), eugenol acetate, cinnamaldehyde, benzyl benzoate, linalol.

Properties

Antimicrobial, antiseptic, antispasmodic, antiputrescent, cardiac stimulant, carminative, circulatory stimulant, digestive, emmenagoguic, febrifugal, haemostatic, parasiticidal, stomachic, vermifugal.

Aromatherapeutic Uses

Cinnamon oil (bark or leaf) can be vaporised as an antidepressant room scent or as a fumigant during infectious illness.

Blends Well With

Citrus essences, clove, elemi, ginger, frankincense. Both bark and leaf oils are highly odoriferous, so use sparingly.

Price and Availability

Cinnamon bark: medium to high price range. Cinnamon leaf: low to medium price range. These two essences are most easily obtained by mail order from essential oil suppliers.

Cautions

Cinnamon oil (especially cinnamon bark) is highly irritant to skin and mucous membranes. Avoid skin applications of the oil and also steam inhalations. However, the oils may be used in low concentrations in a vaporiser as a room scent or fumigant.

CLARY SAGE
(*Salvia Sclarea*)

Plant Family
Lamiaceae (Labiatae)

Synonyms
Clary, clary wort, clear eye, common clary, see bright, eye bright, muscatel sage, orvale, toute-bonne.

Description and Distribution
A strongly aromatic, shrubby herb reaching up to 3 feet (1 m) with spikes of white, violet or pink flowers. Clary is native to the Mediterranean, but is cultivated worldwide. The highest quality oil is produced in France, Britain and Morocco.

Extraction Method
Steam distillation of the flowering tops and leaves.

Nature of the Oil
A colourless to pale yellow liquid. The aroma is sweetly herbaceous and nutty with a floral tinge. Its odour effect is uplifting and relaxing; a reputed aphrodisiac.

Main Constituents
Linalyl acetate, linalol, pinene, myrcene, sclareol, phellandrene.

Properties
Anticonvulsive, antidepressant, anti-inflammatory, antiseptic, antispasmodic, astringent, bactericidal, carminative, cicatrisant, deodorant, digestive, emmenagoguic, hypotensive, sedative, stomachic, tonic.

Aromatherapeutic Uses
High blood pressure, muscular aches and pains, respiratory problems, irregular menstruation, pre-menstrual syndrome, depression, migraine, nervous tension and stress-related disorders.

Blends Well With
Most oils, especially bergamot, jasmine, mimosa, juniper berry, lavender, neroli, petitgrain, pine, frankincense, vetiver.

Price and Availability
Medium to high price range; widely available.

Cautions
Not to be used in pregnancy. Although the oil is commonly believed to cause excessive drowsiness when used immediately before or after drinking alcohol, I have not found clary to be especially potent in this respect. In fact, any form of relaxing massage (with or without sedative or intoxicating essences) will intensify the effects of alcohol.

CLOVE
(*Syzygium aromaticum*)

Plant Family
Myraceae

Synonyms
Eugenia aromatica, E. caryophyllata, E. caryophyllus.

Description and Distribution
A slender evergreen tree with brilliant red flowers, attaining a height of about 20 feet (6 m). When dried, the flower buds turn reddy-brown and are rich in essential oil. The tree is believed to be native to Indonesia, but is extensively cultivated in other tropical countries such as the Philippines, the Molucca Islands, Madagascar and the West Indies.

Extraction Method
Steam distillation of the buds. Lower grade oils are also extracted from the leaves, stalks and stems.

Nature of the Oil
Clove bud: a pale yellow liquid. The aroma is sweet and spicy with a pleasantly sharp top-note. Clove leaf: a dark amber liquid with a harsh dry odour. Clove stem: a pale yellow liquid whose odour is reminiscent of clove bud oil. The odour effect of clove bud oil is warming and stimulating; a reputed aphrodisiac.

Main Constituents
Clove oils contain an extremely high proportion of the potentially caustic eugenol. Clove bud (the preferred oil for aromatherapy): eugenol (up to 90 per cent), eugenyl acetate, caryophyllene. Clove leaf: eugenol (up to 90 per cent), little or no eugenyl acetate (the leaf oil is used by the chemical industry to extract eugenol). Clove stem: eugenol (up to 95 per cent), with other minor constituents.

Properties

Analgesic, antibiotic, anti-emetic, antirheumatic, anti-neuralgic, antispasmodic, antioxidant, antiseptic, antiviral, carminative, expectorant, larvicidal, stimulant, stomachic, vermifugal.

Aromatherapeutic Uses

Although some aromatherapists use clove bud oil on the skin for conditions such as acne, athlete's foot and as an insect repellent, I would not recommend this (see 'Cautions'). However, it can be used in a vaporiser as a room scent or fumigant, or as a first-aid measure for toothache while awaiting dental treatment.

Blends Well With

Citrus essences, other spices, rose, vanilla, ylang ylang. The oil is highly odoriferous, so use sparingly.

Price and Availability

Medium to high price range; the highest quality clove bud oil is more easily obtained by mail order from essential oil suppliers.

Cautions

Clove oil is highly irritating to skin and mucous membranes. Therefore, it is advisable for the home user to avoid skin applications and steam inhalations of any type of clove oil. However, it can be used in a vaporiser as a fumigant or room scent.

CORIANDER
(*Coriandrum sativum*)

Plant Family

Apiaceae (Umbelliferae)

Description and Distribution

An annual herb reaching a height of about 3 feet (1 m) with umbels of white or pink flowers. The seeds are green at first, turning brown on ripening. Coriander is native to southern Europe and western Asia. Most of the oil is now produced in Eastern Europe.

Extraction Method

Steam distillation of the seeds.

Nature of the Oil

A colourless to pale yellow liquid. The fragrance is light, sweet and spicy with a faintly musky undertone. Its odour effect is warming, uplifting and stimulating; a reputed aphrodisiac.

Main Constituents

Linalol, decyl aldehyde, borneol, geraniol, carvone, anethole.

Properties

Analgesic, aperitif, antioxidant, antirheumatic, antispasmodic, bactericidal, circulatory stimulant, depurative, digestive, carminative, fungicidal, larvicidal, restorative, stomachic.

Aromatherapeutic Uses

Arthritis, muscular aches and pains, poor circulation, digestive problems, colds and 'flu, mental fatigue, nervous exhaustion.

Blends Well With

Other spices, citrus essences, cypress, jasmine, juniper berry, petitgrain, neroli, pine, frankincense, sandalwood.

Price and Availability

Lowest price range; widely available.

Cautions

Generally believed to be non-irritant and non-sensitising.

CYPRESS
(*Cupressus sempervirens*)

Plant Family

Cupressaceae

Synonyms

C. stricta, *C. lusitanicus*, Italian cypress, Mediterranean cypress.

Description and Distribution

An evergreen conifer reaching a height of 80–150 feet (25–45 m).

The tree is native to the eastern Mediterranean. Most of the oil comes from trees cultivated in France, Spain and Morocco.

Extraction Method

Steam distillation of the needles, twigs and cones.

Nature of the Oil

A pale greenish-yellow liquid. The aroma is fresh, woody and balsamic. Its odour effect is cooling and calming.

Main Constituents

Pirene, camphene, sylvestrene, cymene, sabinol.

Properties

Antirheumatic, antiseptic, antispasmodic, astringent, deodorant, diuretic, hepatic, restorative for the nerves, sudorific, tonic (to veins), vasoconstrictive.

Aromatherapeutic Uses

Skin care (oily skin), acne, haemorrhoids, varicose veins, poor circulation, cellulite, excessive perspiration, gum disorders, wounds, bronchitis, spasmodic coughs, rheumatism, excessive menstruation, menopausal problems, nervous tension and stress.

Blends Well With

Bergamot and other citrus essences, clary sage, frankincense, petitgrain, pine, juniper berry, lavender, sandalwood.

Price and Availability

Medium price range; widely available.

Cautions

Although people who have been exposed to cypress wood have developed contact dermatitis, the essential oil is generally regarded as non-irritant and non-sensitising.

ELEMI
(*Canarium commune*)

Plant Family

Burseraceae

Synonyms

C. luzonicum, Manila elemi

Description and Distribution

A tall tree reaching up to 180 feet (30 m), indigenous to the Philippines and the Molucca Islands. When the bark is incised it exudes a highly aromatic oleoresin (a gummy substance composed mainly of essential oil and resin). The substance is at first fluid and white, becoming waxy and yellow as it ages.

Extraction Method

Steam distillation of the gummy exudate.

Nature of the Oil

A pale yellow or colourless liquid. The aroma is tenacious, dry and slightly spicy with a geranium-like overtone. The odour effect is warming and stimulating.

Main Constituents

Phellandrene, dipentene, elemol, elemicin, terpineol, limonene, pinene.

Properties

Antiseptic, cicatrisant, expectorant, stimulant, stomachic.

Aromatherapeutic Uses

Muscular aches and pains, respiratory disorders, skin infections, aids healing of broken bones, nervous exhaustion.

Blends Well With

Citrus essences, coriander, frankincense, rosemary, lavender, cinnamon, clove, geranium. The oil is highly odoriferous, so use sparingly.

Cautions

Even though elemi is generally regarded as non-irritant and non-sensitising, the oil may cause contact dermatitis in hypersensitive individuals.

EUCALYPTUS, BLUE GUM
(*Eucalyptus globulus*)

Plant Family

Myrtaceae

Description and Distribution

A very tall evergreen tree reaching up to 400 feet (90 m). The mature leaves are blue-green and roughly sword-shaped. The tree is a native of Australia and Tasmania and is also cultivated in Spain, Portugal, Brazil, California, Russia and China, from where much of the world's supply of eucalyptus oil originates.

Extraction Method

Steam distillation of the leaves and young twigs.

Nature of the Oil

A colourless liquid. The aroma is piercing and camphoraceous with a woody-sweet undertone. Its odour effect is head-clearing and cooling.

Main Constituents

Cineol, pinene, limonene, cymene, phellandrene, terpinene, aromadendrene.

Properties

Analgesic, antineuralgic, antirheumatic, antiseptic, antispasmodic, antiviral, balsamic, cicatrisant, deodorant, depurative, diuretic, expectorant, febrifugal, parasiticidal, prohylactic, rubefacient, stimulant, vermifugal, vulnerary.

Aromatherapeutic Uses

Burns, blisters, chickenpox, measles, cold sores, cuts, insect bites and stings, insect repellent, headlice, skin infections, wounds, arthritis, muscular aches and pains, sprains, poor circulation, cystitis, hay fever, colds and 'flu, headaches, neuralgia.

Blends Well With
Cedarwood, lavender, lemon, marjoram, pine, rosemary, thyme.

Price and Availability
Lowest price range; widely available.

Cautions
Eucalyptus oil is generally regarded as non-irritant and non-sensitising. However, it is advisable for allergy sufferers to carry out a patch test before use (see page 23).

FENNEL, SWEET
(*Foeniculum vulgare*)

Plant Family
Apiaceae (Umbelliferae)

Description and Distribution
A short-lived perennial reaching a height of around 6 feet (2 m) with feathery leaves and umbels of small yellow flowers. All parts of the plant smell strongly of aniseed. The plant is native to the Mediterranean, but has become naturalised throughout Europe. Most of the oil is produced in Eastern Europe, Germany, France, Italy and Greece.

Extraction Method
Steam distillation of the crushed seeds.

Nature of the Oil
A virtually colourless liquid. The strong aroma is reminiscent of aniseed, but with a camphor-like undertone. The odour effect is warming and stimulating.

Main Constituents
Anethol, anisic acid, anisic aldehyde, pinene, camphene, estragol, fenone, phellandrene.

Medical Actions
Aperitif, anti-inflammatory, antimicrobial, antiseptic, antispasmodic, carminative, circulatory stimulant, depurative, diuretic, emmenagoguic, expectorant, galactagoguic, tonic, vermifugal.

Aromatherapeutic Uses
Bruises, gum disorders, halitosis, cellulite, rheumatism, respiratory ailments, colic, indigestion, loss of appetite, nausea, loss of menstruation outside pregnancy,

menopausal problems, insufficient milk in nursing mothers.

Blends Well With
Lavender, geranium, sandalwood. The oil is highly odoriferous, so use sparingly.

Price and Availability
Low to medium price range; obtained more easily from essential oil suppliers by mail order.

Cautions
The oil may irritate sensitive skin. There is a remote possibility that fennel may provoke an epileptic attack in prone subjects. Avoid during pregnancy. Use in the lowest recommended concentration of around 0.5 per cent.

FRANKINCENSE
(*Boswellia carterii*)

Plant Family
Burseraceae

Synonyms
Boswellia thurifera, olibanum, incense.

Description and Distribution
A small tree or shrub native to north-east Africa and the Red Sea region. It produces an oleo gum resin which is collected by making incisions into the bark. The substance is at first fluid and milky-white, solidifying into pea-sized amber 'tears'. Although the raw material is mainly produced in Somalia and Ethiopia, most of the oil is distilled in Europe.

Extraction Method
Steam distillation of the 'tears'.

Nature of the Oil
A colourless to pale yellow liquid. The fragrance is warm and balsamic with a hint of lemon and camphor. The aroma improves as the oil ages. The odour effect is warming, head-clearing and calming. A popular oil for use during meditation.

Main Constituents
Pinene, dipentene, limonene, thujene, phellandrene, cymene, myrcene, terpinene.

Properties
Anti-inflammatory, antiseptic, astringent, carminative, cicatrisant, cytophylactic, digestive, diuretic, emmenagoguic, expectorant, sedative, tonic, uterine, vulnerary.

Aromatherapeutic Uses

Skin care (particularly ageing skin), acne, abscesses, scars, wounds, haemorrhoids, respiratory ailments such as asthma, bronchitis, coughs, catarrh and laryngitis, cystitis, painful menstruation, uterine bleeding outside menstruation, pre-menstrual syndrome, nervous tension and stress-related disorders.

Blends Well With

Citrus oils, spice oils, basil, cedarwood, cypress, elemi, galbanum, juniper berry, lavender, neroli, patchouli, rose, sandalwood, vetiver.

Price and Availability

High price range. May be available in small quantities from health shops and other retail outlets. Otherwise, it can be obtained by mail order from essential oil suppliers.

Cautions

Generally regarded as non-irritant and non-sensitising. Since the oil is an emmenagogue (stimulates menstruation) it is advisable to avoid during the first trimester of pregnancy.

GALBANUM
(Ferula galbaniflua)

Plant Family
Apiaceae (Umbelliferae)

Synonym
F. Gummosa

Description and Distribution

A large perennial herb reaching up to 6 feet (2 m) with umbels of small white flowers. When incisions are made in the thick stalks, the plant exudes a brownish oleoresin or gum which becomes viscous when in contact with the air. The plant is native to the Middle East and western Asia. Distillation usually takes place in Europe or the USA.

Extraction Method
Steam distillation of the oleoresin.

Nature of the Oil

An olive green, slightly viscous liquid. The powerful aroma is reminiscent of dense green undergrowth with a dry earthy quality. The odour effect is essentially calming; a reputed aphrodisiac.

Main Constituents
Carvone, cadinene, myrcene, cadinol, limonene, pinene.

Properties

Analgesic, anti-inflammatory, antimicrobial, antiseptic, antispasmodic, balsamic, carminative, cicatrisant, diuretic, emmenagoguic, expectorant, hypotensive, restorative.

Aromatherapeutic Uses

Skin care (especially ageing skin), abscesses, acne, boils, scars, cuts and sores, inflamed skin, skin ulcers, insect stings and bites, wounds, poor circulation, muscular aches and pains, rheumatism, respiratory ailments, indigestion, delayed menstruation outside pregnancy, nervous tension, stress-related conditions.

Blends Well With

Bergamot, cedarwood, cypress, lavender, frankincense, geranium, oakmoss, pine. The oil is exceptionally odoriferous, so use sparingly (as little as one drop to 30 ml of base oil, blended with other essences).

Price and Availability

High price range. Obtainable by mail order from essential oil suppliers.

Cautions

Since the oil stimulates menstruation, it is advisable to avoid during pregnancy. The oil is generally regarded as non-irritant and non-sensitising.

GARLIC
(Allium sativum)

Plant Family
Liliaceae

Synonyms
Common garlic, allium

Description and Distribution

A highly pungent herb with grass-like leaves rising from a collection of bulbets or cloves. The country of origin is not known for certain, but it is believed to have spread from Siberia through to Europe and central Asia. The plant is cultivated worldwide, but Egypt, Bulgaria and France are the major oil-producing countries.

Extraction Method
Steam distillation of the fresh, crushed bulbs.

Nature of the Oil

A colourless to pale yellow liquid. It has an overpowering sulphurous odour which can only be described as 'garlicky'.

Main Constituents

Allicin, various sulphides such as allylpropyl disulphide, citral, geraniol, linalol, phellandrene.

Properties

Antibiotic, antimicrobial, antiseptic, anti-tumour, antiviral, bactericidal, carminative, cholagogue, cytophylactic, depurative, diuretic, expectorant, febrifugal, fungicidal, hypoglycaemic, hypotensive, insecticidal, larvidical, prophylactic, sudorific, vermifugal.

Aromatherapeutic Uses

Because of its offensive odour and skin irritant properties, garlic oil is best taken orally in the form of garlic capsules for conditions such as gastrointestinal infections, intestinal worms, respiratory ailments, heart and circulatory disorders, and as a prophylactic against infectious illness such as colds and 'flu.

Price and Availability

Medium price range; widely available in capsule form from chemists and health shops.

Cautions

Garlic in any shape or form is contra-indicated for those suffering from eczema or irritation of the stomach or intestines, or for breastfeeding mothers (it may cause colic in the infant). Applied externally, the oil can burn or irritate the skin.

GERANIUM
(Pelargonium graveolens)

Plant Family

Geraniaceae

Synonyms

Rose geranium, pelargonium.

Description and Distribution

A spreading shrub growing to a height of 3 feet (1 m) with rose-pink flowers. The whole plant is aromatic. It is a native of South Africa, but cultivated worldwide. Most of the oil is produced in Egypt and Réunion.

Extraction Method

Steam distillation of the leaves, stalks and flowers.

Nature of the Oil

A greenish liquid. The aroma is piercingly sweet and rosy with an unexpected hint of mint. The odour effect is refreshing and uplifting.

Main Constituents

Geraniol, borneol, citronellol, linalol, terpineol, limonene, phellandrene, pinene.

Properties

Antidepressant, antihaemorrhagic, anti-inflammatory, antiseptic, astringent, cicatrisant, deodorant, diuretic, fungicidal, haemostatic, stimulant of the adrenal cortex, tonic, vermifugal, vulnerary.

Aromatherapeutic Uses

Skin care (most skin types), burns, eczema, headlice, ringworm, neuralgia, cellulite, haemorrhoids, poor circulation, engorgement of the breasts, menopausal problems, pre-menstrual syndrome, nervous tension, stress-related disorders.

Blends Well With

Bergamot (and other citrus essences), black pepper, clary sage, coriander, clove, elemi, jasmine, juniper berry, lavender, neroli, patchouli, petitgrain, rosemary, sandalwood, vetiver.

Price and Availability

Medium price range; widely available.

Cautions

Generally regarded as non-irritant and non-sensitising, though it may irritate very sensitive skin.

GINGER
(Zingiber officinale)

Plant Family

Zingiberaceae

Synonym

Jamaican ginger

Description and Distribution

A perennial plant growing to a height of about 2 feet (1 m), with long narrow reed-like leaves stemming from tuberous rhizomes. Ginger is a native of southern Asia and is cultivated commercially in the West Indies and Africa. Most of the oil is distilled in Britain, China and India.

Extraction Method

Steam distillation of the dried, ground rhizomes.

Nature of the Oil

A pale amber liquid The aroma is pungent, warm and spicy. However, it lacks the fruity odour nuance found in the raw plant material because the process of steam distillation distorts the aroma. The odour effect is warming and stimulating; a reputed aphrodisiac.

Main Constituents
Gingerin, linalol, camphene, phellandrene, citral, cineol, borneol.

Properties
Analgesic, antioxidant, antiseptic, antispasmodic, aperitif, bechic, bactericidal, carminative, cephalic, expectorant, febrifugal, rubefacient, sudorific, stimulant.

Aromatherapeutic Uses
Arthritis, muscular aches and pains, poor circulation, rheumatism, catarrh, coughs, sore throats, diarrhoea, colic, indigestion, loss of appetite, nausea, travel sickness, colds and 'flu, infectious illness, mental fatigue, nervous exhaustion.

Blends Well With
Cedarwood, coriander, cinnamon, citrus essences, neroli, patchouli, petitgrain, rose, sandalwood, vetiver, ylang ylang. The oil is highly odoriferous, so use sparingly.

Price and Availability
Medium to high price range. More easily obtained by mail order from essential oil suppliers.

Cautions
May irritate sensitive skin. Use in the lowest concentrations. The oil is mildly phototoxic, but only if it is applied to the skin neat or in high concentrations.

GRAPEFRUIT
(Citrus x paradisi)

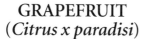

Plant Family
Rutaceae

Description and Distribution
A cultivated tree attaining a height of 35 feet (10 m) with glossy leaves and large yellow fruits. This hybrid cultivar is thought to be a cross between *C. grandis* and *C. sinensis*. All citrus trees are native to tropical Asia, but are extensively cultivated throughout the world. Most of the oil is produced in California.

Extraction Method
Cold expression of the fresh peel of the fruit. A lower grade oil is obtained by steam distillation of the peel and fruit pulp.

Main Constituents
Limonene, paradisiol, neral, geraniol, citronellal.

Properties
Antiseptic, antitoxic, astringent, bactericidal, diuretic, depurative, digestive, tonic.

Aromatherapeutic Uses
Cellulite, muscle fatigue, chills, colds and 'flu, depression, nervous exhaustion.

Blends Well With
Other citrus essences, cardamom, coriander, cypress, juniper, lavender, neroli, petitgrain, pine, geranium, rosemary.

Price and Availability
Low to medium price range. More easily obtained by mail order from essential oil suppliers.

Cautions
Unlike most other citrus essences, grapefruit oil is non-phototoxic. However, the oil has a very short shelf-life and must be used within six months of purchase. Once it begins to oxidise, it can cause skin irritation and sensitisation.

HOPS
(Humulus lupulus)

Plant Family
Cannabaceae

Description and Distribution
A perennial creeping herb which twines through other plants or up supports to a height of 30 feet (8 m). The greenish-yellow male and female flowers are on separate plants. The male flowers hang in loose bunches or panicles; the female flowers are cone-like catkins known as 'stobiles'.

Extraction Method
Steam distillation of the recently dried stobiles. If the stobiles are left for too long, the aroma becomes objectionable because the soft resin (present in hops) oxidises and valerianic acid forms.

Nature of the Oil
A yellowish liquid with a sweet, warm and spicy aroma. The odour effect is soothing and soporific.

Main Constituents
Humulene, myrcene (only in the fresh oil), caryophyllene, farnesene.

Properties

Analgesic, anaphrodisiac (quells sexual desire) in men, antimicrobial, antiseptic, antispasmodic, astringent, bactericidal, carminative, diuretic, oestrogenic properties, hypnotic, nervine, sedative.

Aromatherapeutic Uses

Asthma, spasmodic coughs, nervous indigestion, headaches, menstrual irregularity, menstrual cramps, menopausal symptoms, insomnia, nervous tension, stress-related conditions.

Blends Well With

Bergamot, cypress, juniper berry, lavender, nutmeg, pine.

Price and Availability

Highest price range. Obtainable by mail order from a few specialist suppliers.

Cautions

The fresh oil can cause sensitisation in some people. This is thought to be due to its myrcene content. As the oil ages, this substance begins to oxidise and the oil becomes more benign to skin. Nevertheless, the essence should always be used in the lowest concentrations. Hops in any shape or form should be avoided by those suffering from depression and lethargy.

JASMINE ABSOLUTE
(*Jasminum officinale*)

Plant Family

Oleaceae

Synonyms

Jasmin, jessamine

Description and Distribution

An evergreen climber which produces an abundance of white star-shaped blooms whose rich fragrance intensifies after dusk. Jasmine is native to China, northern India and the Middle East, but is cultivated worldwide. The absolute is mainly produced in France and Egypt. Other species of jasmine commonly used for oil production include *J. grandiflorum, J. paniculatum, J. auriculatum*.

Extraction Method

Solvent extraction of the flowers which must be picked after dusk when the essential oil is at its highest concentration.

Nature of the Oil

An orangey-brown, viscous liquid. The tenacious fragrance is richly floral with a pronounced musky note.

The odour effect is warming and intoxicating; a reputed aphrodisiac.

Main Constituents

Jasmone, benzyl acetate, benzyl alcohol, indol, linalol, linalyl acetate, phenylacetic acid, methyl jasmonate.

Properties

Analgesic, antidepressant, anti-inflammatory, antiseptic, antispasmodic, cicatrisant, expectorant, parturient, sedative, uterine tonic. Sometimes listed as a galactagogue, but is much more likely to have the opposite effect.

Aromatherapeutic Uses

Muscular aches and pains, catarrh, coughs, laryngitis, painful menstruation, labour pains, depression, premenstrual syndrome, stress-related disorders.

Blends Well With

Other floral essences, citrus essences, clary sage, oakmoss, sandalwood. The oil is highly odoriferous, so use sparingly.

Price and Availability

Extremely costly. Often available from health shops diluted in a base oil. The absolute is easier to obtain by mail order from essential oil suppliers.

Cautions

Avoid during pregnancy. Unfortunately, because of the high price of jasmine absolute it is especially susceptible to adulteration. Therefore, it may be advisable to regard the oil as a perfume material rather than an aromatherapy grade oil. It may irritate sensitive skin.

JUNIPER BERRY
(*Juniperus communis*)

Plant Family

Cupressaceae

Synonym

Common juniper

Description and Distribution

A small evergreen conifer tree which reaches up to 12 feet (4 m). It has bluish-green prickly needles and produces an abundance of bluish-black berries. Juniper has a wide natural distribution and can be found growing wild in North America, Europe (including Britain), northern Asia, Korea and Japan. The oil is mainly produced in eastern Europe, France, Italy, Austria, Germany and Canada.

Extraction Method

Steam distillation of the crushed, dried (or partially dried) berries. A cheaper, inferior quality oil is also distilled from the needles and wood. An even lower grade oil is produced from berries that have been fermented and distilled in the making of gin. The juniper oil recommended throughout this book refers to the superior grade oil distilled from virgin berries.

Nature of the Oil

The oil captured from the needles and wood is not recommended for aromatherapy, neither is that extracted from fermented berries (see 'Cautions'). The highest grade juniper berry oil is virtually colourless. The aroma is fresh and woody with a pleasant peppery overtone. Its odour effect is uplifting to the spirits and yet also warming and calming; a reputed aphrodisiac.

Main Constituents

Pinene, myrcene, borneol, camphene, thugene, terpenic alcohol.

Properties

Antirheumatic, antiseptic, antispasmodic, astringent, carminative, cicatrisant, depurative, diuretic, emmenagoguic, nervine, parasiticidal, rubefacient, sedative, sudorific, tonic, vulnerary.

Aromatherapeutic Uses

Skin and hair care (oily), acne, weeping eczema, haemorrhoids, wounds, cellulite, arthritic and rheumatic complaints, muscular aches and pains, loss of periods outside pregnancy, painful menstruation, cystitis, pre-menstrual syndrome, nervous tension, stress-related disorders.

Blends Well With

Bergamot, cedarwood, cypress, elemi, frankincense, geranium, lavender, neroli, petitgrain, rosemary, sandalwood.

Price and Availability

Medium to high price range. To ensure the highest quality juniper berry oil, it is advisable to purchase from a reputable mail order supplier.

Cautions

Although juniper oil is often cited as being irritant to skin, this may be due to the fact that the market is flooded with adulterated juniper oils masquerading as 'pure'. The lower grade oils extracted from the wood or the berries are often adulterated with turpentine. Juniper in any shape or form should be avoided by those with kidney disease as it may be nephrotoxic if used without specialist knowledge. Avoid during pregnancy.

LAVANDIN
(*Lavandula x intermedia*)

Plant Family

Lamiaceae (Labiatae)

Description and Distribution

A hybrid lavender developed in the late 1920s by crossing true lavender (*L. angustifolia* with spike lavender *L. latifolia*, it reaches a height of about 2–2½ feet (60–80 cm). The flowers may be bluish-mauve like true lavender or greyish-mauve like spike lavender. The plant is hardy, easy to cultivate and produces twice as much oil as true lavender, which is why it is increasingly preferred by growers. Although it is sometimes used in aromatherapy, most of the oil is used by the perfume industry to extract linalol. Unfortunately, lavandin is also used as an adulterant to 'bulk' the more expensive true lavender. Most of the oil is produced in France and Eastern Europe.

Extraction Method

Steam distillation of the fresh flowering tops.

Nature of the Oil

A pale to deep yellow liquid. The strong aroma is similar to true lavender, but less sweet and more camphoraceous with a woody undertone. Its odour effect is uplifting, head-clearing and refreshing.

Main Constituents

Borneol, camphor, cineol, geraniol, linalol, linalyl acetate. Compared with true lavender, the oil contains a greater proportion of borneol and a lesser proportion of linalol.

Properties

Similar to true lavender, though perhaps a little more stimulating to the nervous system.

Aromatherapeutic Uses

The oil has properties similar to the sweeter-smelling true lavender. Being less expensive than other lavenders, lavandin could be used as a room scent or fumigant during infectious illness.

Blends Well With

Cedarwood, citrus essences, clove, cinnamon, cypress, petitgrain, pine, geranium, thyme, patchouli, rosemary.

Price and Availability

Lowest price range. It may be easier to obtain the oil by mail order from an essential oil supplier.

Cautions

Compared with true lavender essence, lavandin is marginally more likely to irritate sensitive skin. I have come across a number of comparatively expensive lavender oils labelled 'L. officinalis' (true lavender) which smell suspiciously like the less expensive lavandin. It is therefore important to seek out a reputable supplier. Admittedly, this can be difficult for the newcomer to aromatherapy.

Price and Availability
Low price range. More easily obtained by mail order from essential oil suppliers.

Caution
Generally regarded as a non-irritant and non-sensitising, though it can cause skin reactions if used in high concentrations or applied neat.

LAVENDER, SPIKE
(*Lavandula latifolia*)

Plant Family
Lamiaceae (Labiatae)

Synonyms
Aspic, *L. spica*

Description and Distribution
Spike lavender looks very similar to true lavender, although its leaves are broader and rougher and the flowers, which are greyish-mauve, grow more closely together on the stem. Spike lavender is native to the mountainous regions of France and Spain. These two countries still produce most of the world's supply of the essence.

Extraction Method
Steam distillation of the flowering spikes.

Nature of the Oil
A colourless to pale yellow liquid. The aroma is fresh and camphoraceous, reminiscent of true lavender and rosemary combined. Unlike most other lavender essences, whose odour effect is somewhat sedating, spike lavender tends to be much more head-clearing and awakening.

Main Constituents
Cineol, camphor, linalol, linalyl acetate.

Properties
Similar to true lavender essence, though as it has a more camphoraceous aroma it is preferable for respiratory complaints. It is interesting to note that French aromatherapy doctors often mix up to 30 per cent of spike lavender to true lavender oil in order to 'activate' the former (see also the information on synergy, page 44).

Aromatherapeutic Uses
See True Lavender.

Blends Well With
Bergamot, cypress, eucalyptus, juniper berry, lemon, petitgrain, pine, rosemary.

LAVENDER, TRUE
(*Lavandula angustifolia*)

Plant Family
Lamiaceae (Labiatae)

Synonyms
L. officinalis, L. Vera

Description and Distribution
An evergreen shrub with a height and spread of 3–4 feet (1 m) whose bluish-mauve flowers are carried in spikes at the end of thin stems. The plant is native to the Mediterranean area of southern Europe. Most of the oil is produced in France, Spain and Bulgaria.

Extraction Method
Steam distillation of the flowering tops.

Nature of the Oil
A colourless to pale yellow liquid. The aroma is sweet floral–herbaceous. Its odour effect is uplifting, calming and refreshing.

Main Constituents
Linalol, linalyl acetate, lavandulol, lavandulyl acetate, terpineol, limonene, caryophyllene.

Properties
Analgesic, anticonvulsive, antidepressant, antimicrobial, antirheumatic, antiseptic, antispasmodic, antitoxic, carminative, cholagogue, cicatrisant, cordial, cytophylactic, deodorant, diuretic, emmenagoguic, hypotensive, insecticidal, nervine, parasiticidal, rubefacient, sedative, sudorific, tonic, vermifugal, vulnerary.

Aromatherapeutic Uses
Skin care (most skin types), acne, allergies, athlete's foot, boils, bruises, eczema, dandruff, dermatitis, burns, chilblains, psoriasis, ringworm, scabies, insect bites and stings, as an insect repellent, asthma, earache, coughs, colds and 'flu, catarrh, laryngitis, nausea, colic, cystitis, painful menstruation, depression, headache, insomnia,

migraine, nervous tension, pre-menstrual syndrome, stress-related disorders.

Blends Well With
Citrus essences, cedarwood, clove, clary sage, coriander, cypress, frankincense, geranium, juniper, mimosa, neroli, rose, oakmoss, petitgrain, pine.

Price and Availability
Lowest price range; widely available.

Cautions
Generally regarded as non-irritant and non-sensitising. However, there are reports of contact dermatitis as a result of over-use of the oil, especially amongst aromatherapists themselves. It is also possible to be sensitive to one particular brand of lavender oil and not to another, even though both types may be labelled 'L. officinalis'. This may suggest that the oil has been adulterated or that it has oxidised. The oil is much more likely to irritate skin when used neat or in high concentrations.

LEMON (*Citrus limon*)

Plant Family
Rutaceae

Synonym
C. limonum

Description and Distribution
A small evergreen tree growing up to 15 feet (5 m), producing white flowers tinged with pink followed by the bright yellow fruit. Lemon is native to Asia, but has become naturalised in the Mediterranean region. It is also cultivated extensively in many parts of the world, with most of the oil being produced in Italy, Cyprus, Israel and California.

Extraction Method
Cold expression of the peel of the fruit. A distilled oil is also available, but this has an inferior aroma.

Nature of the Oil
A pale yellow liquid. The aroma is fresh and sharp just like the fresh fruit. The odour effect is uplifting and cooling.

Main Constituents
Limonene, terpinene, pinene, myrcene, citral, linalol, geraniol, citronellal.

Properties
Anti-anaemic, antimicrobial, antirheumatic, antiseptic, antispasmodic, antitoxic, astringent, bactericidal, carminative, cytophylactic, cicatrisant, depurative, diuretic, febrifugal, haemostatic, hypotensive, insecticidal, rubefacient, sudorific, tonic, vermifugal.

Aromatherapeutic Uses
Skin care (oily skin), acne, boils, chilblains, warts, cellulite, arthritis, high blood pressure, poor circulation, rheumatism, asthma, sore throat, bronchitis, catarrh, indigestion, colds and 'flu.

Blends Well With
Other citrus essences, chamomile (Roman), elemi, frankincense, juniper berry, lavender, myrrh, neroli, petitgrain, rose, sandalwood, ylang ylang.

Price and Availability
Lowest price range; widely available.

Caution
Like most other expressed citrus essences, lemon oil is phototoxic. Do not apply to the skin shortly before exposure to natural or simulated sunlight as it may cause pigmentation. The distilled oil is non-phototoxic. Lemon oil has a short shelf-life and should be used within six months of purchase. Once oxidised, it is much more likely to irritate the skin. Use in low concentrations.

LEMONGRASS, WEST INDIAN (*Cymbopogon citratus*)

ALSO, EAST INDIAN LEMONGRASS (*C. flexuosus*)

Plant Family
Poaceae (Gramineae)

Description and Distribution
A fast-growing aromatic grass native to tropical Asia, though cultivated in India, Sri Lanka, Indonesia, the West Indies and Africa. Most of the oil, whether 'West Indian' or 'East Indian', is produced in Guatemala and India.

Extraction Method
Steam distillation of the fresh and partially dried grass.

Nature of the Oil
West Indian lemongrass is reddish amber. The aroma is sweet and lemony with an earthy undertone. The East Indian type is yellowish with a similar consistency to the West Indian type, but with a lighter fragrance. The odour

effect of both types of lemongrass is uplifting and slightly cooling. Some people find the aroma relaxing, others regard it as a 'wake up' essence.

Main Constituents
Citral, dipentene, linalol, geraniol.

Properties
Analgesic, antidepressant, antioxidant, antiseptic, bactericidal, astringent, carminative, deodorant, febrifugal, fungicidal, galactagoguic, insecticidal, nervine, rubefacient, tonic.

Aromatherapeutic Uses
Athlete's foot, insect repellent, scabies, muscular aches and pains, poor circulation, insufficient milk in breast-feeding mothers, colitis, indigestion, fevers, infectious illness, headaches, nervous exhaustion and other stress-related disorders.

Blends Well With
Bergamot, cardamom, chamomile (Roman), clove, eucalyptus, geranium, ginger, lavender, myrrh, palmarosa, patchouli, petitgrain, rosemary. The aroma is highly odoriferous, so use sparingly.

Price and Availability
Lowest price range; widely available.

Cautions
The oil may irritate sensitive skin. Use in the lowest recommended concentration of 0.5 per cent or even less.

LIME
(*Citrus aurantifolia*)

Plant Family
Rutaceae

Synonyms
C. medica var acida, C. latifolia.

Description and Distribution
A small evergreen tree growing to 8 feet (2 m), crooked and prickly with small white flowers followed by yellowish-green fruit about half the size of a lemon. The tree is native to Asia, but is extensively cultivated in other parts of the world. Most of the oil is produced in the USA and Italy.

Extraction Method
Cold expression of the peel of the unripe fruit. There is also a distilled oil with an inferior aroma captured from the crushed whole fruit, a by-product of the fruit juice industry. Most aromatherapists favour the expressed oil.

Nature of the Oil
A pale yellow or green liquid. The strong aroma is sharp and refreshing, just like the fruit. The odour effect is uplifting and cooling.

Main Constituents
Limonene, pinene, camphene, citral, cymene, cineol, linalol. The expressed oil also contains coumarins.

Medical Actions
Antiseptic, antiviral, aperitif, bactericidal, febrifugal restorative.

Aromatherapeutic Uses
Colds and 'flu, depression, nervous exhaustion and other stress-related disorders.

Blends Well With
Other citrus essences, neroli, petitgrain, lavender, rosemary, clary sage, ylang ylang. The oil is highly odoriferous, so use sparingly.

Price and Availability
Lowest price range. The oil may be easier to obtain by mail order from an essential oil supplier.

Cautions
The expressed oil is highly phototoxic and must never be applied to the skin shortly before exposure to natural or simulated sunlight. However, the distilled oil is non-phototoxic because it is free from coumarins. Both types of oil are potentially irritant to skin, so use in low concentrations. The oil has a short shelf-life and is therefore best used within six months of purchase.

MANDARIN
(*Citrus reticulata*)

Plant Family
Rutaceae

Synonyms
C. noblis, C. madurensis, C. deliciosa, tangerine

Description and Distribution
A small evergreen tree growing to about 20 feet (6m) with glossy leaves and fragrant white flowers followed by an abundance of small, loose-skinned orange-like fruits. The mandarin is a native of Southern China. At one time, tangerines were a little larger than mandarins, but nowa-

days growers have developed cultivars which produce fruits of a similar size to the original mandarin. The word 'tangerine' is commonly used in the USA, whereas most other countries prefer 'mandarin'.

Extraction Method
Cold expression of the peel of the fruit.

Nature of the Oil
A yellowish-orange liquid. The aroma is delicately sweet and citrus. Its odour effect is soothing, uplifting and cheery.

Main Constituents
Limonene, geraniol, citral, citronellal.

Properties
Antiseptic, antispasmodic, carminative, digestive, diuretic, laxative, sedative, tonic.

Aromatherapeutic Uses
Scars, a preventative of stretch marks (especially during pregnancy), digestive problems, insomnia, nervous tension and other stress-related disorders.

Blends Well With
Other citrus essences, chamomile (German), coriander, geranium, lemongrass, neroli, petitgrain, rose, rosemary. Incidentally, when mandarin oil is mixed in equal proportions with lemongrass oil it acts as a 'quencher' of the potentially skin-irritant element of the lemongrass.

Price and Availability
Low price range; widely available.

Cautions
Generally regarded as non-irritant and non-sensitising. However, it can cause allergic reactions in those who have a sensitivity to citrus fruits. The oil is mildly phototoxic, so do not apply to the skin shortly before exposure to natural or simulated sunlight. It has a short shelf-life and is therefore best used within six months of purchase.

MELISSA
(Melissa officinalis)

Plant Family
Lamiaceae (Labiatae)

Synonym
Lemon balm

Description and Distribution
A bush perennial herb with bright green aromatic leaves, having a height and spread of about 2 feet (60 cm). The plant is native to the Mediterranean, but has become common throughout Europe, parts of Asia, North America and North Africa. Most of the oil is produced in France, Spain, Germany and Russia.

Extraction Method
Steam distillation of the leaves and flowering tops.

Nature of the Oil
A pale yellow liquid. The aroma is light, fresh and distinctly lemony. Its odour effect is uplifting and calming.

Main Constituents
Cital, citronellol, eugenol, geraniol, linalyl acetate.

Properties
Antidepressant, antihistaminic, antispasmodic, bactericidal, carminative, emmenagoguic, febrifugal, nervine, sedative, sudorific, uterine, vermifugal.

Aromatherapeutic Uses
Allergies (skin and respiratory), cold sores, eczema, asthma, bronchitis, indigestion, nausea, irregular menstrual cycle, insomnia, migraine, anxiety, nervous exhaustion and other stress-related disorders.

Blends Well With
Citrus essences, chamomile (Roman), lavender, petitgrain, neroli, geranium, rose. The oil is highly odoriferous, so use sparingly.

Price and Availability
Very high price range; available by mail order from specialist suppliers.

Cautions
It is very difficult to obtain the genuine oil. Many of the so-called melissa oils on the market are blends of cheaper lemon-scented essences such as lemon, lemongrass and citronella, sometimes with the addition of synthetic chemicals. Although true melissa oil is popular with aromatherapy doctors in Germany, it is a relative newcomer to aromatherapy and has not been thoroughly tested on humans. Available data indicates that the oil can irritate skin and provoke sensitisation reactions in a few people. Always use in the lowest recommended concentrations.

MARJORAM, SWEET
(*Origanum marjorana*)

Plant Family
Lamiaceae (Labiatae)

Synonyms
Marjorana hortensis, knotted marjoram

Description and Distribution
An annual, or sometimes biennial, herb with greyish leaves and small white or purplish flowers arranged in roundish clusters or 'knots'. The plant is native to the Mediterranean region, but is cultivated throughout the world. Most of the oil is produced in France, North Africa, Eastern Europe and Germany.

Extraction Method
Steam distillation of the dried flowering herb.

Nature of the Oil
A light amber liquid. The aroma is warm, woody and camphoraceous. The odour effect is warming and calming; a reputed anaphrodisiac (quells sexual desire).

Main Constituents
Carvacrol, thymol, camphor, borneol, origanol, pinene, sabinene, terpineol.

Properties
Analgesic, antioxidant, antiseptic, antispasmodic, antiviral, bactericidal, carminative, digestive, emmenagoguic, expectorant, fungicidal, hypotensive, laxative, nervine, sedative, sudorific, vasodilator, vulnerary.

Aromatherapeutic Uses
Chilblains, bruises, arthritis, muscular aches and pains, rheumatism, sprains and strains, respiratory ailments, colic, constipation, absence of periods outside pregnancy, painful menstruation, pre-menstrual syndrome, colds and 'flu, headache, high blood pressure, insomnia, migraine, nervous tension, stress-related disorders.

Blends Well With
Bergamot, cypress, eucalyptus, juniper berry, lavender, rosemary, tea tree.

Price and Availability
Low to medium price range; widely available.

Cautions
Avoid during pregnancy. There are no significant reports in the dermatological literature of adverse skin reactions to sweet marjoram oil. This oil is not to be confused with the less expensive, Spanish marjoram (*Thymus mastichina*) which, as the botanical name confirms, is actually a species of thyme and therefore has a different chemical composition. Almost all chemovars of *T. mastichina* are highly irritant to the skin and mucous membranes and are therefore not recommended for home use.

MIMOSA ABSOLUTE
(*Acacia dealbata*)

Plant Family
Leguminosa

Description and Distribution
An evergreen tree with attractive fern-like leaves and fragrant yellow flowers borne in long panicles. The tree is native to Australia and Tasmania. Most of the oil is produced in southern France.

Extraction Method
Solvent extraction of the flowers and twigs.

Nature of the Oil
A pale yellow slightly viscous liquid with a woody-floral scent reminiscent of violets. Its odour effect is uplifting, cooling and calming.

Main Constituents
Palmic aldehyde, enathic acid, anisic acid, acetic acid and phenols.

Properties
Apart from being antiseptic and astringent, the oil is regarded as being of minimal importance medicinally.

Aromatherapeutic Uses
Being an absolute rather than an essential oil, mimosa is not often used by aromatherapists. It is included here as a mood-enhancing natural perfume material. However, its light, soothing aroma can be helpful for those suffering from pre-menstrual syndrome, anxiety and stress-related disorders.

Blends Well With
Bergamot, cedarwood, coriander, geranium, lavender, neroli, oakmoss, petitgrain, rose, sandalwood. The oil is highly odiferous, so use sparingly.

Price and Availability
Very high price range. Obtainable by mail order from essential oil suppliers.

Cautions

The oil may cause dermatitis in hypersensitive individuals. Always use in low concentrations not exceeding 1 per cent.

MYRRH
(Commiphora myrrha)

Plant Family

Burseraceae

Synonym

Balsamodendrom myrrha

Description and Distribution

A small tree or shrub growing up to about 9 feet (3 m), with knotted branches and branchlets that stand out at right angles in a sharp spine. The wood secretes a pale yellow oleoresin which flows out from natural fissures, or when the bark is incised. The oleoresin hardens into walnut-sized reddish-amber 'tears'. Myrrh is native to the Middle East, North Africa and Northern India.

Extraction Method

Steam distillation of the crude myrrh or 'tears'.

Nature of the Oil

A reddish-amber viscous liquid. The aroma is strong and bitter with just a hint of camphor. Its odour effect is head-clearing and warming.

Main Constituents

Heerabolene, limonene, dipentene, pinene, eugenol.

Properties

Anti-inflammatory, antimicrobial, antiseptic, astringent, balsamic, carminative, cicatrisant, emmenagoguic, expectorant, fungicidal, sedative, stomachic, uterine, vulnerary.

Aromatherapeutic Uses

Skin care (oily skin, ageing skin), athlete's foot, chapped and cracked skin, eczema, dermatitis, ringworm, scars, wounds, arthritis, respiratory ailments, gum infections, mouth ulcers, sore throat, diarrhoea, haemorrhoids, loss of menstruation outside pregnancy, thrush.

Blends Well With

Cedarwood, coriander, cypress, elemi, frankincense, geranium, juniper, lemongrass, oakmoss, palmarosa, patchouli.

Price and Availability

High price range. Most easily obtained by mail order from an essential oil supplier.

Cautions

Generally regarded as non-irritant and non-sensitising. Avoid during pregnancy.

NEROLI
(Citrus aurantium var amara)

Plant Family

Rutaceae

Synonyms

C. vulgaris, *C. bigaradia*, orange flower, Seville orange

Description and Distribution

An evergreen tree growing up to 34 feet (10 m), with intensely fragrant white flowers. The fruit is earth-shaped, a little rougher and darker than the sweet orange. The tree is native to Asia, but cultivated extensively in the Mediterranean region. Most of the oil is produced in Italy, Tunisia, Morocco, Egypt and France.

Extraction Method

Steam distillation of the freshly picked blooms. Orange flower water is produced as a by-product of the distillation process.

Nature of the Oil

A pale yellow liquid. The aroma is sweet and floral with a bitter undertone. Its odour effect is uplifting and calming; a reputed aphrodisiac.

Main Constituents

Linalol, linalyl acetate, limonene, pinene, nerolidol, geraniol, nerol, indole, citral, jasmone.

Properties

Antidepressant, antiseptic, antispasmodic, bactericidal, carminative, cicatrisant, deodorant, digestive, mild hypnotic, nervine, cardiac and circulatory tonic.

Aromatherapeutic Uses

Skin care (most skin types), stretch marks, palpitations, poor circulation, diarrhoea, pre-menstrual syndrome, depression and other stress-related disorders.

Blends Well With

Citrus essences, chamomile (Roman), clary sage, coriander, geranium, jasmine, lavender, rose, ylang ylang.

Price and Availability

Very high price range. Often available from health shops diluted in a base oil. The concentrated essence is more easily obtained by mail order from an essential oil supplier.

Cautions

Generally regarded as non-irritant, non-sensitising and non-phototoxic. However, there are some very rare reports of contact dermatitis and photosensitivity as a result of using neroli essence.

NUTMEG
(*Myristica fragrans*)

Plant Family
Myristicaceae

Synonyms
M. officinalis, M. aromata, Nux moschata

Description and Distribution
A tropical evergreen tree growing up to 80 feet (24 m). The tree does not bear fruit until it is about seven or eight years old. The fruits of the nutmeg tree are large and fleshy, like an apricot, splitting open when ripe to reveal the kernel wrapped in its bright red, net-like arils or mace. Nutmeg is native to the Moluccas and islands in the West Indies.

Extraction Method
Steam distillation of the crushed nutmegs. Oil from the islands is re-distilled in France to improve the quality. An oil can also be obtained from the dried aril or mace, but this is rarely available for aromatherapy or perfumery work. More often the arils are removed from the nutmegs and sold for culinary purposes.

Nature of the Oil
A pale yellow liquid. The aroma is very warm, sweet and spicy. Its odour effect is warming and comforting; a reputed aphrodisiac.

Main Constituents
Borneol, camphene, cymol, dipentene, eugenol, geraniol, linalol, pinene, sapol, terpineol, myristicin, safrol.

Medical Actions
Analgesic, anti-emetic, antioxidant, antirheumatic, antiseptic, antispasmodic, carminative, digestive, emmenagoguic, stimulant.

Aromatherapeutic Uses
Arthritis, rheumatism, muscular aches and pains, flatulence, indigestion, neuralgia, nervous exhaustion.

Blends Well With
Citrus essences, coriander, geranium, neroli, petitgrain, ylang ylang. Nutmeg is highly odoriferous, so use sparingly.

Price and Availability
Medium to high price range. More easily obtained by mail order from essential oil suppliers.

Cautions
Over-use of nutmeg essence (or the whole spice) can cause nausea, hallucinations, over-rapid heartbeat and stupor. The oil may also irritate sensitive skin. Always use in very low concentrations of 0.5 per cent or even less. Avoid during pregnancy.

OAKMOSS ABSOLUTE
(*Evernia prunastri*)

Plant Family
Usneaceae

Description and Distribution
A lichen, usually found growing on oak trees, and sometimes on other species such as spruce and pine. The raw material is collected mainly in France, Greece, Morocco and Eastern Europe. Most of the oil is extracted in France and the USA. Other species used for oil extraction include E. furfuracea, Usnea barbata, Sticta pulmonaceae.

Extraction Method
Solvent extraction of the lichen, which is first sprayed with hot water and kept wet overnight to promote fermentation.

Nature of the Oil
A dark green viscous liquid with an extremely tenacious aroma reminiscent of a damp forest floor. The odour effect is uplifting, cooling and calming; a reputed aphrodisiac.

Main Constituents
Evernic acid, d-usnic acid, atranorine, chloratronorine.

Properties
Antiseptic, expectorant.

Aromatherapeutic Uses
It is not advisable to use this oil for professional aromatherapy (see 'Cautions'), but it can be used as a mood-enhancing skin perfume or environmental fragrance.

Blends Well With
Cedarwood, citrus essences (especially bergamot), coriander, clary sage, cypress, floral oils (especially mimosa), galbanum, juniper berry, lavender, patchouli, petitgrain, pine, vetiver. The oil is extremely odoriferous, so use sparingly.

Price and Availability

Medium price range. Available by mail order from essential oil suppliers.

Cautions

It is an excellent oil for perfumery purposes, for those who like fern-like fragrances, but it is a pity that it is especially susceptible to modification or adulteration. This is usual practice in the perfume industry where a standardised odour nuance is important; however, modified oils cannot be regarded as medicinal agents. None the less, the pleasing fragrance of oakmoss does have psychotherapeutic potential. It can be used as a personal fragrance or to perfume rooms. The oil can irritate sensitive skin and provoke sensitisation reactions in some people, so always carry out a patch test before use (see page 23) and use in very low concentrations of 0.5 per cent or even less.

ORANGE, SWEET
(*Citrus sinensis*)

Plant Family

Rutaceae

Synonyms

C. aurantium, var. sinensis, C. aurantium var. dulcis

Description and Distribution

An evergreen tree which can grow to a height of 13–33 feet (4.5–10 m), producing an abundance of fragrant white flowers followed by fruit. Since it can take up to a year for the fruit to be formed, there is often blossom and fruit on the tree at the same time. The orange tree is native to China, but is extensively cultivated in many parts of the world. Most of the oil is produced in France, Italy, Israel, Cyprus and the USA.

Extraction Method

Cold expression of the skin of the fruit. An inferior essential oil is steam distilled from the fruit pulp, a by-product of orange juice manufacture.

Nature of the Oil

The expressed oil is yellowy-orange. The aroma is sweet and refreshing. The distilled version has a paler yellow hue and lacks the fresh aromatic top notes found in the expressed oil. The odour effect of orange oil (the expressed oil in particular) is uplifting and cheery.

Main Constituents

Limonene, citral, citronellal, geraniol, linalol, terpinol. The expressed oil also contains bergapten, auraptenol and acids.

Properties

Antidepressant, antiseptic, bactericidal, carminative, choleretic, hypotensive, tonic.

Aromatherapeutic Uses

Palpitations, bronchitis, colds and 'flu, indigestion, depression, nervous tension, stress-related disorders.

Blends Well With

Other citrus essences, clary sage, coriander (and other spices), frankincense, geranium, lavender, myrrh, neroli, patchouli, rosemary.

Price and Availability

Lowest price range; widely available.

Cautions

Some reports suggest that both the expressed and distilled oils are phototoxic; other studies indicate otherwise. It appears that the oil extracted from the bitter orange (*C. aurantium var. amara*) is much more likely to provoke phototoxicity. Nevertheless, it is advisable to err on the side of caution by avoiding skin applications of sweet orange oil shortly before exposure to natural or simulated sunlight. Certainly, the oil can irritate sensitive skin, especially if used in concentrations above 1 per cent. The potential of all citrus oils to cause skin irritation and sensitisation increases once the oil begins to oxidise. Orange essence deteriorates very quickly, so it is best to use it within six months of opening the bottle.

PALMAROSA
(*Cymbopogon martinii var. motia*)

Plant Family

Gramineae

Synonyms

East Indian geranium, Turkish geranium, Indian rosha, motia

Description and Distribution

A fragrant grass related to lemongrass and citronella. Palmarosa is native to India, though cultivated in Africa, Madagascar, Indonesia, Brazil and the Comoros Islands, where most of the oil is produced.

Extraction Method

Steam distillation of the fresh or dried grass.

Nature of the Oil

A yellowish-green liquid. The strong, sweet aroma is

geranium-like but with an earthy undertone. Its odour effect is uplifting and stimulating.

Main Constituents

Mainly geraniol (between 75 and 95 per cent) with citronellal, citral, farnesol, limonene, dipentene.

Properties

Antidepressant, antiseptic, bactericidal, cicatrisant, circulatory stimulant, digestive, febrifugal, tonic.

Aromatherapeutic Uses

Skin care (especially oily or dehydrated skin), acne, boils, wounds, loss of appetite, digestive upsets, feverish conditions, nervous exhaustion and other stress-related disorders.

Blends Well With

Cedarwood, citrus essences, chamomile (Roman), coriander, lavender, patchouli, petitgrain, sandalwood. The oil is highly odoriferous, so use sparingly.

Price and Availability

Low price range. Most easily obtained by mail order from essential oil suppliers.

Caution

Generally regarded as non-irritant to skin, but only if used in low concentrations of around 1 per cent.

PATCHOULI
(*Pogostemon cablin*)

Plant Family

Lamiaceae (Labiatae)

Synonym

P. patchouly

Description and Distribution

An herbaceous perennial which grows up to 3 feet (90 cm), with white flowers tinged with purple. The soft 'furry' egg-shaped leaves give out the peculiar earthy fragrance of patchouli when rubbed. The plant is native to Malaysia, but is cultivated for its oil in other regions such as India, China and South America. Most of the oil is distilled in Europe and the USA from the dried leaves.

Extraction Method

Steam distillation of the dried and fermented leaves.

Nature of the Oil

A dark amber viscous liquid. The highly tenacious aroma is earthy-musky, becoming sweeter as the harsh topnotes begin to wear off. Unlike most other essences, patchouli oil improves with age. Its odour effect is warming and stimulating; a reputed aphrodisiac.

Main Constituents

Patchoulol, pogostol, bulnesol, nor patchoulenol, bulnese, patchoulene.

Properties

Antidepressant, anti-inflammatory, antimicrobial, antiseptic, antiviral, bactericidal, cicatrisant, deodorant, diuretic, febrifugal, fungicidal, nervine, stimulant, stomachic, tonic.

Aromatherapeutic Uses

Skin and hair care (especially oily skin and scalp conditions), abscesses, acne, athlete's foot, bed sores, cracked and sore skin, dandruff, dermatitis, weeping eczema, insect repellent, wounds, depression, nervous exhaustion, stress-related disorders.

Blends Well With

Bergamot (and other citrus essences), cedarwood, clary sage, clove, lavender, geranium, palmarosa, petitgrain, rose, neroli, sandalwood, vetiver. The oil is highly odoriferous, so use sparingly.

Price and Availability

Low price range; widely available.

Cautions

Generally regarded as non-irritant and non-sensitising.

PEPPERMINT
(*Mentha piperita*)

Plant Family

Lamiaceae (Labiatae)

Description and Distribution

A perennial herb growing up to 3 feet (1 m) and spreading prolifically by rhizomes. The dark green leaves and hairy stems contain the oil-secreting glands. Peppermint is thought to be a hybrid between water mint (*M. aquatica*) and spearmint (*M. spicata*). The plant is native to the Mediterranean and Western Asia, but has naturalised throughout Europe and America. Most of the world's supply of peppermint oil is produced in the USA.

Extraction Method
Steam distillation of the flowering tops.

Nature of the Oil
A pale yellow liquid. The aroma is fresh, piercing and minty. Its odour effect is awakening, cooling and head-clearing.

Main Constituents
Menthol, carovne, cineol, limonene, menthone, pinene, thymol.

Properties
Analgesic, anti-inflammatory, antigalactagoguic, antimicrobial, antiseptic, antispasmodic, astringent, antiviral, carminative, cephalic, cholagogue, emmenagoguic, expectorant, digestive, diuretic, febrifugal, hepatic, nervine, parasiticidal, stimulant, stomachic, sudorific, vermifugal.

Aromatherapeutic Uses:
Bruises, sprains and strains, swellings, ringworm, scabies, toothache, neuralgia, muscular aches and pains, respiratory disorders, halitosis, colic, indigestion, irritable bowel syndrome (oil taken internally in the form of peppermint capsules – dosage according to manufacturer's instructions), flatulence, mouth ulcers, mouth thrush, nausea, feverish conditions, colds and 'flu, fainting, headache, mental fatigue, migraine.

Blends Well With
Clary sage, eucalyptus, geranium, lavender, lemon, rosemary. The oil is highly odoriferous, so use sparingly.

Price and Availability
Lowest price range; widely available.

Cautions
Use in the lowest concentrations as it may irritate sensitive skin. Since the oil promotes menstruation, it is best avoided during the first trimester of pregnancy.

PETITGRAIN
(Citrus aurantium var. amara)

Plant Family
Rutaceae

Synonyms
C. bigaradia, bitter orange

Description and Distribution
Petitgrain oil is ostensibly obtained from the leaves and twigs of the same tree that produces bitter orange oil and neroli. However, this classification is outdated as many varieties and hybrids of orange and lemon trees are used for oil called 'petitgrain'. Most of the oil is produced in Paraguay, though the supplies from Italy, Egypt and Tunisia are considered superior.

Extraction Method
Steam distillation of the leaves and twigs.

Main Constituents
Linalyl acetate, geranyl acetate, linalol, nerol, terpineol.

Properties
Antiseptic, antispasmodic, deodorant, digestive, nervine, stomachic, tonic.

Aromatherapeutic Uses
Skin and hair care (oily), indigestion, flatulence, insomnia, pre-menstrual syndrome, nervous exhaustion and other stress-related disorders.

Blends Well With
Bergamot (and other citrus oils), cedarwood, clary sage, clove, coriander, cypress, elemi, frankincense, geranium, lavender, neroli, oakmoss, rose, vetiver.

Price and Availability
Lowest price range; widely available.

Cautions
Generally regarded as non-irritant, non-sensitising, non-phototoxic.

PINE
(Pinus sylvestris)

Plant Family
Pinaceae

Synonyms
Scotch pine, Norway pine

Description and Distribution
A tall evergreen conifer reaching up to 120 feet (36 m), the only pine which is indigenous to the British Isles. It is also native to Russia, Scandinavia, Finland and the Baltic states. Most of the oil is produced in the eastern USA and Canada.

Extraction Method
Steam distillation of the needles. An inferior grade oil is also extracted from the cones, twigs and wood chippings, but this is not recommended for aromatherapy.

Nature of the Oil

A colourless to pale yellow liquid. The aroma is strong, dry and balsamic with a camphoraceous undertone. The odour effect is refreshing, cooling and enlivening.

Main Constituents

Bornyl acetate, citral, cadinene, dipentene, phelladrene, pinene, sylvestrene.

Properties

Antimicrobial, antirheumatic, antiseptic (pulmonary, urinary, hepatic), antiviral, bactericidal, balsamic, chola-gogue, circulatory stimulant, deodorant, insecticidal, restorative, rubefacient, stimulant of the adrenal cortex and the nerves, vermifugal.

Aromatherapeutic Uses

Cuts and abrasions, wounds, headlice, scabies, excessive perspiration, arthritis, gout, muscular aches and pains, poor circulation, rheumatism, respiratory ailments, cystitis, colds and 'flu, neuralgia, fatigue, stress-related disorders.

Blends Well With

Bergamot, cedarwood, cypress, eucalyptus, frankincense, juniper, lavender, lemon, rosemary, tea tree.

Price and Availability

Medium price range; widely available.

Cautions

Generally regarded as non-irritant, though there are many reports indicating that pine essence is a sensitising agent. Oils which are old and oxidised are much more likely to cause problems with irritation and sensitisation. The oil should be avoided by those with sensitive skin. Always use in low concentrations of around 1 per cent.

ROSE
(Rosa centifolia and r. damascena)

Plant Family

Rosaceae

Synonyms

R. centifolia: Cabbage rose, Moroccan rose, Indian rose; *R. damascena*: Damask rose, Bulgarian rose, Turkish rose. These are the two main varieties of rose used for oil extraction. There are also numerous sub-varieties and cultivars within these two groups which are used commercially and there is the new English Rose Phytol oil (see page 00) which cannot be pinned down to a single rose variety since a number of cultivars are used. At pre-sent, the use of Rose Phytol oil is in its infancy, and so it is not discussed here.

Description and Distribution

A small deciduous shrub with prickly stems and large fragrant flowers. The cabbage rose is pale pink with numerous petals, whereas the Damask rose is deep pink and has fewer petals. The birthplace of the cultivated rose is believed to be Persia, but they are now extensively cultivated worldwide. The oil of *R. centifolia* is mainly produced in Morocco, Tunisia, Italy, France and China. The best oil of *R. damascena* comes from Bulgaria, though excellent oils are also produced in Turkey and France.

Extraction Method

There are two main types of rose oil commonly used in aromatherapy: rose otto, captured by steam distillation of the fresh petals, and rose absolute which is obtained by solvent extraction of the fresh petals. The distilled version, which is always labelled 'otto', is the preferred oil for aromatherapy. Rosewater is produced as a by-product of the distillation process.

Nature of the Oil

Rose otto is a virtually colourless liquid which becomes semi-solid at cooler temperatures. The aroma is sweet and mellow with a hint of cloves and vanilla. Rose absolute is a yellowy-orange viscous liquid with a similar, sweet–mellow, fragrance to rose otto, though much lighter and lacking in the rich spicy-vanilla nuance. The odour effect of rose otto is warming and intoxicating. The odour effect of rose absolute is warming and uplifting, but not quite as heady. Both oils are reputed to be aphrodisiacs.

Main Constituents

The chemical compositions of rose absolute and rose otto are very complex, with over 300 constituents identified. However, most rose oils contain appreciable quantities of citronellol, geraniol, phenyl ethanol, nerol and stearopten.

Properties

Antidepressant, anti-inflammatory, antiseptic, antispasmodic, antiviral, astringent, bactericidal, choleretic, cicatrisant, depurative, emmenagoguic, haemostatic, hepatic, laxative, sedative, stomachic, tonic, uterine.

Aromatherapeutic Uses

Skin care (most skin types), thread veins, conjunctivitis (rosewater), eczema, palpitations, respiratory ailments, liver congestion, nausea, irregular menstruation, excessive menstruation, depression, insomnia, headache, premenstrual syndrome, nervous tension and other stress-related disorders.

Blends Well With

Citrus and floral oils, cedarwood, coriander, chamomile (Roman and German), clary sage, frankincense, petitgrain, sandalwood, vanilla. Rose otto is extremely odoriferous, so use sparingly.

Price and Availability

High price range. Rose otto is even more expensive than the absolute. Although sometimes available diluted in a base oil such as almond or grapeseed, the undiluted oils are easier to obtain by mail order from a specialist supplier.

Cautions

Both oils are generally regarded as non-irritant, non-sensitising and the least toxic of all aromatic oils. Of the two oils, rose absolute is more likely to cause skin reactions in hypersensitive individuals.

ROSEMARY
(*Rosmarinus officinalis*)

Plant Family

Lamiaceae (Labiatae)

Synonyms

R. coronarium

Description and Distribution

An evergreen flowering shrub which can grow to a height of 6 feet (1.8 m). The leaves are leathery and needle-like, dark on the outside and pale underneath. The bluish, two-lipped flowers look rather like tiny irises. Rosemary is native to the Mediterranean, but is cultivated worldwide. Most of the oil is produced in Morocco, France and Spain.

Extraction Method

Steam distillation of the flowering tops. Inferior grade oils are distilled from the whole plant.

Nature of the Oil

A colourless to pale yellow liquid. The aroma is slightly camphoraceous with a woody-balsamic undertone. Lower quality oils are highly camphoraceous and somewhat harsh. The odour effect is refreshing and head-clearing, and yet warming and invigorating; a reputed aphrodisiac.

Main Constituents

Borneol, camphene, camphor, cineol, lineol, pinene, terpineol.

Properties

Analgesic, antimicrobial, antidiarrhoeal, antioxidant, antirheumatic, antineuralic, bechic, cardiotonic, carminative, cephalic, cholagogue, cicatrisant, cytophylactic, diuretic, emmenagoguic, fungicidal, hypertensive, parasiticidal, rubefacient, stimulant of the adrenal cortex, sudorific, vulnerary.

Aromatherapeutic Uses

Skin and hair care (oily), dandruff, to promote growth of healthy hair, headlice, insect repellent, scabies, respiratory ailments, muscular aches and pains, rheumatism, poor circulation, painful menstruation, colds and 'flu, headaches, mental fatigue, depression, nervous exhaustion and other stress-related disorders.

Blends Well With

Basil, cedarwood, citrus essences, coriander, elemi, frankincense, lemongrass, lavender, peppermint, petitgrain, pine.

Price and Availability

Medium price range; widely available.

Cautions

Avoid during pregnancy. There is a remote chance that the oil may trigger an epileptic attack in prone subjects. Rosemary essence may irritate sensitive skin, so use in low to medium concentrations.

SANDALWOOD
(*Santalum album*)

Plant Family

Santalaceae

Synonyms

East Indian sandalwood, Mysore sandalwood, sanderswood

Description and Distribution

An evergreen semi-parasitic tree which grows on the roots of other trees during the first seven years of its life, causing the hosts to die. It takes about 30 years to attain its maximum height of about 40–50 feet (12–15 m). The tree is native to tropical Asia, especially Mysore in India where the highest quality oil is produced.

Extraction Method

Steam distillation of the roots and heartwood.

Main Constituents

Santalols, fusanols, borneol, santalone.

Properties

Antidepressant, anti-inflammatory, antiseptic (urinary and pulmonary), antispasmodic, astringent, bactericidal, carminative, cicatrisant, diuretic, expectorant, fungicidal, insecticidal, sedative, tonic.

Aromatherapeutic Uses

Skin care (most skin types), acne, eczema, cracked and chapped skin, respiratory ailments, laryngitis, cystitis, nausea, insomnia, pre-menstrual syndrome, depression, stress-related disorders.

Blends Well With

Bergamot, cedarwood, coriander, cypress, frankincense, juniper berry, jasmine, lavender, patchouli, pine, rose, ylang ylang, vetiver.

Price and Availability

High price range. Most easily obtained by mail order from specialist suppliers.

Cautions

Generally regarded as non-irritant and non-sensitising. However, it has been known to cause contact dermatitis when applied to the skin neat. Occasionally, the oil known as West Indian sandalwood (*Amyris balsamifera*) is sold as an inexpensive alternative to Mysore sandalwood. However, *Amyris* bears no relation to true sandalwood oil. It has an inferior musky-woody aroma of poor tenacity. Moreover, the oil should be regarded as potentially risky, for it has not undergone formal testing on humans.

TAGETES
(*T. patula and T. minuta*)

Plant Family

Asteraceae (Compositae)

Synonyms

Tagette, taget, marigold

Many books wrongly cite this oil as 'calendula', confusing it with the pot marigold or *Calendula officinalis*, which produces too little essential oil to make distillation commercially viable. However, the infused oil of calendula is often used in aromatherapy as a healing base oil.

Description and Distribution

A half-hardy annual of compact and bushy habit. It has dark green deeply cut and divided leaves and an abundance of brownish-orange, daisy-like flowers. The plant is native to Mexico, but extensively cultivated worldwide. Most of the oil is produced in South Africa, South America, Nigeria and France.

Extraction Method

Steam distillation of the fresh flowers and leaves.

Nature of the Oil

A yellowy-orange, slightly viscous liquid. The offbeat aroma is composed of fruity-sweet top notes with a bitter green, murky undertone. It is difficult to offer an objective assessment of the oil's odour effect, except to say that many people find it somewhat disturbing: rather like the resonance of a discordant musical chord.

Main Constituents

Tagetones, ocimene, myrcene, linalol, limonene, pinenes, carvone, citral camphene, valeric acid.

Properties

Antispasmodic, bactericidal, emmenagoguic, fungicidal, sudorific, vermifugal.

Aromatherapeutic Uses

Athlete's foot, ringworm, absence of menstruation outside pregnancy.

Blends Well With

The oil is extremely difficult to work with, for the penetrating aroma has the curious property of becoming stronger when combined with other essences. Nevertheless, it is just about acceptable when blended with bergamot, orange, lemon or lavender. Tagetes should be used in concentrations of less than 0.5 per cent.

Price and Availability

Medium price range. Most easily obtained by mail order from specialist suppliers.

Cautions

The oil may cause skin irritation or provoke sensitisation reactions in some people. Highly phototoxic, so avoid skin applications prior to exposure to simulated or natural sunlight. Avoid during pregnancy. Use in very low concentrations.

TEA TREE
(*Melaleuca alternifolia*)

Plant Family
Myrtaceae

Description and Distribution
A small tree growing to about 23 feet (7 m) with small needle-like leaves and bottlebrush-like yellowy or purplish flowers. The tree is native to New South Wales in Australia.

Extraction Method
Steam distillation of the leaves and twigs.

Nature of the Oil
A pale yellow liquid. The aroma is strong and medicinal, reminiscent of a mixture of juniper and cypress. The odour effect is cooling and head-clearing.

Main Constituents
Terpinene-4-ol, cineol, pinene, terpenes, cymene.

Properties
Antiseptic, anti-inflammatory, antibiotic, antiviral, fungicidal, parasiticidal, immunostimulant.

Aromatherapeutic Uses
Acne, athlete's foot, abscesses, cold sores, dandruff, ringworm, warts, burns, wounds, insect bites and stings, respiratory ailments, colds and flu, thrush, cystitis.

Blends Well With
Eucalyptus, lemon, lavender, marjoram, pine, rosemary.

Price and Availability
Medium price range; widely available.

Cautions
There are many reports of minor skin reactions caused by tea tree. Unfortunately, the market is flooded with adulterated and modified versions of the oil and this may explain why it does not always live up to its benign reputation. Caution should be exercised if the oil is used neat or in high concentration. Formal skin tests carried out on humans involved 1 per cent dilutions of the oil. The potential irritant or sensitising effects of regular applications at higher levels is still unknown.

THYME, SWEET
(*Thymus vulgaris*)

Plant Family
Lamiaceae (Labiatae)

Synonym
Garden thyme

Description and Distribution
Garden thyme is a hardy perennial sub-shrub with small greyish-green leaves and tiny white or pink two-lipped flowers arranged in whorls at the top of upright stems. The plant is native to the Mediterranean, though extensively cultivated worldwide. Most of the oil is produced in Spain, France, Israel, Greece and north Africa.

Extraction Method
Steam distillation of the leaves and flowering tops.

Nature of the Oil
A pale yellow liquid with a sweet herbaceous aroma reminiscent of fresh thyme. The odour effect is gently stimulating and warming.

Main Constituents
Thymol, carvacrol, borneol, cineol, menthone and pinene. Depending on the source, sweet thyme oil may also contain appreciable quantities of geraniol, linalol, thujanol-4 or alpha-terpineol.

Properties
Antimicrobial, antioxidant, antiputrescent, antirheumatic, antiseptic, antispasmodic, aperitif, carminative, cicatrisant, circulatory stimulant, diuretic, emmenagoguic, expectorant, fungicidal, hypertensive, immunostimulant, nervine, rubefacient, sudorific, vermifugal.

Aromatherapeutic Uses
Abscesses, insect bites and stings, scabies, wounds, arthritis, gout, rheumatism, muscular aches and pains, respiratory ailments, gum disorders, halitosis, tonsillitis, indigestion, flatulence, cystitis, colds and 'flu, infectious illness, nervous exhaustion, tiredness, depression.

Blends Well With
Lavender, lemon, marjoram, rosemary.

Price and Availability
Medium price range. It is advisable to obtain the oil from a specialist supplier.

Cautions
Avoid during pregnancy. Aromatherapist Daniel Ryman

points out that thyme has been especially vulnerable to the effects of radioactive fallout from the Chernobyl disaster. However, Israeli versions of the oil are apparently safe in this respect.

There are a number of chemovars (chemotype varieties) of thyme oil available, but only a few are gentle enough for aromatherapeutic use. Those oils broadly categorised as 'red thyme' are high in potentially caustic phenols such as carvacrol and thymol and are therefore not recommended. For example, *T. vulgaris* cv. carvacrol, *T. vulgaris* cv. thymol.

Those oils which are labelled 'sweet thyme' are to be preferred because they are comparatively high in gentle alcohols such as geraniol and linalol. For example, *T. vulgaris* cv. geraniol, *T. vulgaris* cv. linalol. If in doubt, make it clear to your supplier that you require sweet thyme oil. Indeed, it is advisable in this instance to purchase the oil from a specialist supplier who will have a good knowledge of aromatherapy-grade essential oils.

Another commonly used oil is labelled 'Wild Thyme' (*T. serpyllum.*) Unfortunately, wild plants have very different chemical compositions, even though they may be found growing in the same area. Therefore, it cannot be guaranteed that the oil from such plants will be gentle to skin and mucous membranes.

VANILLA
(*Vanilla plantifolia*)

Plant Family
Orchidaceae

Description and Distribution
An exotic climbing orchid with greenish-yellow or white flowers. The green vanilla pod or bean grows to 10 inches (25 cm) and contains a mass of tiny seeds. The plant contains no essential oil: its taste and aroma come from the vanillin crystals which form on the surface of the pod after fermentation. This consists of alternate sweating and drying which can take anything up to five or six months, by which time the pods are soft and very dark brown. Vanilla is native to Central America and Mexico; it is also grown in other tropical areas such as East Africa and Indonesia.

Extraction Method
Solvent extraction of the 'cured' pods or beans. Unlike most other solvent-extracted aromatics, the alcohol used in the process is not evaporated. The final product contains about 30 per cent alcohol and is known as a resinoid rather than an absolute.

Nature of the Oil
A dark brown viscous liquid with a sweet, smooth balsamic aroma, characteristically vanilla. Its odour effect is warming, comforting and gently stimulating; a reputed aphrodisiac.

Main Constituents
Vanillin, acetic acid, ethyl alcohol, cinnamate, eugenol, vanillyl ethyl acid, eugenol, furfural.

Properties
The medicinal value of vanilla is rarely acknowledged today, but it was at one time considered to be a stimulant, an aid to digestion and to arouse sexual desire, especially in women.

Aromatherapeutic Uses
Not usually used in aromatherapy, mainly because it is extremely expensive and also because it is not a true essential oil. However, it can be vaporised as a mood-enhancing room scent. Alternatively, you may wish to make your own infused oil of vanilla which can be used as a base oil for massage (see page 235).

Blends Well With
Citrus essences, cedarwood, coriander, frankincense, jasmine, rose, sandalwood, vetiver, ylang ylang. The substance is highly odoriferous, so use sparingly. Although concentrated vanilla extract is not entirely soluble in vegetable oil, it can be used in oil-based perfumes and massage oils as long as the mixture is shaken each time before use. For professional perfumery work, the substance is usually diluted in pure alcohol.

Price and Availability
Extremely costly. Although the cooking variety of natural vanilla extract (a dilution of the resinoid in alcohol and water) is available at a much more affordable price, the highly concentrated perfumery-grade version is only available by mail order from a few essential oil suppliers.

Cautions
May provoke sensitisation reactions in some people. Always carry out a patch test before use (see page 23).

VETIVER
(*Vetiveria zizanoides*)

Plant Family
Poaceae (Gramineae)

Synonyms
Andropogon muricatus, khus khus, vetivert

Description and Distribution

A tall growing grass with unscented leaves and highly fragrant roots. Vetiver is a close relative of other aromatic grasses such as lemongrass and palmarosa. The plant is native to southern India, Indonesia and Sri Lanka, but is cultivated elsewhere. The highest quality oil is obtained from Réunion and the Comoros Islands.

Extraction Method

Steam distillation of the dried and chopped roots.

Nature of the Oil

A dark brown viscous liquid. The aroma is rich and earthy with a molasses-like undertone. The fragrance improves as the oil ages. The odour effect is calming and warming; a reputed aphrodisiac.

Main Constituents

Vetiverol, vitivone, vetivenes.

Properties

Antiseptic, antispasmodic, circulatory stimulant, depurative, rubefacient, stimulates production of red blood corpuscles and pancreatic secretions, tonic, vermifugal.

Aromatherapeutic Uses

Skin care (oily), acne, arthritis, muscular aches and pains, rheumatism, poor circulation, insomnia, light-headedness (a good 'grounding' essence), pre-menstrual syndrome, nervous exhaustion and other stress-related ailments.

Blends Well With

Clary sage, cedarwood, citrus essences, jasmine, lavender, patchouli, petitgrain, mimosa, neroli, oakmoss, rose, sandalwood, ylang ylang.

Price and Availability

Low to medium price range; widely available.

Cautions

Generally regarded as non-irritant and non-sensitising.

YLANG YLANG
(Cananga odorata var. genuina)

Plant Family

Anonaceae

Synonym

Flower of Flowers

Description and Distribution

A tropical tree which can reach a height of about 100 feet (30 m). The branches are gracefully arched like the weeping willow, bearing large, oval shiny leaves and an abundance of intensely fragrant yellow blooms which appear constantly. Ylang ylang is native to tropical Asia, though most of the oil is produced in Madagascar, Réunion and the Comoros Islands.

Extraction Method

Steam distillation of the flowers. There are four grades of the oil: ylang ylang extra, and ylang ylang one, two and three. Always use the more expensive ylang ylang extra, which has a vastly superior aroma. This is because it is collected from the 'first running' of the distillation process; the plant material is distilled two or three more times to obtain the lower grades.

Nature of the Oil

A pale yellow liquid. The aroma is intensely sweet and floral, reminiscent of almonds and jasmine combined. The odour effect is warming and intoxicating; a reputed aphrodisiac.

Main Constituents

Methyl benzoate, methyl salicylate, linalyl acetate, cadinene, caryophyllene, pinene, cresol, eugenol, linalol, geraniol.

Properties

Antidepressant, antiseptic, hypotensive, nervine, sedative, circulatory stimulant, tonic.

Aromatherapeutic Uses

High blood pressure, palpitations, depression, insomnia, pre-menstrual syndrome, nervous tension, stress-related disorders.

Blends Well With

Other florals, black pepper, citrus essences, frankincense, geranium, vetiver.

Price and Availability

Medium price range; widely available. If in doubt about the quality, the 'extra' grade can be obtained by mail order from specialist suppliers.

Cautions

Generally regarded as non-irritant. However, it can provoke sensitisation reactions in some people. Use in low concentrations of around 1 per cent.

GLOSSARY OF MEDICAL TERMS

Abortifacient	Causes abortion.
Analgesic (also, anodyn)	Pain-relieving.
Anaphrodisiac	Reduces sexual desire.
Anti-allergenic	Prevents allergic reactions.
Anti-anaemic	Prevents or combats anaemia.
Antibiotic	Destroys or inhibits the growth of micro-organisms, especially bacteria.
Anticonvulsive	Helps prevent or arrest convulsions.
Antidepressant	Helps alleviate depression.
Anti-emetic	Helps prevent vomiting.
Antigalactagoguic	Decreases the secretion of milk.
Antihaemorrhagic	Prevents or combats bleeding.
Antihistaminic	Counteracts the effects of histamine. (Histamine is released in the body as part of an allergic response, triggering symptoms such as sneezing, wheezing or skin irritation.)
Anti-inflammatory (also, antiphlogistic)	Counteracts inflammation.
Antimicrobial	Destroys, or hinders the proliferation of, micro-organisms, especially bacteria.
Antineuralgic	Counteracts neuralgia.
Antioxidant	Prevents or delays oxidation or deterioration, especially with exposure to air.
Antiputrescent	Prevents or combats decay or putrefaction.
Antirheumatic	Relieves rheumatism.
Antiseborrheic	Controls the production of sebum, the oily secretion of the skin.
Antiseptic	Destroys micro-organisms.
Antispasmodic	Prevents or eases spasms or cramps.
Antitoxic	Counteracts the effects of poison.
Anti-tumour	Prevents or retards the growth of tumours.
Antiviral	Inhibits the proliferation of viruses.
Aperitif	Stimulates the appetite.
Aphrodisiac	Increases or stimulates sexual desire.
Astringent	Causes contraction of tissues and thus reduces secretions and discharges.
Bactericidal	Destroys bacteria or inhibits their growth.
Balsamic	A soothing medicine, especially for the respiratory system.
Bechic	Soothes or relieves coughs.
Cardiac	Pertaining to the heart.
Cardiotonic	Strengthens the heart.
Carminative	Stimulates the digestive system and relaxes the stomach, thereby preventing flatulence.
Cephalic	A remedy for disorders of the head.
Cholagogic	Stimulates the secretion and release of bile from the gall bladder into the duodenum.
Choleretic	Stimulates the production of bile in the liver.
Cicatrisant	Promotes healing by increasing the regeneration of skin cells and the formation of scar tissue.

Cordial	A stimulant and tonic.
Cytophylactic	Increases the production of white blood cells (which help defend the body against infection).
Deodorant	Masks or removes unpleasant odours.
Depurative	Detoxifying, helps to combat impurities in the blood and organs.
Digestive	Aids the digestion of food.
Diuretic	Increases the flow and excretion of urine.
Emmenagoguic	Stimulates and/or normalises menstruation.
Expectorant	Helps in the removal of excess mucus from the respiratory system.
Febrifugal (also, anti-pyretic)	Reduces or combats fever.
Fungicidal	Destroys fungi or prevents their growth.
Galactagoguic	Increases the secretion of milk.
Genito-urinary	Pertaining to the reproductive organs and urinary tract.
Haemostatic	Arrests bleeding.
Hepatic	Relating to the liver; aids liver functioning.
Hypnotic	Promotes sleep (not hypnotic trance).
Hypoglycaemic	Lowers blood sugar levels.
Hypotensive	Lowers high blood pressure.
Immunostimulant	Strengthens the immune system.
Larvicidal	Destroys larvae.
Laxative (also, aperient)	Promotes evacuation of the bowels.
Nervine	Tones and strengthens the nervous system.
Parasiticidal	Destroys parasites such as fleas and lice.
Parturient	Promotes and eases labour (childbirth).
Prophylactic	Preventative.
Pulmonary	Pertaining to the lungs.
Restorative	Strengthens and revives the mind/body complex.
Rubefacient	When rubbed into the skin, causes the superficial blood vessels (capillaries) to dilate.
Sedative	Calms the nervous system and reduces stress.
Stimulant	Quickens and enlivens the mind/body complex.
Stomachic	Stimulates digestive secretions in the stomach and improves appetite.
Sudorific (also diaphoretic)	Induces or increases perspiration.
Tonic	Strengthens and enlivens either specific organs or the whole body.
Uterine	Pertaining to the uterus; a substance which strengthens and tones the uterus.
Vasoconstrictive	Causes narrowing of the blood vessels.
Vasodilating	Dilates or relaxes the blood vessels.
Vermifugal	Destroys and expels worms.
Vulnerary	Aids the healing of wounds and cuts.

SUGGESTED READING

AROMATHERAPY

DAVIES, P. *Aromatherapy; An A-Z,* C. W. Daniel, 1988
LAWLESS, J. *The Encyclopaedia of Essential Oils,*
  Element Books, 1991
PRICE, S. *The Aromatherapy Workbook,* Thorsons, 1993
TISSERAND, R. *Aromatherapy for Everyone,* Arkana, 1988
WILDWOOD, C. *Create Your Own Perfumes Using Essential
  Oils,* Piatkus, 1994
WILDWOOD C. *The Aromatherapy and Massage Book,*
  Thorsons, 1994

MASSAGE

DOWNING, G. *The Massage Book,* Penguin, 1982
HAROLD, F. *The Massage Manual,* Headline, 1992

HERBAL MEDICINE

HOFFMAN, D. *The New Holistic Herbal,* Element Books,
  1991

HOLISTIC HEALING

SHAPIRO, D. *The Bodymind Workbook,* Element Books,
  1990

HEALTH AND BEAUTY

EARL, L. *Save Your Skin,* Vermilion, 1992
KENTON, L. *The Joy of Beauty,* Century, 1985

FLOWER REMEDIES

WILDWOOD, C. *Flower Remedies,* Element Books, 1992
HARVEY, C.G. AND COCHRANE, A. *The Encyclopaedia of
  Flower Remedies,* Thorsons, 1995

HEALING

MACRAE, J. *Therapeutic Touch,* Arkana (now Penguin),
  1987
REGAN, G. AND SHAPIRO D. *The Healer's Hand Book,*
  Element Books, 1991

NUTRITION

HOLFORD, P. *The Whole Health Manual,* Thorsons, 1981
WRIGHT, C. *The Wright Diet,* Green Library
  (distributed by Element Books), 1991

USEFUL ADDRESSES

Please enclose a stamped addressed envelope with all enquiries.

UNITED KINGDOM

● Essential oils, related products and aromatherapy courses:

Fleur Aromatherapy
Pembroke Studios
Pembroke Road
London
N10 2JE

Clare Maxwell-Hudson
PO Box 457
London
NW2 4BR

Natural By Nature Oils Ltd
Aromatherapy Centre
9 Vivian Avenue
Hendon Central
London
NW4 3VT

Purple Flame Aromatics
61 Clinton Lane
Kenilworth
Warwickshire
CV8 1AS

Shirley Price
Essentia House
Upper Bond St
Hinckley
Leicestershire
LE10 1RS

The Tisserand Institute
PO Box 746
Hove, Sussex
BN3 3XA

● Aromatherapy training courses:

London School of Aromatherapy
PO Box 780
London
NW5 1DY

● Advanced aromatherapy and aromacology courses:

Hygeia School of Holistic Aromatherapy
7 Springfield Road
Altrincham
Cheshire
WA14 1HE

Shirley Price
(address listed above)

Medical Aromatherapy Training Services
    (contact Martin Watt)
7 Elm Court Park
Chelmsford Road
Blackmore
Essex
CM4 OSE

● Essential oils and aromatherapy products:

Aqua Oleum
Unit 3
Lower Wharf
Wall Bridge
Stroud
Gloucestershire
GL5 3JA

Butterbur & Sage
7 Tessa Road
Reading
Berkshire
RG1 8HH

Kittywake Oils
Cae Citty
Taliaris
Llandeilo
Dyfed
SA19 3XA

● Lists of accredited aromatherapists and training schools:

International Federation of Aromatherapists
Stamford House
2–4 Chiswick High Road
London W4

International Society of Professional Aromatherapists
41 Leicester Road
Hinckley
LE10 1LW

● Herbs, oils and cosmetic materials:

Baldwins
171–173 Walworth Road
London
SE17 1RW

Culpeper Ltd
34 The Pavilions
High Street
Birmingham
B4 7SL

Neals Yard Remedies
126 Whiteladies Road
Clifton
Bristol
BS8 2RP

● To obtain rose oil captured by the new Phytonics process (as described on page 20) contact:

Dr Peter Wilde,
91 Front Street
Sowerby
Thirsk
YO7 1JP

● Bach flower remedies (products, books, lists of accredited practitioners):

The Bach Centre
Mount Vernon
Sotwell
Wallingford
Oxon
OX10 OPZ

● Healing (lists of accredited healers and information on training courses):

National Federation of Spiritual Healers
Old Manor Farm Studio
Church Street
Sunbury-on-Thames
Middlesex
TW16 6RG

● Nutritional therapy (information and consultations):

The Institute of Optimum Nutrition
Blades Court
Deodar Road
London
SW15 2NU

Higher Nature Ltd
The Nutrition Centre
Burwash Common
East Sussex
TN19 7LX

Society for the Promotion of Nutritional Therapy
PO Box 47
Heathfield
East Sussex
TN21 8ZX

The Eating Disorders Association
Sackville Place
44 Magdalen Street
Norwich
Norfolk
NR3 1JU

UNITED STATES

● Essential oils, aromatherapy products and information:

Aroma Vera Inc
PO Box 3609
Culver City
California 90231

M. Das Co
888 Brannan Street
San Francisco
California 94103

- Lists of accredited aromatherapists and training schools:

American Society for Phytotherapy and Aromatherapy
PO Box 3679
South Pasadena
California 91031

National Association for Holistic Aromatherapy
PO Box 17622
Boulder
Colorado 80308

- Herbs, oils and cosmetic materials:

Neal's Yard USA
284 Connecticut St
San Francisco
California 94107

- Bach flower remedies:

Dr Edward Bach Healing Society
644 Merrick Road
Lynbrook
New York 11563

AUSTRALIA

- Essential oils, related products and aromatherapy courses:

Essential Therapeutics
58 Easey Street
Collingwood
Victoria 3066

In Essence Aromatherapy
3 Abbott Street
Fairfield
Victoria 3078

- Information on accredited aromatherapists and training courses:

International Federation of Aromatherapists
1st Floor
390 Burwood Road
Hawthorn
Victoria 3122

GENERAL GLOSSARY

Absolute (*see also* Concrete) A highly concentrated aromatic material, usually captured by alcohol extraction from the waxy concrete. The alcohol is then removed by means of vacuum distillation, leaving behind the viscous or semi-viscous absolute.

Aromatherapy The therapeutic use of essential oils with or without massage.

Aura (*also* electro-magnetic field, energy field, subtle body) An emanation surrounding a person, animal or plant, and other natural substances such as water and stone. Usually invisible, though some people claim to see auras. Aura is also another word for the fragrance of a plant.

Aromatology The use of essential oils for their pharmacologial properties without the complement of massage.

Base/carrier oil A vegetable oil such as almond or sunflower seed in which essential oils are diluted for massage.

Chemotype Plants within a given botanical species whose chemical composition is somewhat different from average, usually as a result of growing conditions such as soil type, climate etc. Other chemotypes are more accurately termed genotypes (derived from the word gene), for their unusual chemical composition is inherited, irrespective of growing conditions.

Chemovar Another word for chemotype meaning 'chemical variety'.

Concrete A highly odoriferous, solid, waxy substance extracted from aromatic plant material by means of hydrocarbon-type solvents.

Decoction A herbal remedy extracted from fibrous plant material, such as roots, bark and seeds, by simmering in water.

Distillation The process of evaporating a liquid and condensing its vapour. The classic method for obtaining plant essences.

Endorphin (*also* enkephalin, beta endorphin, casomorphin and dynorphin) A morphine-like family of molecules produced in body cells, especially in parts of the brain and spinal cord. They block pain and lift mood. Feelings of relaxation and/or joy raise the level of these 'happiness chemicals' which also stimulate our immune defences.

Essential oil (*also* aromatic oil, essence, ethereal oil, volatile oil) The odoriferous, volatile (i.e. evaporates in the open air) component of an aromatic plant, usually captured by steam distillation or expression.

Expression A method employed for capturing the essential oils of citrus fruits. The oil is found in the outer skin and is obtained by pressure. Although this was once carried out by hand, machines using centrifugal force are now used instead.

Fixative An aromatic material which slows down the evaporation rate of more volatile aromatics used in an aromatheraphy or perfume blend.

Fixed Oil Ordinary vegetable oil such as olive or almond which, unlike an essential oil, does not evaporate in the open air.

Fractionated Oil An essential oil or vegetable oil which has had part of its chemical structure removed.

Free radicals Unstable waste products of cellular metabolism which trigger a chain reaction of cellular damage and may increase the risk of heart disease and certain cancers.

Genotypes *see* Chemotype

Hormone According to the classical definition, a chemical secreted in the blood which acts on cells elsewhere in the body. However, the revised definition is a chemical secreted by body cells (including brain cells) which diffuses into the body fluids to act on other cells both nearby and distant (*see also* Neurotransmitters).

Infused Oil (*also* herbal oil, macerated oil) Plant material is placed in vegetable oil and gently heated until the aroma has permeated the oil. It is then strained and used as a massage oil or healing agent for skin complaints.

Infusion (*also* tisane, tea) A herbal remedy prepared by steeping the plant material in hot water.

Inunction The application of an ointment or oil to the skin, especially by rubbing to facilitate absorption.

Neurotransmitters Brain chemicals which transmit specific messages from one neuron (cell in nervous system which transmits nerve impulses) to another. Until recently, hormones were defined as substances which deliver their message to glands and neurotransmitters to nerves, but definitions are evolving. Neutrotransmitters are now classified as brain hormones.

Oleo gum resin An odoriferous exudation from trees and plants consisting of essential oil, gum and resin (e.g. frankincense).

Oleoresin A natural odoriferous exudation from trees and plants consisting of essential oil and resinous material (e.g. myrrh). Also, a prepared resin from which the essential oil has been removed (*see* Resinoid).

Oxidation A process whereby a substance is chemically combined with oxygen and its original structure is altered or destroyed.

PEA (phenylethylamine) a mood-altering chemical produced in the brain and body cells. It is said to be part of tender feelings, specifically 'falling in love'.

Pheromone A volatile hormone-like secretion, the subtle odour of which evokes a response in another member of the same species. Often, but not exclusively, sexual.

Phenylethylalcohol The 'happiness chemical' with a rose odour, related to PEA and found in chocolate, cheese, rosewater, and also in rose otto and rose Phytol oils.

Phytohormones Plant substances with a similar chemical composition to certain hormones secreted by the human organism.

Phytotheraphy Another term for herbal medicine.

Psychoneuroimmunology The study of the interrelationship of body and mind, especially the influence of emotion upon the body's immune defences.

Rectified Oil An essential oil which has been re-distilled to remove impurities or a fraction of its chemical composition.

Resin An exudation from certain trees which becomes solid or semi-solid on exposure to air (e.g. mastic).

Resinoid A viscous, highly odoriferous substance (e.g. benzoin), extracted from resinous plant material by means of hydrocarbon-type solvents. Resinoids are also called oleoresins.

Synergy Agents working harmoniously together; the effect of the whole is greater than the sum total of its separate parts.

Tincture A herbal remedy or perfumery material obtained by macerating plant material in alcohol.

Unguent A soothing or healing salve. Also, an oil-based or fat-based perfume used in ancient times, especially in Egypt, Greece and Rome.

BIBLIOGRAPHY

ACKERMAN, D. *The Natural History of the Senses*, Chapmans, 1990

ANNAND, M. *The Art of Sexual Ecstasy*, Aquarian, 1991

BAHR, R. *Good Hands, Massage Techniques for Health*, Thorsons, 1984

BALASKAS, J. *Active Birth*, Unwin, 1989

BYLINSKY, C. *Mood Control*, Charles Scribners (USA), 1978

CAMPION, K. *A Woman's Herbal*, Century 1987

CASTLETON, V. *The Handbook of Natural Beauty*, Rodale Press (USA), 1975

CHOPRA, D. *Quantum Healing*, Bantam Boooks, 1989

COLLINGS, J. *Life Forces*, New English Library, 1991

DAVIS, P. *Aromatherapy: An A–Z*, C.W. Daniel, 1988

DOWNING, G. *The Massage Book,* Penguin, 1982

EARL, L. *Vital Oils*, Ebury Press, 1991

EARL, L. *Save Your Skin*, Vermilion, 1992

FAWCETT, M. *Aromatherapy for Pregnancy and Childbirth*, Element Books, 1993.

FERUCCI, P. *What We May Be*, Aquarian, 1982

FISCHER-RIZZI, S. *Complete Aromatherapy Handbook*, Sterling (USA), 1990

GAIER, H. *What Doctors Don't Tell You*, Vol. 4, No. 9

GAIER, H. *Journal of Alternative Medicine*, September 1993

GATTEFOSSÉ, R. M. *Gattefossé's Aromatherapy*, C. W. Daniel, 1993

GIMBEL, T. Form, *Sound and Colour Healing,* C. W. Daniel, 1987

GRANT, D. AND JOICE, J. *Food Combining for Health*, Thorsons 1990.

GREER, G. *The Change*, Penguin, 1992

GREGORY, R.L. *The Oxford Companion to the Mind*, 1987

GRIEVES, M.A. *A Modern Herbal*, Penguin, 1982

GRIGGS, B. *Green Pharmacy*, Jill Norman and Hobhouse, 1982

GUILD PUBLISHING (no named author), *The Family Medical Encyclopaedia*, 1986

HOFFMAN, D. *The New Holistic Herbal*, Element Books, 1991

HOLFORD, P. *The Whole Health Manual,* Thorsons 1981

INTERNATIONAL SCHOOL OF AROMATHERAPY, *A Safety Guide on the Use of Essential Oils*, privately published, 1993

JELLINEK, DR. P. *The Practice of Modern Perfumery*, Leonard Hill, 1959

KENTON, L. *The Joy of Beauty*, Century, 1985

LAKE, M. *Scents and Sensuality*, Futura Publications, 1989

LAWLESS, J. *The Encyclopaedia of Essential Oils*, Element Books, 1992

LAWLESS, J. *Aromatherapy and the Mind*, Thorsons, 1994

LAUTIE, R. AND PASSEBECQ A. *Aromatherapy*, Thorsons, 1979

LE GUÉRER, A. Scent: *The Mysterious Power of Smell*, Chatto & Windus, 1993

MACRAE, J. *Therapeutic Touch*, Arkana, 1987

MAURY, M. *Marguerite Maury's Guide to Aromatherapy*, C. W. Daniel, 1989

MAXWELL-HUDSON, C. *The Complete Book of Massage*, Dorling Kindersley, 1990

MESSEGUE, *Health Secrets of Plants and Herbs,* Pan Books, 1979

NIELSEN, G. AND POLANSKY, J. *Pendulum Power*, Excalibur Books, 1981

PLESHETTE, J. *Health on Your Plate*, Hamlyn, 1983

PRICE, S. *The Aromatherapy Workbook*, Thorsons, 1993

READER'S DIGEST ASSOCIATION (no named author) *The Reader's Digest Encyclopaedia of Garden Plants and Flowers*, 1978

RYMAN, D. *Aromatherapy*, Piatkus, 1992

SHAPIRO, D. *The Bodymind Workbook*, Element Books, 1990

TISSERAND, R. *The Art of Aromatherapy*, C. W. Daniel, 1977

TISSERAND, R. *Aromatherapy for Everyone*, Arkana, 1988

TORTORA, G. AND ANAGNOSTAKOS, N.P. *The Principles of Anatomy and Physiology*, HarperCollins, 1990

UNIVERSITY OF CALIFORNIA, BERKELEY *The Wellness Encyclopedia*, Houghton Mifflin Company (USA), 1991

VALNET, J. *The Practice of Aromatherapy*, C. W. Daniel, 1980

VAN TOLLER, S. AND DODD, G. H. (edited by) *Perfumery, The Psychology and Biology of Fragrance*, Chapman & Hall, 1991

WATT, M. *Plant Aromatics, Set 4: Effects on the Skin of Aromatic Extracts*, privately published, 1994

WATT, M. An unpublished paper entitled *Some Thoughts on Where Aromatherapy Training is Going Wrong*

WEINER, M. A. *Maximum Immunity*, Gateway Books, 1986

WHITTON, S. *Wild About The Rose*, an article which appeared in *Aromatherapy Quarterly*, No 38, Autumn 1993

WILDWOOD, C. *Create Your Own Perfumes Using Essential Oils*, Piatkus, 1994

WILDWOOD, C. *Holistic Aromatherapy*, Thorsons, 1992

WILDWOOD, C. *The Aromatherapy and Massage Book*, Thorsons, 1994

WILDWOOD, C. *Flower Remedies for Women*, Thorsons, 1994

WILDWOOD, C. *Sensual Massage*, Headline, 1994

WILLS, P. *Colour Therapy*, Element Books, 1993

WINTER, R. *The Smell Book*, J. B. Lippincott (USA), 1976

WOLF, N. *The Beauty Myth*, Vintage, 1991

WORWOOD, V. *The Fragrant Pharmacy*, Bantam Books, 1990

WORWOOD, V. *Aromantics*, Bantam Books, 1993

WRIGHT, C. *The Wright Diet*, Green Library, 1991

INDEX